2003

Cloning and the Future of Human Embryo Research

Cloning and the Future of Human Embryo Research

Edited by
PAUL LAURITZEN

OXFORD
UNIVERSITY PRESS

2001

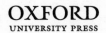

OXFORD

UNIVERSITY PRESS

Oxford   New York
Athens   Auckland   Bangkok   Bogotá   Buenos Aires   Calcutta
Cape Town   Chennai   Dar es Salaam   Delhi   Florence   Hong Kong   Istanbul
Karachi   Kuala Lumpur   Madrid   Melbourne   Mexico City   Mumbai
Nairobi   Paris   São Paulo   Shanghai   Singapore   Taipei   Tokyo   Toronto   Warsaw

and associated companies in

Berlin   Ibadan

Copyright © 2001 by Paul Lauritzen

Published by Oxford University Press, Inc.,
198 Madison Avenue, New York, New York, 10016
http://www.oup-usa.org

Library of Congress Cataloging-in-Publication Data
Cloning and the future of human embryo research / edited by Paul Lauritzen.
    p. cm.   Includes bibliographical references and index.
    ISBN 0-19-512858-3
    1. Human cloning—Moral and ethical aspects.
    2. Human embryo—Research—Moral and ethical aspects.
    3. Human reproductive technology—Moral and ethical aspects.
I. Lauritzen, Paul.

QH442.2 .C566 2000 176—dc21   00-024562

9 8 7 6 5 4 3 2

Printed in the United States of America
on acid-free paper

For Sam and Julia

Acknowledgments

This book was conceived while I was on a leave from John Carroll University that was supported by the George E. Grauel Faculty Fellowship. I am grateful to the University for this award and to Nick Baumgartner, Fred Travis, and Sally Wertheim, who, in their respective roles as Dean of the College, Academic Vice President, and Dean of the Graduate School, have been unwaveringly supportive of my work. Thanks as well to Tom Schubeck, who, as former chairperson of my department and fellow ethicist, helped to create a collegial environment conducive to research and writing. I am also indebted to the ethics writers group that meets regularly at John Carroll University. This group read several chapters of this work and made valuable suggestions for revisions. I am also deeply grateful to several individuals whose encouragement both for this project and for my work generally has been enormously important to me. Thanks to Gil Meilaender, Tom Murray, Jock Reeder, David Smith, and Barney Twiss. Finally, special thanks to Mary Jane Ponyik for help in preparing the manuscript and to Jane Marie Ponyik for help with the index.

One of the scenarios that supporters of cloning offer as legitimating its use involves the effort to replace a loved one who has died tragically. I have been blessed with a wonderful family, and so I can well imagine an almost desperate desire to see a son or daughter or spouse again. In reality, of course, a cloned parent or child or spouse would not be the person you love. I thus try to remind myself daily of the unique good fortune I have in the form of my children, Sam and Julia, and my spouse, Lisa deFilippis. Their love makes everything I do possible.

Contents

Contributors, xi

Introduction, 1
Paul Lauritzen

I Moral Status of the Preimplantation Embryo

1 Respect for Human Embryos, 21
Bonnie Steinbock

2 Source or Resource? Human Embryo Research as an Ethical Issue, 34
Courtney S. Campbell

3 Creating Embryos for Research: On Weighing Symbolic Costs, 50
Maura A. Ryan

4 Casuistry, Virtue, and the Slippery Slope: Major Problems with Producing
Human Embryonic Life for Research Purposes, 67
James Keenan, S.J.

5 Every Cell is Sacred: Logical Consequences of the Argument from
Potential in the Age of Cloning, 82
R. Alta Charo

II Debates Surrounding Cloning and Embryo Research

6 Cloning Human Beings: An Assessment of the Ethical Issues Pro
  and Con, 93
  Dan W. Brock

7 Much Ado About Mutton: An Ethical Review of the Cloning
  Controversy, 114
  Ronald M. Green

8 Born Again: Faith and Yearning in the Cloning Controversy, 132
  Laurie Zoloth

III Public Policy Issues

9 Responsibility and Regulation: Reproductive Technologies, Cloning, and
  Embryo Research, 145
  Carol A. Tauer

10 Consensus, Ethics, and Politics in Cloning and Embryo Research, 162
  Jonathan D. Moreno and Alex John London

11 Morality, Religion, and Public Bioethics: Shifting the Paradigm for the
  Public Discussion of Embryo Research and Human Cloning, 178
  Brian Stiltner

12 The Law Meets Reproductive Technology: The Prospect of Human
  Cloning, 201
  Heidi Forster and Emily Ramsey

Notes, 222

Appendix 1 Human Embryo Research Panel Report: Executive Summary, 251

Appendix 2 National Bioethics Advisory Commission Report on Cloning:
  Executive Summary, 264

Appendix 2a National Bioethics Advisory Commission Report on
             Cloning—Excerpts from Chapter 2, The Science and
             Application of Cloning, 269

Index, 287

Contributors

DAN W. BROCK, Ph.D.
Department of Philosophy
Brown University
Providence, Rhode Island

COURTNEY S. CAMPBELL, Ph.D.
Department of Philosophy
Oregon State University
Corvallis, Oregon

R. ALTA CHARO, J.D.
School of Law and School of Medicine
Program in Medical Ethics
University of Wisconsin
Madison, Wisconsin

HEIDI P. FORSTER, J.D.
Department of Clinical Bioethics
National Institutes of Health
Bethesda, Maryland

RONALD M. GREEN, Ph.D.
Department of Religious Studies
Dartmouth College
Hanover, New Hampshire

JAMES F. KEENAN, S.J.
Weston Jesuit School of Theology
Cambridge, Massachusetts

ALEX J. LONDON, Ph.D.
Department of Philosophy and
Center for the Advancement of
Applied Ethics
Carnegie Mellon University
Pittsburgh, Pennsylvania

JONATHAN D. MORENO, Ph.D.
Center for Biomedical Ethics
University of Virginia Health
Sciences Center
Charlottesville, Virginia

EMILY RAMSEY
Attorney Grievance Commission
Detroit, Michigan

MAURA A. RYAN, Ph.D.
Department of Theology
University of Notre Dame
Notre Dame, Indiana

BONNIE STEINBOCK, Ph.D.
Department of Philosophy
University at Albany/State
University of New York
Albany, New York

BRIAN STILTNER, Ph.D.
Sacred Heart University
Fairfield, Connecticut

CAROL A. TAUER, Ph.D.
Department of Philosophy
College of St. Catherine
St. Paul, Minnesota

LAURIE ZOLOTH, Ph.D.
College of Humanities
San Francisco State University
San Francisco, California

Introduction

PAUL LAURITZEN

In February 1997, scientists from the Roslin Institute near Edinburgh, Scotland, announced that they had successfully cloned an adult sheep. Because many scientists had been skeptical about the possibility of such cloning, and because the particular technique that Ian Wilmut and his colleagues used to create the clone promised tremendous advances in knowledge about mammalian cell development and cell differentiation, the birth of Dolly received intense, international attention. Dolly's birth also generated enormous controversy. Could this technology be extended to humans? If it could, would cloning humans be morally acceptable? Even the apparently remote possibility of human cloning conjured apocalyptic visions for many commentators, and so Wilmut's announcement was met almost everywhere with a sense of alarm and moral urgency. Certainly in the United States there was a sense of urgency, for, the day after the story broke, President Clinton instructed the National Bioethics Advisory Commission (NBAC) to "undertake a thorough review of the legal and ethical issues associated with the use of this technology" and to do so within 90 days.[1] The President was not alone: The United States House of Representatives convened hearings on cloning the following week, as did the United States Senate the week after that.

In retrospect, the reaction of alarmed surprise that Dolly's birth generated in so many quarters is itself somewhat surprising. Embryologists have been studying early cell development in non-human animals for at least a century, and there has been growing, if sporadic, progress toward somatic cell nuclear transplant cloning in animals since at least the 1950s, when Robert Briggs and Thomas King first cloned tadpoles from undifferentiated cells taken from early frog embryos. For example, in 1986, Steen Willadsen published a paper in the journal *Nature* that described his successful effort to clone sheep from early sheep embryos. In 1987, Neal First announced that he had cloned cows from early cow embryos. Indeed, in 1993 Hall and Stillman reported that they had cloned human embryos through blastomere separation. Even the much more difficult task of cloning differentiated cells was not completely unprecedented, because Campbell and Wilmut had, in 1996, reported success in cloning using sheep embryos that had started the process of differentiation.[2]

Nor was discussion of the general cultural and moral significance of cloning absent before Dolly's birth. In 1963, the well-known British biologist J. B. S. Haldane publicly and explicitly endorsed the idea of human cloning, as did Nobel laureate Joshua Lederberg a few years later.[3] In 1971, James Watson testified before the United States Congress about the need to think carefully about the implications of human cloning. Each of these public discussions of cloning by a prominent scientist elicited vigorous moral discussion, in some cases by ethicists as prominent in their fields as the scientists were in their own.[4] So, when Wilmut and coworkers announced their accomplishment, the possibility of human cloning was neither new nor previously undiscussed.

In fact, since at least the 1970s, when the possibility of in vitro fertilization (IVF) in humans was beginning to be seriously discussed, cloning has been a subject of considerable attention. Thus, instead of treating the birth of a cloned sheep as the beginning of serious discussion and debate about human cloning, it is better to see Dolly's birth as an intermediate step—perhaps the penultimate step—leading from the birth of the first IVF baby, Louise Brown, toward the birth of the first cloned human baby. That, at least, is the frame that structures the essays in this volume. Although the focus is on the philosophical, ethical, and policy issues raised by human cloning, throughout the volume cloning is considered in the context of general considerations about human embryo research, which any attempt at cloning humans will inevitably involve. Hence the title.

Although Leon Kass now highlights what he considers to be the essential differences between cloning and IVF, I believe he was closer to the truth when he wrote a number of years ago that

[w]ith IVF, the human embryo emerges for the first time from the natural darkness and privacy of its own mother's womb . . . into the bright light and utter publicity of the scientist's laboratory where it will be treated with unswerving rationality, before the clever and shameless eye of the mind and beneath the obedient and equally clever touch of the hand.[5]

We need not accept the implied condemnation of Kass's observation to recognize the truth of the connection he marks between access to human embryos and the many manipulations of the embryo that assisted reproduction has wrought. Seen in this light, cloning appears little different from other forms of embryo manipulation, from freezing embryos to screening them for genetic defects. All require access to early embryos or to the sperm and egg that will become the embryo, and all involve manipulation of the embryo to serve human ends.

Once we recognize the continuity between cloning and human embryo research, we are also in a position to see that there are two obvious points of departure for this volume. The first I have already mentioned. When President Clinton directed the NBAC to consider the issue of cloning, he assured that one point of departure for future discussions of cloning would be the NBAC's report on the matter. Indeed, although there has been a mixed response to many of the Commission's recommendations, almost all commentators applaud the NBAC's call for "widespread and continuing deliberations" on the ethical and social implications of this technology in order to arrive at a long-term policy on human cloning. This volume represents one such effort.

The second point of departure is also a government-sponsored report, namely, the 1994 Human Embryo Research Panel (HERP) Report.[6] This report was issued by a committee convened by the director of the National Institutes of Health (NIH) to make recommendations about federal funding for research involving experimentation on preimplantation human embryos. Like the NBAC, the HERP was asked to help in the formulation of public policy in an area of scientific research spawned by assisted reproductive technologies, and, like the NBAC, it took up the issue of cloning. Because most of the essays in this volume discuss one or both of these reports, it is worth saying a bit more about each. I begin with the HERP Report.

The Human Embryo Research Panel report

I have suggested that whatever distinctive or new issues may be raised by the prospect of human cloning, it is also important to consider cloning in the context of the history of the development of assisted reproductive technology. The report of the HERP is one significant milestone in that history.[7] The origins of the panel report can be traced back to 1974, when the United States Congress established the National Commission for the Protection of Human Research Subjects of Biomedical and Behavioral Research. One of the first mandates given to the National Commission by Congress was to review federal funding of fetal research.

After reviewing the research, the Commission recommended that the NIH fund certain kinds of fetal research, subject to approval by an Ethics Advisory Board

(EAB). In 1978, the EAB was established and a year later it recommended NIH funding for IVF research. Before the EAB could approve any federal funding for such research, however, the board was allowed to expire. Without EAB approval, no federal funding could take place, and both the Reagan and Bush administrations refused to appoint an EAB, effectively creating a moratorium on federal funding of IVF research.

This situation changed in June 1993, when the United States Congress passed the NIH Revitalization Act. This law nullified the regulatory provision that required EAB approval for any federal funding of research involving preimplantation human embryos. By eliminating this requirement, the NIH Revitalization Act lifted the 18-year-old de facto moratorium on federal funding of IVF research. In response to this regulatory change, the acting director of the NIH sought and received approval to establish the HERP. The panel was charged with the responsibility of sorting potential research into one of three categories, research that is *(1)* acceptable for federal funding, *(2)* problematic but warrants additional review, or *(3)* unacceptable for federal funding. The panel issued its report in October 1994. The executive summary of the panel report is given in Appendix 1.

It is significant that the HERP placed research on cloning in the third category, unacceptable for federal funding, but there are other reasons why the panel report is important for any discussion of cloning. First, the report implicitly highlights the continuity between cloning and other forms of embryo research brought about by the existence of IVF technology, including research on human stem cells.[8] For example, Chapter 2 of the report, entitled "Scientific and Medical Issues in Preimplantation Embryo Research," in which the panel reviews existing and promising research in the field, draws no significant distinction between cloning and any other form of embryo research. Cloning is discussed along with studies of preimplantation genetic diagnosis, oocyte maturation, parthenogenesis, cross-species fertilization, deriving human stem cells, and other forms of embryo research. This observation is salutary because the HERP's rather indifferent classification of cloning as only one among many offshoots of IVF technology suggests that we have no choice but to discuss cloning together with assisted reproduction. Indeed, the connection between cloning and embryo research was dramatically highlighted recently in the announcement that Geron Corporation, the developer of human embryonic stem cells, was forming a $20 million alliance with the Roslin Institute, the laboratory where Dolly was cloned.[9]

Thus, even if we accept the dramatic claims that have been made about the birth of Dolly—"world-transforming," "genuinely revolutionary," and so forth—ultimately, cloning is an outgrowth of IVF technology, and we are unlikely to formulate an adequate view of cloning unless we take this fact into account.[10]

The second reason that the HERP Report is important is that it highlights the fact that, whatever one may think about the status of the preimplantation embryo or about embryo research generally, such research, including research on human cloning, holds the promise of significant clinical benefit. Among the possible benefits, the panel includes the improvement of IVF technology itself, greater understanding of birth defects, the development of safer and more effective forms of birth control, advances in treating cancer, advances in regenerating damaged tissue or organs, and the development of techniques for avoiding or correcting inherited cytoplasmic defects. Although not all of these benefits would flow from research on human cloning, some of them would. The important point for our purposes is that, once again, the HERP has tacitly drawn attention to a key fact: As with embryo research generally, no discussion of cloning will be adequate that fails to take into account the clinical implications of pursuing or prohibiting human cloning.

Finally, the HERP Report is important to debates about cloning because the panel clearly recognized the significance of discussing the moral status of the early embryo to any effort to formulate public policy in this area. Although the panel's discussion of the status of the preimplantation embryo has been sharply criticized, including by authors in this volume, the prominence the panel gave this issue in their chapter on the ethical issues raised by embryo research is striking.

One reason the HERP may have devoted such attention to this issue was the recognition that, at least in the United States, the issue of embryo research is deeply tied to that of abortion. In a paper commissioned by the HERP, Lori Andrews and Nanette Elster compared the policies on embryo research in 11 countries to that in the United States.[11] They concluded that in most other countries laws affecting embryo research are part of a regulatory scheme addressing IVF and assisted reproduction. In contrast, in the United States, laws affecting embryo research have generally been part of abortion legislation. This historic association between embryo research and abortion suggests that any adequate account of the former must inevitably take up the issue of the status of the embryo, an issue that has been fundamental in debates about abortion in the United States. It also follows that, if cloning is best discussed as part of a comprehensive review of the implications of assisted reproduction, including embryo research, then the issue of the status of the embryo is unavoidable when considering cloning.

Perhaps it is because the issue of embryo research has been tied so directly to that of abortion in the United States that the work of the HERP was controversial from the start. Shortly after the HERP was formed, 32 members of Congress wrote to Harold Varmus, the director of NIH, to complain about the composition of the panel and about the process by which members of the panel were selected.[12] A lawsuit was also filed, which attempted to block the work of the panel. In the end, however, the panel completed its work and issued its report, calling for limited federal funding of embryo research within a framework of strict guidelines. Although the report was accepted by both the NIH Director's Advisory

Committee and by President Clinton, at least in part, the recommendations of the HERP have not in fact been implemented.[13] Instead, in January 1996, congressional opponents of embryo research blocked the use of federal funds for such work by passing a continuing resolution that prohibits such funding. A similar prohibition was included in appropriations bills for the Department of Health and Human Services for 1997 and 1998.

The National Bioethics Advisory Commission report on cloning

The NBAC report is an obvious starting point for any discussion of cloning, if for no other reason than the fact that the report was the first sustained effort to address the implications of Dolly's birth for public policy in the United States. There are, however, other reasons as well. I think even critics would acknowledge that the report does a good job both describing the techniques used to clone Dolly and distinguishing between realistic and fanciful concerns raised by the prospect of human cloning. For example, the report provides a very useful discussion of how many fears about cloning are based on a mistaken belief in a kind of genetic determinism, according to which a person's genes are thought to "bear a simple relationship to the physical and psychological traits that compose the individual" (p. 32). The report also provides a helpful review of the positions on cloning taken by various religious traditions, and it effectively summarizes many of the ethical arguments that have been made both for and against cloning.

In addition, the commission made specific recommendations about cloning that continue to shape debates about cloning in the United States. Among the recommendations made by the commission were the following:

- A continuation of the current moratorium on the use of federal funding in support of any attempt to create a child by somatic cell nuclear transfer.
- An immediate request to all firms, clinicians, investigators, and professional societies in the private and non-federally funded sectors to comply voluntarily with the intent of the federal moratorium.
- Federal legislation should be enacted to prohibit anyone from attempting, whether in a research or clinical setting, to create a child through somatic cell nuclear transfer cloning. It is critical, however, that such legislation include a sunset clause to ensure that Congress will review the issue after a specified time period (three to five years) in order to decide whether the prohibition continues to be needed.
- Any regulatory or legislative actions undertaken to effect the foregoing prohibition on creating a child by somatic cell nuclear transfer should be carefully written so as not to interfere with other important areas of scientific research. In particular, no new regulations are required regarding the cloning of human DNA sequences and cell lines, since neither activity raises the scientific and

ethical issues that arise from the attempt to create children through somatic cell nuclear transfer, and these fields of research have already provided important scientific and biomedical advances.[14]

In addition to these recommendations, the commission also urged continued public discussion of the issue and called on federal agencies to support initiatives designed to educate the public about cloning and human genetics.

In acknowledging the real contribution of the NBAC report, it is also important to note some of the report's limitations. It is important to recall the volatile political situation into which the NBAC was thrust when it was given the responsibility of issuing a report on cloning within 90 days of the announcement of Dolly's birth, for some of the limitations flow from the circumstances in which the commission received its charge. For example, it should not be surprising that the commission sought to restrict the scope of its assignment. Given the experience of the HERP, which several of the commissioners knew first hand because they had been on the panel, and given the time pressure under which the NBAC was working, the commission made a strategic decision to limit the scope of its inquiry. Harold Shapiro, the chairman of the commission, made this very clear in the letter he wrote to President Clinton conveying the report to the President. "In this report," Shapiro wrote,

[w]e address a very specific aspect of cloning namely where genetic material would be transferred from the nucleus of a somatic cell of an existing human being to an enucleated human egg with the intention of creating a child. We do not revisit either the question of the cloning of humans by embryo-splitting or the issues surrounding embryo research. The latter has, of course, recently received careful attention by a National Institutes of Health panel, the Administration, and Congress.[1]

Both of these restrictions are important and merit comment.

The decision not to discuss embryo splitting draws attention to the fact that when discussing cloning we must be careful to distinguish among the different types of cloning. In general, *cloning* refers to the process of producing a precise genetic copy of an organism, be it cell, plant, animal, or human. The NBAC, of course, was concerned with the possibility of human cloning, and even here we can distinguish at least three types. The first and least controversial type involves replicating genetic or cellular material. For example, molecular biologists can make copies of DNA fragments in order to have large quantities of identical DNA, which is useful for many kinds of scientific experiments. Alternatively, scientists can replicate particular cells by growing them in culture in a laboratory, creating what is called a cell line, that is, a group of cells that is identical to the original cell from which all subsequent cells are derived. Both molecular cloning and cellular cloning are widespread, and both have produced important clinical advances in the treatment of human diseases. Because neither form of cloning involves the production of a new human being, neither has been, nor is likely to be, controversial.

The second kind of human cloning involves the splitting of a human embryo. Sometimes referred to as *blastomere separation* or *twinning*, this type of cloning involves attempting to get the early embryo to divide into multiple embryos, as sometimes happens naturally when identical twins, triplets, or quadruplets are produced. Because the cells that make up the early embryo are undifferentiated and thus have the potential to develop into any and all of the tissues and organs that are necessary for embryo development, it is possible to separate the blastomeres and to have them continue to develop as separate organisms that are genetically identical (Fig. 1).

Although blastomere separation has been possible in non-human animals for some time, it was not until 1993 that it was successfully tried in humans. At that point, researchers at the George Washington University Medical Center took 22 fertilized eggs, allowed them to divide into two-, four-, or eight-cell organisms, dissolved the protective outer covering of the developing embryos, and placed them in a solution that allowed individual blastomeres to separate and fall apart. They then recorded the divisions of the developing blastomeres that resulted and noted that they ended up with 48 cleaving blastomeres. Although the eggs the researchers used had been fertilized by more than one spermatozoan and were thus not viable, and although the resulting embryos were not transferred to a uterus, the investigators concluded that cloning through blastomere separation in humans was possible.[15]

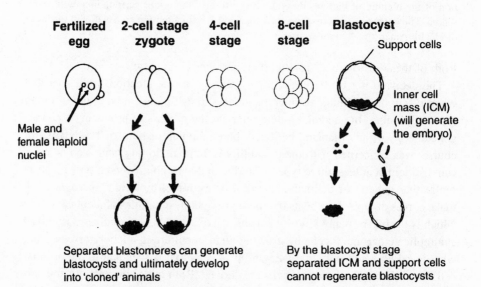

FIGURE 1 Cloning by blastomere separation. The developing embryo is split when it is between the 2-cell stage and the 8-cell stage.

The third type of cloning is what the NBAC calls *somatic cell nuclear transfer cloning*. This form of cloning involves transferring the nucleus from a cell that has two sets of genes into an egg from which the nucleus has been removed. If the egg and the transferred nucleus fuse and if the transferred nucleus begins to direct cell development, an embryo results that is genetically identical to the donor from whom the transferred nucleus came (Fig. 2).

When discussing nuclear transfer cloning, it is also important to note that the nucleus that is transferred can come from different sources. In the early work on nuclear transfer cloning in non-human animals, the procedure was successful only when the nucleus came from a donor cell taken from an early embryo. As we have seen, cells from the early embryo are undifferentiated, and thus the speculation was that undifferentiated cells were necessary for nuclear transplant cloning because only such cells would be capable of directing cell development when fused with an enucleated egg. The significance of Dolly's birth, therefore, was that it proved that a nucleus transferred from a differentiated cell taken from an adult could also produce a viable embryo. It thus demonstrated the possibility of cloning both embryos and adults through nuclear transplantation.

With this as background, we can see the exact scope of the NBAC investigation into human cloning. By limiting its discussion to somatic cell nuclear transfer cloning, the commission chose only to consider the most direct implication of Dolly's birth, namely, the possibility that a somatic cell from a human adult could be transferred into an egg to produce a human clone. Furthermore, the recommendations made by the commission reflect this choice. For example, although the NBAC recommended that federal legislation be enacted to prohibit any attempt to clone through somatic cell nuclear transfer, they did not recommend a similar ban on cloning through blastomere separation, even though many of the concerns they raised about nuclear transfer would apply to embryo splitting as

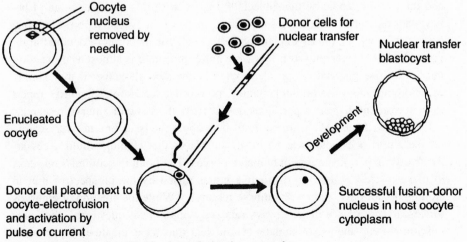

FIGURE 2 Nuclear transfer via electrofusion in mammals.

well. In fact, the commission defined somatic cell nuclear transfer in such a way that transferring a nucleus from an embryo or fetus would not be covered by their proposed ban.

This does not mean that the commission approved of cloning through either blastomere separation or nuclear transplantation using embryos. The NBAC report simply does not address these issues, and this is the point: As valuable as the NBAC report is, it is not comprehensive. By choosing to limit the scope of its inquiry, the commission enhanced its chances of reporting on time, but at a price. Limiting the scope of its inquiry also meant limiting the usefulness of its report.

This trade-off is also evident in the decision not to discuss the relationships between cloning and embryo research. Even more than the decision not to discuss blastomere separation, the choice to avoid discussing embryo research represents a strategic decision to avoid controversy and thus to promote consensus. In this case, the decision represents an understandable effort to sidestep the pitfall of abortion politics in which the HERP Report became mired. As I have already indicated, however, there are good reasons for thinking that cloning should not be discussed in isolation from the general moral issues raised by assisted reproduction and the many kinds of embryo manipulations to which it has given rise.

In a well-known critique of the HERP Report, George Annas, Arthur Caplan, and Sherman Elias have argued that, despite the fact that the panel devoted a substantial portion of the chapter on the ethical implications of embryo research to discussing the status of the preimplantation embryo, the panel failed to avoid the "gridlock" of abortion politics because it was unwilling to defend a position on the moral status of the embryo. "Inability to define the moral status of the embryo convincingly," they wrote, "is the crucial failure of both the panel's report and the overall debate on the subject."[16] I agree with this assessment, and I believe that much the same criticism could be made of the NBAC report. The irony here is that, when Annas, Caplan, and Elias call for much more detailed argument, the NBAC responds as if less were more. Indeed, it is almost as if the commissioners thought that the problem could be avoided altogether if they simply said nothing about the preimplantation embryo. Hence Harold Shapiro's report to the President that the report does not "revisit" the issue of embryo research.

Of course, the NBAC is not entirely silent about the issue of embryo research, for the report does acknowledge in several places that cloning would necessarily involve experimentation on human embryos. The point the commission seeks to make instead is that the distinctive issues raised by the prospect of human cloning do not have to do with embryo research. "While the creation of embryos for research purposes alone always raises serious ethical questions," the commission writes, "the use of somatic cell nuclear transfer to create embryos raises no new issues in this respect. The unique and distinctive ethical issues raised by the use of somatic cell nuclear transfer to create children relate to, for example, serious safety concerns, individuality, family integrity, and treating children as objects" (p. 64). For the reasons cataloged above, therefore, the commission chose to focus on the "unique and distinctive" issues.

Again, this decision is understandable and was probably necessary if the commission was to meet its deadline. Nevertheless, there are two problems with this strategy. First, it allows the NBAC to proceed as if the status of the preimplantation embryo and thus of embryo research generally has already been definitively resolved, which is simply not the case. Second, it gives the impression that the issues that the NBAC identifies as distinctive of cloning are unrelated to the status of the embryo. Although this may be true in some cases, it is not true in all. For example, surely the issue of treating children as objects requires us to think carefully about how we conceptualize the early embryo and whether the treatment of embryos has implications for the treatment of children.

Given the important, if circumscribed, contribution of both the HERP Report and the NBAC report, where should a discussion of cloning begin? If, as I have argued, it is important to consider cloning in the context of wider issues facing assisted reproduction and embryo research generally, then one clear starting point is precisely the moral status of the early embryo. That is in fact where this volume begins. Part I, then, takes up the issue of the status of the early embryo and considers the relationship between cloning and embryo status. One obvious question here is whether the preimplantation embryo has the same moral status as an infant or child. Yet, even when there is agreement that the embryo is not morally comparable to a person with rights, other issues remain vexing. Is there a difference, for example, between using embryos left over from IVF procedures and creating embryos through cloning, solely for research purposes? Is conceptualizing the embryo as not fully a person equivalent to reducing it to a mere object? Does the way in which we think about the early embryo affect how we think about the parent–child relationship? What is the relationship between the issue of embryo research and that of abortion?

The authors in Part I take sharply differing views about the status of the preimplantation embryo, and so they would, in turn, answer these questions very differently. The section begins with a chapter by Bonnie Steinbock in which she defends her well-known and influential view that because the early embryo is incapable of experiencing pain, it cannot be said to have interests. For that reason, killing the early embryo does not have the same moral significance as killing an adult human being or a child. Of course, knowing that killing an early embryo is not morally equivalent to killing a person is not yet to know exactly how we ought to treat the early embryo. According to Steinbock, because the embryo has value, if not interests, it should be treated with respect. At the very least, says Steinbock, respect for the embryo would rule out frivolous or trivial research.

Although Courtney Campbell would certainly agree with Steinbock that trivial research on early embryos should not be allowed, he argues in Chapter 2 that the position of the HERP, which is in many ways similar to Steinbock's, that the early embryo deserves "serious moral consideration" does not in fact ensure the requisite respect. Given the tendency within medicine and within science generally to reduce the person to body parts, and given that embryo research removes the embryo from "its originating context of reproduction," there is a grave danger that embryos will be treated merely as replenishable resources. When embryos become merely resources for research, Campbell argues, they will not be accorded the respect they deserve. Indeed, in such a context, talk of "respect" is deeply misleading.

Campbell's talk about embryos being relocated from reproduction to research is picked up by Maura Ryan in Chapter 3. Like Campbell, Ryan is skeptical that appeals to respect the embryo will actually safeguard the moral values at stake in cloning and human embryo research. Indeed, Ryan responds directly to Steinbock's interest view and argues that the interest view simply cannot do justice to all of the morally important considerations raised by access to embryos. Specifically, says Ryan, focusing on competing rights and interests, as the interest view does, distracts us from considering whether we might be undermining the integrity of human procreation in a way that "may be violating some of the deepest and most basic of human matter—procreation, kinship, [and] marital intimacy. . . ." By moving beyond the interest view, says Ryan, we come to see the need to reconsider what we were doing when we intervened in the process of reproduction in accepting IVF. If, as Ryan suggests, the goal of reproductive interventions should be "the bringing forth of new life in loving and nurturing relationship," then there should be serious constraints on how embryos might be used in research, and no embryos should be created solely for research purposes.

Just as Maura Ryan extends Courtney Campbell's insight that embryo research removes the embryo from its originating context, so too does James Keenan's essay dovetail with Ryan's. In Chapter 4, Keenan agrees with Ryan that debates about cloning and embryo research have not sufficiently attended to the question of what kind of society we become in undertaking such research. According to Keenan, supporters of cloning and embryo research have not provided a positive argument to justify their activities, and the concept of "respect" that they invoke to constrain research is largely without meaning. In Keenan's view, the issues raised by cloning and embryo research are so novel, and traditional moral categories have proved of such limited use in sorting out these issues, that we face a situation analogous to that faced by moralists in the sixteenth century who developed the method of moral reasoning known as *casuistry*. Just as those moralists turned to cases for guidance, so, too, should we reason casuistically in thinking about embryo research.

If the first four chapters are all, in one way or another, focused on the moral status of the preimplantation embryo, Chapter 5 highlights the significance of the fact that so much of the debate about cloning and embryo research is framed in these terms. Given how important the question of embryo status is to debates about cloning and embryo research, it should not be surprising that both issues are readily linked with that of abortion. As Alta Charo points out, however, the argument against abortion is frequently framed as an argument from potential, and the possibility of cloning raises interesting problems for the argument from potential.

Opponents of abortion, for example, typically draw no distinction between embryos in vitro and embryos in vivo. Thus opponents of abortion also typically oppose embryo research. But if in vitro embryos should not be destroyed because they have the potential to develop into adult humans, what will we say about the potential of skin cells to develop into adult humans if cloning is achieved? By examining this question in detail, Charo seeks to drive a wedge between the issues of abortion and embryo research, thereby creating space for a compromise that would allow for public funding of embryo research.

An adequate discussion of cloning cannot, however, be restricted to an examination of the moral status of the early embryo. As the NBAC report points out, cloning raises some distinctive moral issues. For example, questions about individuality, family integrity, and the objectification of children arise in particularly striking or even unique ways if cloning human beings is possible. Part II, therefore, takes up some of the more distinctive issues raised by cloning. It begins with the report written by Dan Brock that the NBAC commissioned to help it sort through the ethical issues raised by cloning. In it, Brock identifies some of the major moral considerations raised by cloning, and he critically examines arguments both for and against cloning. In Brock's view, although there is no urgent human need that cloning uniquely addresses, neither does it violate basic human rights. For example, according to Brock, cloning would violate neither a right to a unique identity nor the right to an open future, both of which have been claimed by critics of cloning. Moreover, although critics of cloning have pointed to a variety of individual and social harms that cloning would produce, Brock argues that many of these harms are entirely speculative. Thus, although Brock concludes that the jury is still out with regard to cloning, the preponderance of evidence he offers appears to support the moral legitimacy of cloning.

If Brock implicitly endorses cloning, Ron Green, the author of the second chapter in Part II, explicitly does so. Unlike most of the authors in this volume, Green is willing to predict that cloning will become a routine part of infertility treatment worldwide. He believes that in 20 years there will be between several hundred and several thousand children born yearly through human cloning. This eventuality should neither shock us nor significantly trouble us morally. Indeed, according to Green, were it not for the rather poor quality of ethical analysis of cloning, we would already have embraced the possibility of cloning as a relatively modest addition to infertility treatment. Alas, says Green, critics of cloning have greatly exaggerated its risks, often invoking wildly implausible nightmare scenarios to sway public opinion against cloning.

Green's chapter thus points to an irony in the cloning debate. Although critics often seek to play on negative visceral responses, the scenarios they envision—sexual reproduction being replaced by commercialized reproduction involving the cloning of desired genotypes—actually discount people's deep commitment to traditional patterns of parenting and reproduction. According to Green, even the NBAC, which generally did a good job of resisting the temptation to paint nightmare scenarios, contributed to the pattern of approaching cloning in alarmist and unhelpful ways. First, by accepting the President's mandate to produce a report in 90 days, the NBAC fueled the sense of urgency and thus alarm. Second, by providing a prominent place for religious responses to cloning, the NBAC chose to highlight testimony from groups that are typically ill-equipped to respond quickly to complex technological innovation. The upshot is that the NBAC issued a more cautious document than its own reasoning supported.

Green observes that the teaching of many religious traditions on sexual ethics developed over centuries and that this fact may impede appropriate reflection on contemporary forms of reproduction, including cloning. This observation may, however, support another conclusion, namely, that religious reflection on cloning may provide a wisdom hard-won over the centuries. This, in any event, is the position that Laurie Zoloth defends in Chapter 8. Drawing on Jewish tradition, Zoloth argues that discussing cloning as a form of assisted reproduction, as even Jewish scholars consulted by the NBAC did, misses the fact that the urge to clone is as much about the desire to avoid death as it is about the need to create life. In fact, she writes, cloning "reflects the deepest of yearnings: for redemption and resurrection into a better, purer, and transformed self. . . ." Yet if cloning is best thought about in the context of confronting our mortality, then Jewish tradition may have much to offer to public debate about cloning, just as other religious traditions may. Specifically, Jewish tradition urges a passionate search for justice in the face of death, not a restrained effort to overcome death through replication.

Finally, the volume takes up the public policy dimension of debates about cloning and human embryo research. Although two specially appointed advisory panels have recommended federal funding of embryo research in the United States, no funding of such research has yet taken place. This history suggests that setting long-term policy on cloning, particularly if the current safety concerns are addressed, is likely to be extremely complicated and divisive. We thus need to think carefully about how to formulate and implement government policies, or laws, on controversial issues like cloning. Part III takes up some of these issues.

Part III begins with a strong indictment of current public policy by Carol Tauer, who sees a peculiar incoherence in public policy on embryo research. On the one hand, moral reservation about such research is sufficiently strong that there is no

public funding allowed for such work. On the other hand, the worries about embryo research have not led to regulation of research in the private sector. The obvious question is how embryo research can be so problematic that we ban it in
the public sphere while at the same time it is so innocuous that it is unrestricted
in the private sphere.

Moreover, says Tauer, the public embraces assisted reproduction that grew out
of embryo research at the same time it denounces embryo research itself. The
consequence is again incoherence. We allow unsafe and unstudied procedures
like IVF, which originally required embryo research, but we will not fund the
kind of embryo research that would make IVF safe and reliable.

According to Tauer, the lesson to be learned from assisted reproduction is that,
if we are going to move forward with cloning and stem cell research, we must
be committed to doing the sort of embryo research that will ensure the safety and
efficacy of procedures based on these techniques. There is, however, an alternative. We could cease using techniques that depend on embryo research for their
safety and efficacy. As Tauer puts it, "Since it is both ethically and scientifically
unacceptable to offer elective procedures whose safety and efficacy are in question, and since adequate testing is unlikely without federal funding and federal
mandates, we have a situation where society as a whole has simply decided not
to take responsibility." Such a situation, Tauer argues, is unacceptable.

The second chapter in Part III examines the role of bioethics panels in the formulation of public policy in the United States. Here Jonathan Moreno and Alex
John London argue that bioethics panels can play an important role in the formulation of a coherent and fair public policy, and to do so they must seek to
forge consensus both within the panel itself and within society as a whole. For
this reason, bioethics panels should not really be understood as ethics bodies;
their job is rather to formulate policy. Although ethical deliberation is necessary
to the process, it is not the goal of the process.

To illustrate their claims about the importance of consensus building for
bioethics panels, Moreno and London examine the experiences of both the NIH
embryo research panel and the NBAC exploration of cloning. According to
Moreno and London, the HERP did an admirable job in achieving internal consensus on embryo research, and their effort to justify their position by stressing
the pluralism of views in American society was well founded. The HERP's fatal
mistake, however, was to present their "consensus compromise" in the form of
an ethical argument for allowing embryo research. The problem, say Moreno and
London, is that, because the real argument to support its recommendation is a
policy argument, not an ethical argument, the panel report was vulnerable to serious criticism about its purported ethical argument.

In contrast, because the NBAC reached an easy consensus on cloning based
on the likelihood (in the short term) of harm to any person created in this way,

it failed to wrestle with some of the substantial long-term moral issues raised by cloning. To its credit, the NBAC took seriously its role as forger of public consensus. For that reason, it sought out the views of religious traditions in a way that the HERP had not. Yet, in grounding the consensus it reached on the issue of safety in the short term, the NBAC ensured that the impact of its report would not be long lasting. As Moreno and London point out, the problems with safety will eventually be overcome. Once we move beyond the issue of safety, we will encounter many of the divisions confronted by the HERP. According to Moreno and London, in the face of the sort of complex and conflicting issues the HERP encountered, the NBAC does little more than acknowledge them and move on.

Writing about the same two ethics bodies as Moreno and London, Brian Stiltner reaches very different conclusions in Chapter 11. Unlike Moreno and London, Stiltner believes that ethics panels should develop substantive moral arguments to support the normative conclusions they inevitably reach. To make his case, Stiltner examines how both the HERP and the NBAC utilized moral and religious arguments in their respective reports.

Interestingly, Stiltner's reading of these two reports is almost completely opposite that of Moreno and London. Where Moreno and London argue that the HERP was effective in promoting a procedural compromise and stymied by its effort to advance ethical arguments, Stiltner suggests that the HERP needed to ground its compromise position much more explicitly and extensively with ethical arguments. Where Moreno and London see the NBAC's attention to the views of religious traditions as opening the door to paralyzing political forces, once consensus around the short-term safety of cloning breaks down, Stiltner urges greater attention to religious views and greater participation by religious communities as necessary to forging a public consensus on cloning. In Stiltner's view, there is no escaping the need for substantive moral argument because all procedural argument ultimately rests on substantive norms. Therefore, it is always a mistake, to use Stiltner's words, to attempt, as Moreno and London do, "to drive a wedge between procedural and substantive argument."

In the end, whether we side with Stiltner or with Moreno and London, there is little question that the work of public ethics bodies is advisory only. Ultimately, public policy will be set by legislation. The final chapter of the volume, therefore, examines efforts to regulate cloning both in the United States and around the world. Canvassing bills introduced in both state legislatures and the United States Congress, Heidi Forster and Emily Ramsey document the kinds of regulations that might determine the direction of cloning and embryo research, at least in the United States. As they note, there are serious and as yet unresolved constitutional questions at stake in efforts to regulate cloning. Once again, we see the connection between cloning and reproductive technology in the question of whether procreative liberty extends to the decision to create a child through cloning.

The moral and legal questions raised by the prospect (and perhaps the eventual reality) of cloning a human being are likely to be with us for a long time to come. No single volume can possibly address the complex issues in their entirety. My hope is that this volume, by attempting repeatedly and consistently to frame the discussion of cloning in the wider context of embryo research and assisted reproduction generally, will provide a helpful corrective to the many works that look at cloning in isolation from the world of reproductive medicine out of which it grows. If this volume broadens the general discussion of cloning to include a consideration of embryo research and assisted reproduction, it may be deemed a success.

I

MORAL STATUS OF THE PREIMPLANTATION EMBRYO

1

Respect for Human Embryos

BONNIE STEINBOCK

How ought we to think about human embryos? Are they due the respect owed to any human person? Do they have the same human rights? These questions are crucial to diverse topics, from abortion and contraception (because some forms of contraception, such as the intrauterine device, work by preventing implantation of a very early embryo) to embryo research, assisted reproductive technology (ART), and germ-line genetic manipulation, in which early embryos are genetically changed, without, it hardly needs to be said, their consent, informed or otherwise. Most recently, the topic of somatic cell nuclear transfer (SCNT) cloning has raised the question of the moral status of human embryos, as this technique, should it prove successful, would in effect turn every cell in the human body into a potential embryo. We need to know, then, what is morally permissible to do to embryos and what is not. To answer this question, we turn to theories of moral status, of which there are basically three.

The first, known as the *species* or *genetic humanity view*, holds that human embryos are human beings, just like you and me. They have all the rights of any human being, including a right to life and the general Kantian right not to be used as a "mere means" to others' ends. This would include a right not to be the subject of experiments that would expose the embryo to significant risks or death, without compensating benefit. Those who accept the genetic humanity view focus on the fact that a human embryo is indisputably human, as human as a newborn

human infant, child, or adult. If all human beings have certain rights independent of their particular characteristics (age, nationality, intelligence, moral good-
ness, and so forth), then the same rights belong to human beings at the earliest
stage of their development, namely, the embryonic stage.

The genetic humanity view is stirring in its commitment to the equal worth of
all human beings. Nevertheless, as Mary Anne Warren has pointed out in a now-
classic article, the genetic humanity view, which is used by conservatives to
demonstrate the wrongness of abortion, begs the question.[1] It maintains that it is
wrong to kill embryos because embryos are human and all humans have a right
not to be killed. This assumes, however, that it is genetic humanity or species
membership that has moral significance. But why should moral status, rights, and
the like be limited to only human beings, that is, members of the species *Homo
sapiens*? Is it not possible that there are non-humans, such as intelligent ex-
traterrestrials, who (if they exist) would be entitled to equal respect and rights?
This suggests that membership in a particular species is not a necessary condition of moral status. But neither does such membership seem to be a sufficient
condition, as can be seen by the example of human beings who have irretriev-
ably lost the ability to think, feel, or experience: patients in a persistent vegetative state. It is far from clear that such individuals have the same moral status
and rights as the rest of us. Their moral status has changed because, while their
bodies continue to live, the persons have ceased to exist.[2] Although the body, living or dead, deserves respect, it is the *person* who has dignity, rights, and a special moral status.[3]

The mistake made by the adherents of the genetic humanity view of moral status, Warren alleges, is that they confuse biological and moral humanity, failing
to see that it is possible to be biologically human without being morally human,
that is, a full-fledged member of the moral community. It is not genetic human
beings who are members of the moral community, but persons. She then goes on
to identify persons as beings who are conscious, self-conscious, thinking, possessed of the ability to use language, and so forth. Clearly, embryos do not have
any of these characteristics, and therefore embryos are not people and do not
have the moral status of persons.

Warren's critics have pointed out that her account of moral status, ironically
enough, suffers from the very same defect she discovered in the genetic humanity account. That is, she maintains that it is persons who are full-fledged members of the moral community and then goes on to define persons in terms of certain cognitive traits. But why should membership in the moral community depend
on these traits? What is the connection between having rights and the ability to
use language, for example? It seems that it is conceptually possible to be a moral
person, a being with rights, entitled to the protection of and respect from the
moral community, without having all, or even most of, the psychological traits
we typically ascribe to persons. Moreover, the person view notoriously leaves

out of the moral community many individuals who most of us firmly believe are members: severely mentally retarded people, people with senile dementia, and infants.

To summarize, the person view has two problems. It does not provide an explanation of the connection between "descriptive personhood" and "normative personhood," and thus it seems as guilty of arbitrariness as the species criterion of moral status. It is also too restrictive, leaving out individuals most people are convinced are moral persons, with the same rights and status as the rest of us. Both problems could be fixed if we could explain the relevance to moral personhood of the traits that confer descriptive personhood. The more ambitious project would be to show why the abilities for abstract thought and language use are conditions of full moral status, but here I will focus only on the minimal condition for having moral status, or sentience.[4]

Strictly speaking, *sentience* is the ability to experience pain or pleasure. The relevance of the capacity to experience pain (or pleasure) to moral status is relatively straightforward: If a being can feel pain, then that provides us with some reason not to inflict pain on it. It is only sentient beings who can suffer and therefore only sentient beings to whom the injunction against needless cruelty can apply.[5]

Additionally, I would argue that sentience is a condition of having any interests at all.[6] Non-sentient beings, whether mere things (like cars and rocks and works of art) or living things without nervous systems (like plants), do not have interests of their own. This is not to say that they cannot be cared for, fed, protected, repaired, and healed, or killed, injured, made sick, and destroyed. It is rather to say that it does not matter to the non-sentient beings whether we care for them or not. We can preserve their existence, and even promote their welfare (in a sense), but we cannot promote their welfare for *their own sake*, out of concern for their feelings, for they do not have any. The view that links moral status to interests and restricts interests to sentient beings I call *the interest view*.[7]

Critics of the interest view ask why a being has to feel or experience anything to have interests. A bicycle left out in the rain will rust, which will affect adversely both its appearance and its performance. Why can we not say that this is contrary to its interests? Stripping the bark off a tree will cause it to die. Why can we not say that this is against the tree's interest? Limiting interests to sentient beings (namely, animal, human, and otherwise) seems to limit unduly the arena of our concern. What about rivers and forests and mountains? What about the environment?

This objection, however, misconceives the interest view. The claim is not that we should be concerned to protect and preserve only sentient beings, but rather that only sentient beings can have an interest or a stake in their own existence. It is only sentient beings to whom anything matters, which is quite different from saying that only sentient beings matter. The interest view can acknowledge the value of many non-sentient beings, from works of art to wilderness areas. It recognizes that we have all kinds of reasons—economic, aesthetic, symbolic, even moral—to protect or preserve non-sentient beings. The difference between sentient and non-sentient beings is not that sentient beings have value and non-sentient ones lack value. Rather, it is that because non-sentient beings cannot be hurt or made to suffer, it does not matter to them what is done to them. In deciding what we should do, we cannot consider their interests because they do not have any. The wrongness of defacing a work of art, for example, cannot be expressed in terms of how it affects the work of art. Nor can we explain why it is wrong by saying, "How would you like it if you were a painting and someone slashed you?"

If sentience is both a necessary and sufficient condition of moral status, then, because embryos are non-sentient, embryos lack moral status. Precisely when in fetal development the ability to experience pain begins is controversial, with estimates ranging from 6 weeks to 6 months. It is clear, however, that very early embryos, which do not have even a rudimentary nervous system, cannot feel pain, be hurt, or made to suffer. Admittedly, they can be killed, but killing an embryo does not have the moral significance that killing a person or an animal has. To kill a sentient being is to take away its life. An embryo is not deprived of its life by being killed. In an important sense, it does not have a life to lose.

Now this claim undoubtedly will strike many people as odd. If the embryo is alive, then surely it has a life to lose? But this is just what I am denying. It seems to me that unless there is conscious awareness of some kind, a being does not have a life to lose. The use of a spermicide kills millions of sperm. Surely it would be absurd to speak of all of them as losing their lives or being deprived of their lives (much less that the loss of their lives provides us with some reason not to use this form of contraception). This suggests that it is not biological life that matters, but rather conscious existence. Killing a non-sentient embryo deprives it of nothing. To put it another way, an embryo has a biological life, but not (yet) a biographical life.[8] The interest view suggests that it is *prima facie* wrong to deprive beings of their biographical lives but not wrong to end merely biological lives, especially when there are good reasons for doing so.

Don Marquis[9] argues that killing a non-sentient fetus[10] does deprive it of its life and that this is precisely what makes abortion seriously wrong, as wrong as killing an adult human being. It is irrelevant that the fetus is unconscious and unaware of its life; the same is true for someone in a coma. What matters is that most fetuses (except those with serious anomalies) have valuable futures. If they are not killed, they will come to have lives they will value and enjoy, just as you and I value and enjoy our lives. Therefore, abortion is seriously wrong for the same reason that killing an innocent adult human being is seriously wrong: It deprives the victim of his or her valuable future.

Marquis thinks that his view is superior to other accounts of moral status in that it is able to explain what is wrong with killing people who are temporarily unconscious, something the interest view seems incapable of doing. If it is morally permissible to kill non-sentient beings, why is it wrong to kill someone in a reversible coma? Such a person is not now conscious or sentient. Furthermore, if we appeal to his future conscious states, the same argument seems to apply to the fetus, who will become conscious and sentient if we just leave it alone.

In response, let me point out an important difference between a temporarily unconscious person and a fetus. The difference is that the person who is now unconscious has had beliefs, desires, and interests that are compounded out of these beliefs and desires. The desire not to be killed while sleeping or comatose is one of my desires, even though I am rarely (if ever) conscious of this desire. This desire or preference is the basis for saying that I have an interest in not being killed should I fall into a coma. By contrast, this is not a desire or preference that can be ascribed to a non-sentient fetus.

It might be objected, however, that even if a fetus lacks preferences and desires about being killed, it nevertheless has an interest in not being killed. Our interests, after all, are not limited to what we take an interest in. Our interests also include what is in our interest, whether or not we are interested in it. For example, getting enough sleep, eating moderately, and foregoing tobacco might be in the interest of a person who has no interest in following such a regime. Now, even if the non-conscious fetus is not interested in continuing to live, could we not say that continued existence is in its interest? If the fetus will go on to have a valuable future, is not that future in its interest?

This is the case, however, only if the valuable future in question belongs to the fetus, whether the future in question is its future, and this is not obvious. It depends on the theory of identity that one accepts. According to one plausible theory of identity, personal identity requires some degree of psychological continuity. A certain set of past experiences is what makes me the person I am and the experiences that I have, my experiences. What makes experiences at two different times experiences of the same person is that they are appropriately related by a chain of memories, desires, intentions, and the like.

On this account of personal identity, then, there is an important difference between someone who is temporarily unconscious and a fetus. When unconscious people regain consciousness, they will remember their past experiences as things that happened to them. It is this chain of memory that allows us to view our experiences, as well as subsequent ones, as ours. Memory is not, however, the only sort of psychological connection. After all, most people have very few memories about anything that occurred before the age of 4 or 5 years, yet most of us are convinced that we are the same individuals we were when very young. A sophisticated psychological theory of identity will account for this, maintaining that one's identity is formed in part by early experiences whether or not one remembers them.

Someone who is toilet trained too early may become an "anal-retentive" type even though he or she has no memory of being toilet trained. Someone who has

a secure relationship with a caregiver in early infancy will become a more confident and happy adult than someone who is neglected, regardless of whether
there are any memories of early infancy. A sophisticated theory of personal identity may also be capable of explaining amnesiacs, either by assimilating them to
the infant case, or by maintaining that, in fact, there are two different persons se-
quentially existing in the same body.

It is possible that there are experiences in utero that also shape personality. If
this is so, and some version of a psychological theory of identity is true, then the
born individual is identical to the fetus, as well as to the infant and very young
child. If psychological experiences are what unify the self, however, then the born
person cannot be identical with the embryo because embryos do not have experiences. Although brain waves are present at about 6 weeks after conception,
more development of the cerebral cortex is necessary for there to be awareness
of painful stimuli, arguably the most basic form of awareness. The neural pathways are not sufficiently developed to transmit pain messages to the fetal brain
until 22 to 24 weeks of gestation. Thus, although we may be identical with sec-
ond- or third-trimester fetuses in a sophisticated psychological theory of personal
identity, we cannot be identical with early-gestation fetuses, much less embryos,
for there are no experiences in early-gestation fetuses or embryos that can shape
the personality of the born human being.

Of course, a psychological theory of identity may not be the correct one. It
may be that a theory of physical continuity provides the better account of personal identity. In that case, because there is a continuous development from the
embryo to the born person, we can view them as the same individual. The embryo is the beginning, the very first stage in the development of a human person.
It is important for Marquis's account that the wrongness of killing stop at embryos. Otherwise, it could be applied to gametes and to the sperm and ovum that
conjoin to make the embryo. If that were the case, then it would be true that gametes as well as embryos have "a future like ours" (FLO) and therefore that contraception (at least the kinds that involve killing gametes) would be seriously
wrong, as seriously wrong as killing an adult human being. This is, of course,
the *reductio ad absurdum* to which all potentiality theories are vulnerable.

Marquis says that his account of the wrongness of killing does not apply to
contraception because, before fertilization, there is no entity that has a future. It
is only after fertilization, when there is a being with a specific genetic code, that
there is an individual with a future, who can be deprived of that future by being
killed.[11] Even if we accept that the particular person who I am is not identical
with either the sperm or the egg and is (in some sense) identical to the embryo
out of which I developed, why should this deprive gametes of having FLO and
therefore of being the sorts of beings it is wrong, on Marquis's account, to kill?
Admittedly, a gamete cannot have a future all by itself. Unless certain things happen to a gamete (like combining with another gamete), it will just die. But that's

also true of the embryo that cannot develop all by itself. Unless certain things happen to the embryo (like implantation in a uterus), it too will die. Admittedly, the future a sperm will have is not its future alone; it shares its future with the ovum it fertilizes. If you prevent the sperm and ovum from conjoining, you deprive each of them of the future they would have had if fertilization had taken place. The sharing of a single future makes the situation of gametes unusual, perhaps unique, but does not seem to provide a reason why gametes cannot have futures, indeed valuable futures like ours, if the criterion of identity is physical continuity. For the embryo does not arise *ex nihilo*; its physical history begins with the conjoining of the sperm and the egg.

Sometimes it is said that a sperm is not a unique individual in the way that a fetus is. For who the sperm turns out to be depends on which ovum it unites with. Why should this lack of uniqueness deprive the sperm of being a potential person, or, to use Marquis's language, why should its lack of uniqueness prevent it from having "a future like ours"? Although we cannot ordinarily specify which future existence the sperm will have, if it is allowed to fertilize an egg, it will become somebody and that somebody will have a valuable future. In the case of intracytoplasmic sperm injection (ICSI), it *is* possible to conjoin a particular sperm and egg and thus to give, or deprive, the gametes of a particular, though shared, future.

To summarize, if a psychological theory of identity is correct, then killing an embryo cannot be wrong on the grounds that such killing deprives the embryo of its future, because before having experiences, an embryo does not have a personal future. If, on the other hand, a physical continuity theory is correct, then it is not only killing embryos that is seriously wrong. Killing gametes is also wrong, because this deprives them of the future they might have had. This conflicts with the very plausible view that there is *nothing* wrong with contraception.[12] The interest view avoids both of these difficulties. It maintains that neither gametes nor embryos are harmed or wronged or deprived of anything by being killed. More generally, nothing can be done for *their* sake because, without sentience or consciousness or awareness of any kind, they do not have sakes of their own. They do not have human rights because they are not the kind of beings who logically can have rights. Neither, and for the same reason, do they have moral status or standing.

Nevertheless, it does not follow that abortion is morally justified. The fact that a being lacks moral status and rights does not automatically justify killing it. In general, there should be a good reason for killing something, and what counts as a "good reason" depends on the kind of thing it is. A fly's irritating buzzing may justify swatting it; a dog's irritating barking would not justify killing it. In the case of abortion, the justification typically alludes to the reasons why the pregnant woman does not want to continue this pregnancy and bear a child. Those who are pro-life regard very few reasons as sufficiently important to justify killing the embryo or fetus.[13] Those who are pro-choice think that, because of the burdens imposed by unwanted childbearing and childrearing, almost any reason a woman has for not wanting to bear a child justifies terminating a pregnancy. This is not the place to explore the sufficiency of reasons for abortion[14]; my point is rather that an adequate justification of abortion will refer *both* to the moral status of the unborn (or rather its lack thereof) *and* to the pregnant woman's right to bodily self-determination.[15]

Abortion is probably the most hotly contested topic having to do with the moral status of embryos and fetuses,[16] but it is by no means the only topic, as I noted at the beginning of this essay. What are the implications of the interest view for areas like assisted reproductive technology, embryo research, germ-line engineering, and cloning? In particular, does the interest view imply that it is morally permissible to do anything you like to embryos? Or are there limits to the ways in which embryos may be treated?[17] In particular, can we make sense of the idea of having respect for embryos if we deny that they have interests, rights, and moral status?

The view that embryo research, while acceptable in principle, should nevertheless be restricted to demonstrate "profound respect" for embryos as a form of human life has been taken by several important official bodies, including the Ethics Advisory Board (EAB) in the United States[18] and the Warnock Committee in Great Britain.[19] This was also the position taken in 1994 by the Human Embryo Research Panel of the National Institutes of Health (NIH) in its report on the ex utero preimplantation embryo. It concluded that the preimplantation embryo "deserves special respect" and "serious moral consideration as a developing form of human life."

Giving meaning to this concept of "special respect" or "serious moral consideration," however, remains problematic. As John Robertson[20] incisively describes the difficulty: "If the embryo has no rights or interests, how can it be owed 'special respect'? On the other hand, if the embryo is owed special respect, is it not then a holder of rights, including the right not to be the subject of research? What does 'special respect' mean?"

Unless we can give a convincing account of "special respect," the suspicion will remain in many minds that this phrase merely allows us to kill embryos and not feel so bad about it.

If giving embryos "serious moral consideration" meant taking seriously their interests or advancing their welfare, then it would be impossible to show them serious moral consideration because, on the view I have been advancing (the interest view), embryos do not have interests or a welfare of their own.

There is another sense of showing "serious moral consideration," however, which does not imply that the entity in question has interests or rights or a welfare of its own. Consider, for example, a proposal to build a shopping center or a baseball field on a sacred burial ground. Most people would find this morally offensive, not because the piece of land is harmed or wronged by this usage (which is absurd) or even because the bodies buried there would be harmed or wronged. Rather, the wrongness is explained by saying that the interests served by building a shopping center or baseball field—that is, commercial and entertainment purposes—are insufficiently important to justify the destruction of a place that has solemn religious significance.

It might be objected that it is wrong to say, in advance, that commercial or entertainment purposes are inevitably "trumped" by things that have religious significance. After all, a shopping center may employ hundreds of people and contribute significantly to their welfare and the welfare of the community. Why should we think that this is less important than preserving burial grounds, however sacred they may be to some?

I readily concede that economic interests may be pressing and, indeed, more important than religious interests. Insofar as the conflict is between two sets of interests, there is no guarantee that one set of interests will prevail. The point of the example of a burial ground is not that symbolic or religious significance is always more important than other kinds of interests. Rather, it is intended to show that things that lack moral status can nevertheless have moral value. It makes no sense to talk about the interests or rights of a burial ground, but perfectly good sense to talk about its moral significance, which stems from its connection with a value that is clearly moral, namely, respect for the dead.

Respect for the dead is a moral value in virtually every culture. It seems likely that it is also what Ronald Dworkin[21] calls an *intrinsic* value. That is, the value of respecting the dead is independent of what people happen to enjoy or want or need or of what is good for them. Dworkin suggests that great paintings, wilderness areas, human cultures, languages, some species, traditional crafts, and human life itself all have intrinsic value. Respect for the dead also seems to fall into this category. If a culture lacked respect for its dead (had no death rituals, for example) we would probably regard it as considerably less evolved, even not quite human.[22] As Feinberg[23] explains:

It would be wrong, for example, to hack up Grandfather's body after he has died a natural death, and dispose of his remains in the trash can on a cold winter's morning. That would be wrong not because it violates Grandfather's rights; he is dead and no longer has the same sort of rights as the rest of us, and we can make it part of the example that he was not offended while alive at the thought of such posthumous treatment and indeed even consented to it in advance. Somehow acts of this kind if not forbidden would strike at our respect for living human persons (without which organized society would be impossible) in the most keenly threatening way.

Just as disrespect for dead bodies can strike at our respect for living human persons, so, too, I want to suggest, can inappropriate treatment or use of embryos. Embryos, as much as dead bodies, are a "potent symbol of human life"[24] and for that reason have moral value and deserve respect, even though they lack interests, rights, and (therefore) moral status. Let us consider the implications of this for research and disposition of frozen embryos.

Respect for embryos as a form of human life does not rule out using embryos in important medical research, for example, in reproductive medicine, genetics, or cancer and other diseases, as these are endeavors with the potential for enormous human benefit. What would be impermissible is frivolous or trivial research on human embryos, such as using embryos to teach high school science classes, to test the safety of new cosmetics,[25] or to create jewelry. These are situations in which there is no pressing need to use human embryos, and their use displays contempt rather than respect for human life.

Daniel Callahan has charged that the NIH Human Embryo Research Panel, while paying lip service to the idea of respect for embryos, failed to support this with a clear demonstration that progress in scientific research depends on using human embryos. Instead, its members simply gave a blank check to scientific research. He writes:

Duly reverential, the panel satisfied itself with simply listing all the research possibilities, including the improvement and increased safety of IVF, the creation of cell lines that might someday be useful for bone marrow transplantation, repair of spinal cord injuries, skin replacement and, naturally, the hint of a greater understanding of cancer.[26]

Callahan thinks that more skepticism was called for, including a more thorough examination of the ways in which knowledge might be gained without using human embryos.

Callahan's point, I take it, is not that respect for embryos entails that they never be destroyed or used in research. Rather, it is that the interests or goals to be accomplished by using human embryos in research must be shown to be compelling and unreachable by other means. For if *any* purposes can justify the destruction of embryos, in what sense are they being shown "profound respect"? The very idea appears hollow.

Although Callahan's point is a good one, it is surely too stringent to ask that researchers know what results embryo research will yield before the research is done. A lot of research is promissory in the sense that it is impossible to predict which research will have beneficial results. Advances in reproductive medicine are, however, hard to envisage if researchers are not permitted to use human embryos. In any event, the principle elaborated by the panel is the correct one: that research using human embryos should be limited to research likely to result in significant benefit to people, as only such research demonstrates respect. Callahan would have liked to see more evidence of the benefit and of the fact that this research could not be done without using human embryos. Because the panel was not charged with determining which specific research projects should be permitted or funded, the criticism seems misapplied.

Another area in which the question of respect for embryos occurs is in the disposition of frozen embryos no longer needed or wanted for reproduction by the individuals who created them. Tens of thousands of embryos are steadily accumulating in tanks of liquid nitrogen in the United States alone.[27] Ideally, their progenitors should decide what to do with them, whether, once they are no longer needed for reproduction, they should be discarded, used in research, or donated (if they are still viable) to other couples. Some couples are unwilling to make this decision, however, preferring to keep the embryos frozen indefinitely rather than discard them. In some cases, the clinic loses touch with the gamete donors.

In August 1996, scientists at fertility clinics in Great Britain "reluctantly destroyed several thousand abandoned human embryos"[28] under the Human Fertilization and Embryology Act, which limits storage to 5 years. The destruction of the embryos was greeted with outrage in some quarters; some officials in the Catholic Church referred to the event as "a prenatal massacre."[29] Italian doctors offered to pay to "adopt" the embryos, with the intention of bringing them to Italy to implant them in women there. Some Catholics argued that the embryos be given a proper funeral and others that the embryos be allowed to die naturally.

It seems to me that these attitudes make sense only if one thinks of preimplantation embryos as human persons who deserve the same respect in death as any other person. (Even if one does take this view of pre-embryos, it is hard to imagine how such respect would be shown. How does one give a proper funeral to something smaller than the period at the end of a sentence?) But suppose one does not regard embryos as very tiny human persons, but instead takes the view that, while not persons, they are forms of human life and, as such, deserving of respect. What would be required to show respect for embryos no longer wanted by their progenitors for reproduction? In particular, may they be discarded? It is hard to see why keeping them frozen in perpetuity shows more respect than discarding them or using them in valuable research. Of course, they could be donated to other couples wishing to use them to reproduce. This certainly should be an option for the individuals who created the embryos. To use them in this way without the knowledge or consent of the gamete donors would, however, violate the principles of informed consent and procreative autonomy. This idea was forcefully expressed by Ruth Deech, chairman of the Human Fertilization and Embryology Authority (HFEA). She writes:

It would not be appropriate to either human dignity or the autonomy of the individual to give these embryos away or use them for research without the informed consent of the parents.
   I would not regard letting them perish as a waste of human life as Life [a British anti-abortion organization] does, because an embryo is not a little baby in the freezer.[30]

It might be objected that even if preimplantation embryos are not "babies in the freezer," nevertheless their destruction *is* a waste of human life and that it is intrinsically bad when human life, once begun, is deliberately ended.[31] This could be so even though embryos have no stake in their own existence and cannot be harmed or wronged or deprived of anything if they are discarded, killed, or allowed to die. In response, I suggest that this intrinsic badness is heavily outweighed by the wrongness of using people's embryos for procreative purposes without their consent. Respect for embryos does not justify violating the rights of persons. Respect is demonstrated by placing limits on the uses to which human embryos may be put, not on the methods for disposing of them when such use is no longer possible.

In Chapter 2 of this collection, "Source or Resource? Human Embryo Research as an Ethical Issue," Courtney Campbell argues that a lack of serious moral consideration may be manifested, not so much in the destruction of embryos, orphaned or otherwise, but rather in the way embryos are destroyed. Referring to a fertility clinic in the United States that sought preliminary approval to use nuclear transfer techniques to move polar bodies into the cytoplasm of donor oocytes and then to discard any developing embryos after 6 days, Campbell writes:

The embryos were to be created from eggs retrieved from "consumers," who would have given their informed consent were [an Institutional Review Board] subsequently forthcoming. As such, the embryos were understood and even described by the research team and the clinicians as "surplus," that is, as a unit of property or resource commodity. Not surprisingly, the discourse of the advisory panel often proceeded as though a business decision were needed about whether to initiate or discontinue a product line. The language of utility, efficiency, and responsiveness to "consumer" demands, especially for genetically related children, had discursive prominence. Such a paradigm diminishes the embryo's status to something equivalent to an office product, whose existence, use, and continuation are contingent on the preferences of the consumer.

It seems to me that Campbell has several different objections to the decision making surrounding the research project he describes. One objection is to treating the gamete donors as "consumers." This eliminates the doctor–patient relationship, with its ethic of confidentiality, trust, and concern for the welfare of the patient, and replaces it with a purely commercial transaction in which those elements are missing. This is offensive, but it has nothing to do with the moral status of the embryos. However embryos are regarded, patients or clients should not be treated as mere consumers. Moreover, concern for the preferences of the gamete donors does not imply, as Campbell suggests, that they are regarded as consumers, but rather expresses the reasonable moral view that they have dispositional authority over their gametes and embryos.

Campbell also suggests that the fact that researchers would so cavalierly dispose of the embryos after six days shows that they treat embryos as they would boxes of cereal that had exceeded their "sell-by date," thus reducing them to mere products, like boxes of Cheerios. Certainly, it displays a lack of respect to treat human embryos like mere products, but it is not clear why the recognition that embryos cannot be safely used for implantation implies regarding them as consumer goods. Nor do I understand why Campbell thinks it important to display some ambivalence or anguish or regret at the loss of the embryos when deciding to discard them. To require anguish only at the moment of discard seems more sentimental than respectful.

What then are the implications for debates about human cloning of treating early embryos as forms of life that deserve respect? To answer this question, we need to keep in mind that somatic cell nuclear transfer (SCNT) has applications other than creation of human beings. For example, SCNT cloning might provide knowledge about how cells grow, divide, and become specialized, which not only has intrinsic interest but also may have implications for cancer therapies and other disease treatments. Additionally, SCNT cloning might be used to create organs for transplant and skin for burn victims. These applications would involve cloning human cells, but not the cloning of a human being. The report of the National Bioethics Advisory Commission (NBAC)[32] was careful to direct its recommendations for a moratorium only to cloning human beings, not to other kinds of human cloning.

The objections to cloning human beings rest largely on the possibility of harm to them. Although this remains controversial because of an ongoing debate about whether a person can be harmed by a technique on which his or her very existence depends,[33] most people would regard the risk of serious defects in offspring as an obvious reason to ban a technique. Yet, this concern about cloning refers to harm to future persons and has nothing to do with respect for embryos.

Some critics argue that the very idea of creating a human clone reflects narcissism, obsession with control, loss of the capacity for awe, and "Frankensteinian hubris."[34] Like respect for dead bodies and human embryos, these are symbolic concerns, ones about which reasonable people can differ. Is creating a child by cloning necessarily any more narcissistic than ordinary reproduction? Would developing cloning reflect hubris any more than any other novel branch of medicine? These questions are no less important for being extremely difficult to answer, perhaps being unanswerable. Even if we agree that human embryos deserve respect, we may not be able to come to consensus on the appropriate ways of showing that respect or on how to balance the good of scientific and medical research, or the reproductive interests of individuals, against that respect. Our only hope is to continue to formulate, as precisely as possible, our views on these symbolic, intangible issues and to listen carefully to those who have opposing views.[35]

2

Source or Resource? Human Embryo Research as an Ethical Issue

COURTNEY S. CAMPBELL

A central consideration in the debate about the ethics and policy of research on human embryos is the moral status of the preimplantation embryo.[1] Broadly speaking, three philosophical views of this question have been articulated. The first two views do not see human embryo research as an ethical issue as such, but rather as a scientific, political, or ideological question. One view contends that the early embryo has full moral status, especially in light of its possession of the necessary and sufficient genetic complement for biological development into a human being or person. Those who affirm such a perspective are characteristically opposed to biomedical research on the unimplanted human embryo on the grounds that it violates the moral respect and humanity of the embryo. A second position holds that the developing embryo, at least during the period immediately after fertilization and for some time thereafter (e.g., until attainment of sentience) has negligible moral status.[2] As a cluster of developing cellular materials, the embryo is an "object" for medical research and manipulation. On this understanding, research on the unimplanted human embryo is primarily a technical question under the domain of the scientific method because the embryo is not vested with moral value or may be assessed as "property."

In philosophical and policy debates about embryo research and disposition, an intermediate view has emerged on the status of the human embryo. According to this view, the early human embryo does not hold full status in the moral community; yet, as a developing biological entity with the potential to become a human being, the embryo warrants what the National Institutes of Health (NIH) Human Embryo Research Panel (HERP) refers to as "serious moral consideration" or "moral respect".[3] Such a claim means that research on the embryo *can be* justified because of the potential for human benefits from the research and because such research does not violate a human life. It also, however, entails that such research must be justified because an entity with some moral value is used in the research. This ascription of moral status further means that the embryo cannot be treated as morally indifferent; thus, such research must be limited as well, not simply by the imprecision of scientific technique and procedure but also by ethical and policy restrictions. Thus, the third view claims that research on the human embryo is an ethical issue, that reasonable arguments can be offered in favor of research or against, and that some research is permissible under an appropriate ethical framework of justification and limitation.

As with any form of research, the principal ethical justification for embryo research should be the generation of generalizable knowledge, for example, insights about cellular differentiation and division or causes of infertility, that we cannot obtain in any other way but by direct research on the embryo. One prospective result of the new knowledge generated may be potential development of therapies for infertility, cancers, or genetic diseases. It is important, however, not to offer prospective therapeutic developments as a justification for research on the embryo; otherwise, the ethics of research are conflated with the ethics of therapeutic experimentation.

The principal ethical limitation on embryo research proposed by various policy bodies, including the HERP, is one of time. That is, embryo research up to 14 days after fertilization and the development of the primitive streak in the embryo is widely, although not universally, accepted as a limit on biomedical research proposals. The HERP also suggests a limit to research based on public views about the beginning and ending of life, although it is unclear how these values are to be ascertained or monitored.

My interpretive overlay is of course not unique to embryo research. Similar kinds of positions seem to be embedded in virtually any dispute when the moral status of a biological entity is contested, whether it be non-human species of plants, animals, or ecosystems or human embryos and fetuses. We find ourselves engaging in disputes about the boundaries of and qualifications for membership in the moral community; at the core of that community is the human person (to be sure, historically envisioned as a white male). The philosophical method involves identification and analysis of the distinguishing characteristics of that moral core (e.g., rationality or sentience), and casuistic application of those characteristics to boundary cases like that of animals, fetuses, or unimplanted human embryos.[4] Once these determinations are made, then moral judgments about, for example, the ethics of animal research or of embryo research, while remaining complex, can be arrived at with some degree of definitive justification.

This anthropocentric methodology and its assumptions are not immune from criticism. The anthropocentric paradigm may be critiqued and an alternative proposed, such as biocentrism or theocentrism. Alternatively, and this seems to be the current approach in much contemporary discourse in biomedical ethics, the paradigm may be subjected to rigorous internal evaluation and revision; if we are to begin ethical analysis by presuming a philosophical conception of the human self, we must accommodate a fuller and thicker picture of the self than, for example, previous portraits of the self as an autonomous rational individual.

It is the latter approach that I take in this chapter. I do so because I seek to contest many (though not all) of the arguments for research on the unimplanted human embryo while remaining within the general anthropocentric paradigm that contemporary biomedical science and biomedical ethics presumes. In particular, I want to claim that, when we consider the ethics of embryo research, the paradigm precludes certain sentiments, attitudes, and experiences from "counting" morally. In so doing, the idea that the human embryo warrants serious moral consideration seems increasingly difficult to sustain. Instead, the biomedical research enterprise is permeated by a reductionist ideology under which the human embryo becomes little more than a replenishable research resource.

The difficulty with the "resource" characterization of the embryo is that it risks diffusing the ethical question about research altogether. To be sure, we can and do engage in moral debates about whether or not a resource should be used (e.g., protection of natural resources) or how resources should be distributed (a matter of justice in the allocation of scarce resources). Yet, it becomes very difficult in such debates to treat the resource under question as anything but a mere instrument to the achievement of certain scientific or social goods. The resource is rather readily divested of intrinsic worth or value.

Diffusing the ethical issues over embryo research may perhaps make good political sense, as polemically contested as the NIH panel's recommendations were by critics on seemingly all sides, and especially so on an issue that stands in the inescapable shadow of the abortion controversy. I think it is important to keep the ethical question alive, however, and to keep our collective and personal moral consciences awake. Such an approach helps maintain the integrity of scientific research and cultivates a critical citizenry.

Thus, I seek to show how the pervasive influence of scientific reductionism presents a substantial challenge to a policy affirmation of the human embryo's "serious moral consideration." This approach should illustrate and enhance not only understanding what is at stake in human embryo research but also self-definition, particularly as manifested in our experiences as embodied persons in familial relationships. I contend that understanding embryo research as an ethical issue, and not (only) a political or scientific issue, requires us to consider carefully whether the embryo is a source of life or a re-source of science. The moral conundrum lies in the prefix.

Resources for research

I serve on an ethics advisory panel of a fertility clinic that provides ethical consultation on research proposals in reproductive technology preliminary to Institutional Review Board (IRB) review. Recently, the panel was asked to consider the science and ethics of a research proposal involving the use of nuclear transfer technology to move polar bodies (a cell that separates from an oocyte) into the cytoplasm of a donor oocyte. Although such research had been carried out with rhesus monkeys, it had not been conducted with human embryos. The research team maintained that such an approach promised significant benefits in overcoming mitochondrial genetic disease and could increase both the quantity and the quality of embryos available for assisted reproduction. Thus, while not making direct reference to it, thè research proposal seemed to clearly meet the first consideration for justifiable embryo research articulated by the NIH panel: "The promise of human benefit is significant, carrying great potential benefit to infertile couples, and to families with genetic conditions. . . ."[5]

The researchers had convened the advisory panel to address two particular issues of concern with the proposal. First, there was concern over proceeding to studying the nuclear transfer technology in human embryos without extensive research in animals. The researchers had considered further research using mice but maintained that, due to limited resources, both financial and spatial, it was practically infeasible to do additional research with animal embryos. Moreover, as one of the investigators put it, "doing animals is humanly uninteresting"; that is, given the anticipated significant benefits to human beings, there would likely be little gained by developing the research with a mouse model. An underlying issue concerned competition within the research community; the researchers were quite sure that other proposals using nuclear transfer methods in human embryos would soon be initiated, and, if they were limited to animal research, they would "fall behind" with respect to human beings.

Thus it cannot be said that the research proposed to use human embryos as a last resort; given adequate resources and an ethos of collaboration rather than competition, further research with animal embryos certainly could have been pursued that might have been valuable in its own right, as well as lending insights for research with human embryos. Such features are, however, luxuries of a bygone era in biomedical research. As Ziman[6] has recently argued, criteria for success in science have shifted from an exploration or discovery of truth to a pursuit of money and professional and social esteem, with a concomitant compromise in scientific objectivity. In a context of limited resources and an emphasis on the immediacy of practical benefits, a research protocol that moves very quickly from testing a technological method in animal embryos to testing it in human embryos is understandable and perhaps defensible.

Presuming that questions over the resort to use of human embryos could be resolved, the second question of concern to the researchers was the disposition of the embryos that would be created by nuclear transfer technology. The protocol involved using the technology to create embryos that would be permitted to develop to approximately 112 cells, or about 6 days post-fusion. If, as anticipated based on prior research with rhesus monkeys, the embryos created using the technology underwent normal division and developmental processes, at least at a rate comparable with that of 50 normal embryos generated through standard in vitro fertilization (IVF), the study of the procedure would be considered "successful" enough to warrant offering the nuclear transfer method to infertile couples. The 50 embryos would be discarded, along with any embryos that had undergone abnormal development. Should the success threshold be achieved, however, the researchers as well as the clinicians on the panel expected such a method to be welcomed by clients because "the carrot of this approach is that a person can use [his or her] own DNA."

I should reiterate here that this was not a formal research proposal presented for review to an IRB, so some of the questions about timing, development, and criteria for success were not definitively established in the minds of the researchers. Thus, although the researchers sought to limit the number of research embryos that would be used and then discarded, it was actually unclear in advance just how many embryos would be required to achieve the IVF-comparable threshold of success.

In consulting with the advisory panel, comprised of scientists, clinicians, and ethicists, before a full presentation to an IRB, the research team implicitly acknowledged the validity of a second consideration proposed by the NIH panel for permissible embryo research: a need to "provide consistent ethical and scientific review for this area of research."[7] The necessity for review and monitoring is, however, tied by the NIH panel to an ethical presupposition: the claim that "the preimplantation embryo possesses qualities requiring moral respect."

The question that was not addressed by the research protocol, or pursued in the panel meeting, was what qualities does the embryo have that require an attitude of respect. Is scientific and ethical oversight a sufficient manifestation of such respect? Does creating embryos specifically for research purposes treat the embryo with respect? Does discarding the embryo after its research interest has been exhausted constitute respect? Is there a difference between according the embryo respect as a philosophical proposition and giving respectful treatment to the embryo in the course of a practical research investigation? Answers to such questions were not forthcoming in the panel discussion; indeed, the questions themselves were scarcely acknowledged as relevant, although one clinician, in a tangent, dismissed as "laughable" the claim once put forward by Paul Ramsey, among others, that research on embryos constitutes unjustifiable experimentation on the unborn. I suspect the questions were not addressed in part because the discussion focused on a specific research proposal and in part because the gleam of scientific discovery and research progress loomed large in the eyes of both investigators and clinicians.

Yet, as I suggested above, if we do not take seriously what the NIH panel means when it declares that "the preimplantation human embryo warrants serious moral consideration as a developing form of human life," then it is hard to see why embryo research as such would constitute an ethical issue. Legitimate questions may be asked about whether funding to support such research should be diverted to other scientific possibilities or whether additional funds, including federal funds, should be forthcoming for human embryo research. To frame the question in this way, however, transforms the ethical question into one of the allocation of scarce resources and presumes the legitimacy of such research were resources more plentiful. The moral status of the embryo in this context is that of a resource for allocation, which is a quite different appeal than one based on its status as a developing form of human life.

What is required of researchers in order to give serious moral consideration to the un-implanted human embryo, or, perhaps more to the point, what is lacking in the scenario described that manifests an absence of moral respect? The embryos were to be created from eggs retrieved from "consumers," who would have given their informed consent were IRB approval subsequently forthcoming. As such, the embryos were understood and even described by the research team and the clinicians as "surplus," that is, as a unit of property or resource commodity. Not surprisingly, the discourse of the advisory panel often proceeded as though a business decision were needed about whether to initiate or discontinue a product line. The language of utility, efficiency, and responsiveness to "consumer" demands, especially for genetically related children, had discursive prominence. Such a paradigm diminishes the embryo's status to something equivalent to an office product, whose existence, use, and continuation are contingent on the preferences of the consumer.

Moreover, in light of the decision to discard a research-created embryo after its research use is deemed exhausted, serious moral consideration would seem to entail moral anguish about both the initiation of the research and the moral loss incurred through destruction of the embryo. Moral considerability, if it means anything, should mean that the destruction of an embryo has more bearing on our sentiments than, for example, the removal of a box of Cheerios from the grocery shelf because it has exceeded its "best-if-sold-by" date. A sentiment of regret is too much to demand, but certainly some ambivalence, some anguish, some verbal expressions of "it's unfortunate" that the process of scientific discovery requires that the sacrifice of entities of moral value are appropriate acknowledgments of the loss occasioned when human embryos are deliberately discarded.

Yet, until pressed by some members of the advisory panel, the research team seemed oblivious to the need for an end point to the research study and its ethical corollary to limit the loss of moral value. When this issue is framed within a resource or property understanding of the human embryo, however, this moral myopia becomes explicable: A "surplus" commodity enables unrestricted use, and, given the essentially limitless supply of consumers with gametic materials, this "surplus" is unlikely to diminish. In this respect, human embryos become not a "source" of potential life, or even a developing form of human life, but a "resource" commodity for investigation and manipulation.

At this juncture, it might seem that the language of "serious moral consideration" used by the HERP is merely a political facade used to disguise and make publicly palatable scientific interests in having access to embryos for research. Perhaps a more credible course would be to expose the facade, candidly explain that neither researchers nor clinicians treat the embryo as of moral value in research or medical practice, and exclude the embryo from the moral community in the way biomedical research and clinical infertility practices seem to presuppose.

Yet, I am reluctant to dispense with the claim of serious moral consideration regarding the human embryo. The claim captures our intuitive sense that a human embryo is, after all, different from a box of cereal and that research on human embryos not only is a matter of technical expertise but also presents an inescapable ethical dimension structured by a framework of justification and limitation. The attitude of moral consideration, at a minimum, warrants limits on the kind of study undertaken or the length of a particular study. My concern, however, is that the surplus or resource/property understanding of the embryo is so deeply embedded within the ideology of scientific research that a discursive appeal by a public policy body to moral consideration is unlikely to have much, if any, impact on research attitudes and practices. A major issue, then, is whether there are ethical resources within, or available to, science that can cultivate respectful treatment of the embryo in research.

Reproductive reductionism

At least until very recently, the culture and ideology of science, as well as scientific researchers, have been unwilling to acknowledge the presence of a realm of values within research and instead have stressed that values, other than detached objectivity, can be an obstacle to sound science.[8] The observation of Max Weber[9] earlier this century continues to be embedded in science discourse and practice: "Natural science gives us an answer to the question of what we must do if we wish to master life technically. It leaves quite aside, or assumes for its purposes, whether we should and do wish to master life technically, and whether it ultimately makes sense to do so."

In short, scientific inquiry can easily be divested of a sense of broader purpose and meaning and be separated from a vision of the ultimate ends that science ought to pursue. Within a culture of science that is already predisposed to view values with some suspicion, the value claim that a human embryo has serious moral consideration is likely to ring hollow.

This cultural chasm between scientific inquiry and human values is often pronounced in science discourse about procreation and reproduction. It is not uncommon to find reproduction to be scientifically constructed as a process of "replicating genes." (If intention is ascribed to reproduction, the process may be described as "self-reproduction.") From the perspective of evolutionary biology, this is a concise and accurate description to indicate how a species perpetuates itself over time. Yet, I have never encountered any person or couple for whom an interest in species perpetuation or gene replication was important compared with the expression of mutuality, love, and self-giving experienced in procreative meaning. The scientific emphasis on the mechanical and technical aspects of life's beginnings, as reflected in the language of reproduction, is surely alien to anyone who has become, or considered becoming, a parent, an experience that is as generative and meaning-full as any that life offers us.

The chasm of meaning, and the difference between reproduction and procreation, is created in part through constructions that rely on different starting points. The scientific understanding is inherently reductionist: Reproduction is initiated at and occurs through the molecular and genetic level of a biological entity, a level that is differentiated from that of personalized intentionality. Genes are the "building blocks of life," which combine and re-combine in apparently random and arbitrary ways to produce more complex organisms and entities, including human beings. Given this starting point, scientific inquiry at the genetic level is especially compelling. As illustrated by the Human Genome Project, substantial research attention and funding is devoted to understanding the cellular and genetic processes of molecular reproduction, with an expectation that such research will enable a re-direction of medical interventions that can alter the "givenness" of the genetic lottery for the good of persons. In this perspective, a person is conceived, as it were, from the genes up.

That is one way to describe the reproductive process. Such a framework enables a kind of professional detachment that can play itself out in moral indifference toward the human embryo, itself seen as a cluster of dividing cells whose size, to cite a particularly media-friendly sound bite coined by the HERP, is "significantly smaller than the period at the end of this sentence."[10] Such a description is technically and biologically sound and encapsulates the worldview of scientific reductionism concisely. Yet, however fascinating the exploration of the frontiers of molecular reproduction is, as a bare biological description this seems to detach scientific inquiry from the larger context of human reproduction and from the meaning and purposiveness we attribute to this more holistic experience. Furthermore, while a fertilized egg may be simply a cellular dot to the objectively detached researcher, not even the attempt to allude to this larger context by using the language of "preimplantation embryos" can rescue the divorce that has occurred between scientific interest and human purposes.

The problem with this divorce is that it undercuts the primary ethical rationale for engaging in research on the human embryo, which is framed entirely in terms of advancing particular human purposes, such as the relief of infertility, prevention of cancer, alleviation of genetic conditions, and so forth. In so doing, the argument for research breaches the boundary between research and (prospective) therapy. In the case of research, the goal is to generate generalizable knowledge; a human embryo is the "living laboratory" wherein study of cellular replication can be undertaken. In the context of therapy, the goal is to provide benefits, in the way of a cure or prevention of some disease, for certain afflicted persons. The human embryo is thereby merely a means to the achievement of these ends. These are valid and valuable ends, but the conflict between research and therapeutic interests can culminate in a diminished status of moral consideration for the embryo, as occurs when it becomes a mere means.

To summarize the contention here, the ethical justification for engaging in research on the embryo is developed with respect to the advancement of human purposes, some of which are generalizable and some of which involve application to specific medical contexts. The reductionist method of scientific inquiry, in contrast, seeks to divest itself of a context of human purpose or meaning. It should perhaps not be surprising, then, that the research vision appears somewhat incoherent.

Meanwhile, the effort to channel (and ethically justify) embryo research through offering advances in reproductive technologies holds out the prospect that we can achieve technical skill and control, if not what Weber referred to as "mastery," over the contingency of nature, in particular, its arbitrariness regarding human fertility. The holistic and fully embodied experience of sexuality and procreation is reproduced in the laboratory setting, not through imitation of the process but by biomedical reductionism of the persons involved and the product generated. As Paul Lauritzen[11] has expressed it, the world of reproductive technologies "can divide up persons into parts. Even when [the technologies] are used to treat infertility, it is often not men or women who are being treated, but testicles, sperm, ovaries, eggs, wombs, etc."

This degree of reductionism, it bears reiterating, is embedded in the therapeutic setting. It can only intensify when the locus of interest in human embryos is transferred from the fertility clinic to the research laboratory. If we consider the human embryo, not in terms of its utility in facilitating human reproduction, but rather as a complex form of human bodily tissue, the reductionistic pressure that makes it hard to sustain serious moral consideration for the human embryo emerges once again.

Biomedicine and the body

The creation of the human embryo in a laboratory setting requires donation or selling of human body tissue, namely, ova and sperm. It is possible, therefore, to think about using human embryos in biomedical research with respect to attitudes toward the body and alienation of bodily parts. This distinction is important because scientific and research interest in parts of the body, including reproductive tissue, can sometimes conflict with important ethical values about bodily integrity.

Indeed, in a recent study on the value and meaning of the human body and its parts, E. Richard Gold cites the "disparate claims of scientific investigation and religious belief on the body" as the exemplary case of incommensurate values regarding the body. According to Gold,[12]

The body, from a scientific viewpoint, is a source of knowledge of physical development, aging, and disease. From a religious perspective, the body is understood as a sacred object, being created in the image of God. . . . The scientist values the body instrumentally, as a means to acquire knowledge; the believer values the body intrinsically, for being an image of God.

Although Gold presents the conflict as constituted by a clash of scientific reductionism with theological holism, various kinds of secular arguments, such as those developed by Kant, can provide a nonreligious basis for an appeal to bodily integrity as well. The basic question from either a secular or religious perspective that emphasizes embodied holism concerns whether the value of the body is composed of the sum of its parts or whether the bodily totality as a whole is greater than the cumulative sum of the parts.

The research perspective on the body and bodily tissue is reductionist in that interest in the body stems from the prospect of gaining information about human character traits and behaviors through study, analysis, and understanding of the basic components of life. Genes and cells, removed from their originating context of a human body, can provide important insights regarding susceptibility to illness, bodily responses to disease, or possible remedies to organic dysfunction. The body as an organic totality is instrumental to the research objective of deciphering codes, messages, and functions transmitted through cellular signals and genetic information. In this respect, the fundamental components of parts of the body are more scientifically significant than the body totality.

Scientific discourse about the human genome project provides numerous illustrations of a reductionist ideology. Rosner and Johnson[13] identify three basic metaphors about the genome project in science discourse: *(1)* interpretation of a "book" or "library"; *(2)* reparation of a "flawed machine"; and *(3)* the mapping of a mysterious "wilderness." Each of these metaphors places the research scientist in a dominant and active role, while the body, seen primarily in terms of its genetic make-up, is reduced to passive malleability, inherently manipulatable.

DNA is the key to a valid interpretation, a repair of the machine, and domestication of the bodily wilderness. The body is portrayed in genomic science merely as a natural resource for "gene prospectors" to map, "mine," and establish claims regarding property rights, patents, and commercial products. The account of the body in genetic science is, in short, analogous to the political and commercial views adopted toward the land in the nineteenth and twentieth centuries, that is, an exploitable natural resource whose contents are of more interest than the integrity of the whole. The legitimacy of the use of body tissue is assumed; the question for the scientific perspective concerns the appropriate limits to be placed on research to avoid abuse.

Certain forms of body tissue, such as reproductive cells, have an important advantage as a scientific resource over the land because they are already "surplus" in the body. Moreover, sperm are replenishable, and although ova are not, a mature woman has more than enough eggs for personal procreative purposes throughout her life. These tissues can be "harvested" without severe disruption to the well-functioning of the body and can then be developed by researchers with the knowledge and expertise into materials with scientific benefit for the community or therapeutic value for individuals.

Does a human embryo have any different status than body tissue, including reproductive tissue, that has been retrieved from the bodily whole? At first glance, the answer would seem to be yes. The embryo created in culture has the potential for developing into a human being if its biological development is not interrupted, although, as with in vivo embryos, such maturation is far from certain. Moreover, sperm and egg must be joined or fused to create the embryo; a biological change has to occur before an embryo can exist. In these respects, a human embryo seems to have a different biological and moral status than body tissues.

Yet, it is difficult to see that this makes any difference once the embryo is relocated from its originating context of reproduction to technological manipulations of research. As with other body tissue, the human embryo is less a source of life than a resource for knowledge and information. It is "harvested" to enhance research prospects on some of the same issues that scientists study at the cellular or molecular level, albeit now in a more complex organism. Also, upon completion of the research project, the research embryo, like body tissue, is discarded. At the very least, then, the languages of ethical status and research practices seem to be at odds with each other.

I have wanted to affirm the position adopted by the HERP, that the preimplantation human embryo is worthy of "serious moral consideration" or moral respect. That claim makes research on the embryo an ethical and policy question and not only a scientific or technical concern. It legitimates ethical scrutiny of the treatment of the embryo per se, rather than as an adjunct to issues in resource allocation or informed consent. The moral claim provides a framework for both justification and limitation of embryo research. Such research can be justified because of the possible human benefits, but it also must be justified and limited in recognition of the embryo's status of deserving serious moral consideration.

Yet, my analysis of the relevant discourse and practices of scientific inquiry indicates that sustaining such status is problematic, especially in the research setting. A first eroding pressure comes from the ideology of reductionism that permeates contemporary scientific and biomedical research inquiry. Microscopic entities, be they genes, cells, or the embryo, are the keys to understanding the more complex responses and interactions that occur at a macrolevel of biological functioning. A second pressure that works against the moral considerability of the embryo is the "resource" paradigm of scientific study. The human embryo may be viewed as "surplus" or as scarce, but in either instance it takes on the features of a replenishable resource, distanced from, if not divested of, its human significance as a source of new life. Generated from body tissue, it is nonetheless treated merely as body tissue, subject to objectification, manipulation, and destruction.

The question is whether these background assumptions of scientific inquiry and method, which are manifested in research practices and in clinical therapeutic settings, make the claim of serious moral consideration of the human embryo simply untenable. Alternatively, is there some medium to reconcile the interests of research and of respect? I think the latter is possible, although this will require (1) the incorporation of a foundational sentiment for scientific inquiry and (2) the adoption of a holistic view of the purposes of science to counteract its reductionist tendencies. Such an approach makes it possible to consider embryo research, and treatment of the embryo, as a legitimate issue for ethical discussion.

Standing in awe

The scientific quest to understand the inner workings of life must be mediated by a foundational sentiment that life is a wondrous mystery, albeit a mystery amenable to our discovery. This sense of awe and wonder in the face of mystery can readily be lost by the routines of demystification that occur in biomedical research and clinical practice. If it is diminished significantly, it will be hard to cultivate and maintain a view of moral status regarding the human embryo.

In describing his self-identification as a "religious" person, Albert Einstein[14] commented:

The most beautiful thing we can experience is the mysterious. It is the source of all true art and science. He to whom this emotion is a stranger, who can no longer pause to wonder and stand rapt in awe is as good as dead; his eyes are closed. This insight into the mystery of life, coupled though it be with fear, has also given rise to religion.

Although Einstein's observation stemmed from his reflections on the mysteries of the cosmos, which his scientific theories did much to de-mystify, the passion he describes can no doubt be experienced in relation to the many microworlds of scientific inquiry, such as wonder at the cellular division process in an embryo or the differentiation of cells from DNA instructions. In Einstein's account, "true art and science," as well as religion, require these sentiments of awe and wonder; they are foundational, not dispensable. The cultivation of awe and wonder, moreover, requires a "pause," a stepping back from one's professional trees to absorb the fullness of the forest. The rationalistic routines and reductionism of research projects risk lessening and perhaps deadening the emotive element of the scientific conscience.

Indeed, when these sentiments are absent, the result is deformed science and deformed religion, a pattern of intellectual thought that is severed from its emotional roots. Although one can certainly participate in sound science without such sentiments, an engagement or "feeling for the organism" provides motivation and direction for scientific inquiry.[15] Awe, wonder, and experience of mystery need to stand behind and permeate ongoing research, lest the routinization of professional practices culminate in describing what actually is a mystery of life, the developing human embryo, as a surplus product or as a resource for allocation and manipulation.

My position, then, is that before a decision is made about whether and how we should apply the scientific method to embryo research, there needs to be a human recognition of the fundamental wonder of life itself, encoded in the embryo. This recognition, which as suggested earlier is not merely an expression of an intellectual claim but is emotively experienced as well, should carry over and inform scientific research. The journey of an organism of microscopic size through various developmental phases to the flourishing of a human person is a source of amazement and should be an occasion for "pause" and reflection on the remarkable fact that life *is*. This pre-research sentiment is, in my view, necessary to the cultivation of an attitude that ascribes serious moral consideration to the human embryo. It can generate in researchers, inculcated with a methodology of objectification and reductionism, a disposition to see the embryo as a resource of moral value and not merely a resource of research material.

Another way to understand my claim is that awe and wonder enable resistance against the compartmentalization of professional life. The chasm between technical mastery of nature and inattentiveness to the meaning of mastery of which Weber warns is particularly endemic to scientific study, but is less likely to occur through attentiveness to these prescientific sentiments.

It is no less important that, as Einstein noted, these sentiments provide a means of connecting science and religion. Rooted in a foundation of awe and wonder at the mysteries of life embedded within and unfolding through embryonic development, embryo research need not be construed as promoting science that is hostile to religion. Nor would opposition to research necessarily be "anti-scientific." In a pluralistic society, it is vital to explore the content and boundaries of the "overlapping consensus" that provides the texture of social morality. An understanding that, at bottom, science and religion share a foundational sentiment in their experience of the world can work to diffuse some of the polarization of science and religion that biomedical research frequently engenders. Religious critics of contemporary biomedicine, for example, have indicated their endorsement of a Baconian approach to science and nature, which sets scientific inquiry within a broader framework of meaning, in contrast to a model that posits science as socially and ideologically autonomous, a realm that is immune from social and moral influence.[16]

I do not mean to understate the substantive differences in this regard, which emerge especially at the level of particular moral judgments. It is mistaken and counterproductive, however, for public discourse to proceed with caricatures of scientists as callous and of members of faith communities as technological Luddities or reactionaries. I do not dispute that the source or content of awe and wonder in a scientific worldview may ultimately differ from that embedded in a religious worldview, but I do maintain that the potential attitudinal overlap can promote substantive dialogue rather than divisiveness.

It follows that a disposition of awe, to be sustained, needs to be supplemented by a holistic vision of scientific research, a vision of professional work that situates research on embryos within a broader vision of the goods of human life and of a good society. The chasm delineated above between technical mastery of nature and the meaning of mastery perpetuates the social isolation and autonomy of science. Its vision is blurred by moral myopia, wherein important questions of science, of ethics, and of meaning are never engaged in common dialogue. A holistic understanding of biomedical research will integrate features of science, ethics, and society. This means, as a corollary, that in certain instances it will be possible to have a meaningful ethical veto over the scientific imperative.

I have articulated above some of the realms in embryo research in which reductionism holds sway. Put within a holistic perspective, the embryo will be seen not only as a resource for science but also a source of life. Indeed, the embryo is a life source before it is a research resource; its originating context is human reproduction, not laboratory replication. Thus, ethical justification is required of scientific proposals to transform the embryo's status to that of resource. Additionally, the status of life source carries a residual moral weight such that, even within the research setting, the language of "surplus" will not do justice to the moral respect due the embryo.

A holistic view of research also resists the tendency to treat the human body and body tissue as inherently alienable, that is, as a form of "property." The body in its biological totality is a source of mystery and awe. Thus, a research approach to the body must begin with a presumption of bodily integrity. Body parts, organs, and tissues can also shape a sense of self. Visible parts of the body, as well as the heart, have a strong correlation with a sense of self-identity.[17] For these reasons, ethical justification is required for research on human body tissue; otherwise disrespect is rendered to the embodied self that is the source of the research resource.

Human embryos are typically not designated "property" within the research setting; such nomenclature seems to arise when the disposition of embryos is contemplated or disputed. Still, under a resource paradigm not infused with sentiments of awe and a holistic understanding of the aims of science, it would not be surprising for the embryo to be treated as though it were property, an exploitable commodity that can be owned, used, alienated, and destroyed without moral reservation. The holistic perspective I advocate would not view human embryos either as property or as persons, that is, as entirely excluded or completely included within the moral community. Human embryos hover on the communal boundaries, evoking serious, but not full moral consideration. The ethical use of human embryos as a research resource must then be constrained by recognition of the embryo as a life source and by an integration of research interests with broader social interests in the extrinsic goods of scientific practice.

To illustrate these constraints, I now wish to return to the research proposal with which I began, involving the use of nuclear transfer technology to transfer a polar body from one cell into host cytoplasm of a donor oocyte. I think it is difficult to defend on ethical grounds what appears to be a hasty and perhaps scientifically premature move to study the success of the procedure with human embryos. The main concern for the researchers appears to be one of expediency, but it is arguable whether sound science may be compromised in the pressure to be first among the scientific community. If the proposal does carry "significant" promise of human benefit, then the moral burden weighs heavily in the direction of proceeding cautiously and carefully with the science and ensuring that the preliminary studies with animal models, however "uninteresting" from the standpoint of human benefit, provide the grounds for a judgment that there is a reasonable expectation of success when the technology is used with human embryos. Such a claim about human benefit also entails a research obligation to find the means to procure the financial, spatial, and temporal resources necessary to do the animal research that could be done—and would be done—but for the concerns about delaying the human embryo research. In short, I think that in research of this kind, it is important that researchers adhere to a criterion of "last resort" with respect to human embryos. They should not be a first or intermediate resort simply because they can be easily obtained, are more scientifically interesting, or are a means to winning a research race within the scientific community.

It is also important in this context to examine whether the prospective human benefits respond to a significant human need. The use of embryos in research that seeks to overcome diseases transmitted through the genetic lottery fits within the basic goals of medicine and medical research. It is harder to make a compelling case when the research objective is to improve the quality and quantity of embryos available for assisted reproduction procedures. This is particularly the case when the principal appeal of the proposed method, in the view of researchers and clinicians, is that it would offer a genetically related child. The experience of parenting, and parenting one's biological offspring, is a profound experience of education and meaning. Persons who are unable to have this experience through natural or social reasons unquestionably suffer a deprivation. It does not, however, rise to the level of a "need"; having biologically related children is neither a necessary nor sufficient condition for a good human life. Thus, once the research objectives shift from responding to a human need, such as overcoming genetic disease, to enhancing a human desire, then research on human embryos does seem to treat the embryo with less than serious moral consideration.

Finally, treating the human embryo with moral respect requires imposing some end points on research, including specifying the number of embryos to be used. It is symptomatic of the resource understanding of the embryo that the initial proposal had no indications either as to how many embryos would be used, and the duration of cellular division, in order for the researchers to determine whether their method was scientifically sound and clinically safe. Such omissions are not surprising when the embryo is treated merely as a resource that is infinitely replenishable.

Conclusion

My claim in this chapter has been that understanding embryo research as an ethical issue requires understanding the human embryo as a biological entity with "serious moral consideration." The discourse and rhetoric of biomedical science and therapeutic medicine do not, however, provide much confidence that this moral claim is taken seriously. I have argued that, on human and scientific grounds, there are valid reasons for treating the human embryo as a life source and only secondarily (and never merely) as a research resource. Alternative perspectives, to treat the embryo as only a life source or only as a resource, cannot accommodate a discussion of the ethics of embryo research. In addition, research on the human embryo requires an account of the ends of science that is broader and more holistic than technical mastery. Assuming that these conditions can be satisfied, I am of the view that embryo research can be discussed as an ethical issue within a framework of justification and limitation of the research and that, within such a framework, some human embryo research is morally permissible. Whether this is a realistic expectation should itself be part of the dialogue on embryo research as an ethical issue.

3

Creating Embryos for Research: On Weighing Symbolic Costs

MAURA A. RYAN

Much of the controversy surrounding the release of the report of the Human Embryo Research Panel (HERP) in September 1994 concerned its approval of federal funding for research involving embryos created expressly for experimental use. Critics as diverse as the Ramsey Colloquium and Daniel Callahan joined in accusing the panel of going a step too far[1]; the *Washington Post* pronounced the creation of research embryos "unconscionable"[2]; and President Clinton promptly declared his intention to block the appropriation of federal funds for research of this kind.

For those who object to the experimental use of human embryos under any circumstances, there is no point in asking whether it is ethical to create embryos solely for the purpose of experimentation. If it is wrong to use embryos as experimental subjects, it is wrong to create them so that you can use them. If experimentation on human embryos cannot be conducted without violating obligations of informed consent or violating a human life, as theologian Paul Ramsey argued almost 30 years ago, it makes little difference whether we are contemplating the use of "spare" embryos (embryos generated in the course of assisted reproduction) or embryos created expressly for that purpose. If human potentiality in itself obliges us to act so as to bring it to fruition, any experiment that entails the destruction of early embryos will be immoral.

Alternatively, what if we hold that at least some kinds of embryo research can be justified? Suppose that we agree with the conclusion of the HERP that embryos in the earliest stages of development ought to be respected as a form of potential human life, but that they are not yet persons and that, therefore, at least under some circumstances, experimentation on the preimplantation embryo should be permitted up to the appearance of the primitive streak.

In that case, is there any reason to object to the production of embryos for research use? Are we doing anything different, in a moral sense, when we initiate embryonic life for research use than when we use embryos that exist as by-products of medically assisted reproduction? Does the creation of research embryos weaken or insult our communal respect for the sanctity of human life or the integrity of human reproduction in some way that in vitro fertilization (IVF) or the experimental use of "spare embryos" does not?[3]

In this chapter, I argue that it is possible to draw a valid distinction between research involving the deliberate creation of embryos and research involving by-products of medically assisted reproduction. I argue, further, that we should find the former deeply troubling even if we accept the latter. My position does not rest on claims about the moral status of the preimplantation embryo or assertions concerning the "rights" of embryos. Rather, I show that the most persuasive argument offered in defense of the deliberate creation of embryos for experimental use neglects fundamental questions concerning the proper or just use of procreative technologies. The power to remove conception from women's bodies is hardly a neutral power. Rather, it is a power that poses material risks to women's health and contains the potential to alter profoundly the practices of reproduction and parenthood. I argue that reproductive interventions are justified only insofar as they serve the goals of responsible and human reproduction: the bringing forth of new life in loving and nurturing relationship. Creating embryos for research is incompatible with the goals that legitimate and should direct reproductive interventions.

I take as my starting point the defense of research embryos offered by Bonnie Steinbock[4] in *Life Before Birth*. Her analysis is useful for at least two reasons. First, Steinbock provides the deep theoretical background for the position taken by the HERP.[5] Here, for example, we see laid out the important distinction between moral status and moral value assumed in the panel's report as well as the justification for marginalizing "symbolic issues" in the development of public policy. Second, and more important, anyone who wishes to object to the creation of research embryos on grounds other than the special moral status of the preimplantation embryo must reckon with the "interest view" Steinbock defends.

If, as Steinbock and the HERP would have us accept, the only serious question is whether the preimplantation embryo is harmed by being brought into existence solely to serve research goals, it is difficult indeed to see how those who hold a developmental view of personhood can offer any rational objection to the use of research embryos. If we want to argue that initiating human embryonic life with the sole intention of producing material for research is morally objectionable even if we accept such a view of personhood, we have to be able to show that there are morally important considerations neglected in the interest view.

Although this chapter is concerned with the conduct of embryo research, the questions it raises have implications for our thinking about reproductive and genetic technologies in general. Debates about human cloning, genetic engineering, and collaborative reproduction turn, in large part, on disagreements about the moral status of the embryo and the limits of procreative liberty. As with embryo research, however, a preoccupation with competing rights and interests, especially in policy debate, obscures crucial questions about the ends we are pursuing in developing and employing reproductive and genetic technologies as well as the means. Whether we are dealing with the deliberate creation of embryos for experimentation or the cloning of a deceased child, narrow assumptions about what is morally important blind us to what we really should be asking: What are we doing when we fertilize in vitro or manipulate genetic material or clone a human being? What is the price and for what ends should we be willing to pay it?

Steinbock and the interest view

According to Bonnie Steinbock, "We may choose to respect embryos and preconscious fetuses as powerful symbols of human life, but we cannot protect them for their own sake."[6] (p. 10). It is the failure to acknowledge the distinction between choosing to protect embryos and preconscious fetuses because of what they represent to us and claiming to protect the interests of embryos and preconscious fetuses, argues Steinbock, that accounts for a persistent confusion and inconsistency in our approach to the treatment of the unborn. That we can find the same voices decrying the use of research embryos and insisting on the right to abortion testifies to the fact that we do not have a single or clear sense of what we mean by "respect" for embryonic or fetal life.

It is true that the manipulation or destruction of human embryos awakens deep moral impulses, even in those who wish to remain agnostic on the question of when an embryo or a fetus becomes a person. Protectiveness toward potential human life is a common and reasonable impulse. But there is an important and, in Steinbock's view, frequently neglected difference between acknowledging the moral and social value of human embryos and according embryos moral standing. To have moral standing is to count morally, to be the sort of being whose interests must be considered, whose interests exert a claim on the behavior of others (Steinbock, p. 10). Following Joel Feinberg, Steinbock argues that a "being can have interests only if it can matter to the being what is being done to it . . ." and " . . . if nothing at all can possibly matter to a being, then that being has no interests." Human embryos have the potential to develop into "the kind of being that will have interests," but, lacking conscious awareness, embryos and even presentient fetuses lack interests of their own; that is, they exist—at this stage—as the sort of being "to whom nothing at all can possibly matter. . . ." (p. 15). Because a human embryo or a presentient fetus has no interests, its interests need not, indeed cannot, be taken into account; thus, human embryos and presentient fetuses lack moral status.

In the interest view, sentience is both a necessary and a sufficient condition for moral standing. Only a being that is conscious and aware of its own experience can have a stake in what is or is not done to it. Having interests (and thus moral status) does not, however, depend on a capacity for "higher order consciousness" (e.g., the ability to use language). According to Steinbock, "[s]o long as a being is sentient—that is, capable of experiencing pleasure and pain—it has an interest in not feeling pain, and its interest provides moral agents with *prima facie* reasons for acting" (p. 24). Sentience acts, therefore, as a threshold as well as a dividing line for the interest view: "mere things and non-conscious living things fall below the moral status line; animals and people lie above it."

She grants that there are good reasons to be concerned about what happens to human embryos and fetuses. As potential persons, embryos and fetuses have a symbolic value that precludes, for example, using them in unnecessary experiments or for purely commercial gain (p. 41). In the interest view, however, it does not make sense to talk about moral obligations to avoid harm to or promote the welfare of preconscious or presentient embryos or fetuses or to object to research using preimplantation human embryos on the grounds that we are "experimenting on unconsenting human subjects." Embryos do not have moral status. "[I]t is more accurate to acknowledge their importance for us by ascribing to them moral value" (p. 209).

What exactly is the difference between moral status and moral value? As we have seen, to have moral status is to possess interests that exert claims on the behavior of others. To accord moral status is to recognize the interests of a being as morally obligating. When we acknowledge the moral value of an entity, however, we are simply admitting that there are "moral reasons why [that entity] ought to be preserved." We resist the careless destruction of trees or flags or fine art, argues Steinbock, not because protection is in their interests, but because protection is in our interests. In other words, the moral reasons we give for protecting a flowering tree or a Picasso or a national flag have to do not with obligating features of the thing in question but with the symbolic or material value we have conferred on it. In the same way, when Steinbock argues that embryos or presentient fetuses should not be used in frivolous research or for crassly commercial purposes, it is not because to do so violates the interests of the embryo or presentient fetus or causes harm to them but because of the potentially brutalizing effect of such use on society—the possibility of undermining "commonly held fundamental values" such as respect for human life.

It does not follow that embryos and even presentient fetuses should not be used in the conduct of legitimate research or that it is wrong to create embryos expressly for research. We respect the moral or symbolic value of human embryonic life when we "choose to treat the embryo differently than other human tissue" (p. 209). In determining the boundaries of permissible research, however, the moral reasons for pursuing certain kinds of research must be weighed against the moral reasons for deciding not to pursue them. Obviously, support for frivolous or unnecessary research does not weigh very heavily against the importance of fostering cultural attitudes of respect for human life; neither does simply furthering the financial gain of certain individuals or groups. Yet when we are "likely to be able to use what we learn from [research on human embryos or presentient fetuses] to save many lives and ameliorate many conditions which make life miserable," the reasons for proceeding are far more compelling, in Steinbock's view, than the reasons for not proceeding (p. 209).[7] Whatever the social or symbolic value of the embryo or presentient fetus, it does not outweigh the interests of real persons in access to goods and services they need and desire. Moreover, respect for human life is hardly expressed when embryos or presentient fetuses are protected at the expense of the "vital human interests" of already existing persons.

Steinbock's conclusion is the same whether she is considering the creation of embryos for research purposes or the use of spare embryos. For obvious reasons she rejects arguments for banning the practice based on appeals to the interests of the preimplantation embryo in being brought to viability. She dismisses, as well, "slippery slope" anxieties about the expansion of the practice into routine and invalid research. She grants that the prospect of human embryos being created merely to provide a plentiful and ready source of material for research, no matter what the research, is distasteful. Yet, in the absence of evidence that the practice cannot be regulated effectively, such anxieties are mere conjecture. Invoking "slippery slope" scenarios is rhetorically powerful, but the argument begs the question (p. 210).

Neither is she persuaded by the claim that it is repugnant to treat the preimplantation embryo merely as a means to research ends (p. 211). She rejects the suggestion that there is an important difference between conducting research on embryos that cannot be used for the purpose for which they were created (to establish a pregnancy) and would otherwise be discarded and creating embryos in order to provide material for research.

It is no more repugnant, in the interest view, to create embryos for use in research than to create embryos for use in medically assisted reproduction. It simply makes no sense, according to Steinbock, to argue that having been created merely for research objectifies the preimplantation embryo in a way that being created for implantation does not (p. 210). Embryos and presentient fetuses have no interests. Therefore, they are neither benefited by being brought into existence for the purpose of establishing a pregnancy nor harmed or demeaned by being brought into existence merely to serve research goals. In both cases, embryos are created to serve the purposes of the initiating parties. The only important question, then, is what purposes are legitimate. Surely, argues Steinbock, "saving lives and preventing misery" is no less legitimate than establishing pregnancies.

The argument Steinbock advances is very persuasive. The HERP, through similar logic, overcame (at least in part) the reluctance of panel members to recommend funding for the creation of research embryos. As we will see, however, when we move beyond the narrow issue of whether the preimplantation embryo has interests that can be served or frustrated in embryo research, an additional set of questions emerges: Beyond whether embryos can be harmed is the question of what we are doing when we intervene in the process of reproduction, what we are affirming or denying when we create embryos for research purposes.

Weighing the symbolic

The debate about acceptable limits to embryo research is often cast as a "fight over symbolic issues."[8] At least for those who agree that fertilized ova and early embryos are not fully persons in a moral sense, the controversy over experimentation on human embryos is about what it means to display respect for embryos not as persons but as potent symbols of human life.

Concerns about the implications of embryo research or cloning on deep symbolic understandings of the sanctity of life or the integrity of human reproduction are quickly dismissed as unimportant or inappropriate for public debate in a pluralistic society into which is admitted only the "objective" language of rights and interests. As Gilbert Meilaender reminds us in *Body, Soul and Bioethics*, however, it is a serious mistake to ignore such concerns as "merely symbolic." Human thought and language is inescapably symbolic. Symbols express and shape the deepest levels of human experience, the most crucial matters of human society. To overlook or dismiss the symbolic is to "cut ourselves off from what is most important in the life of human beings who are, after all, symbol-making animals."[9]

In the case of embryo research or human cloning, overlooking or dismissing the symbolic evades what is really at stake in conflicts over where to draw the line. It is only when we recognize our anxieties about what we are doing when we fertilize human eggs in vitro or reproduce asexually as acknowledgments that we are close to, and may be violating, some of the deepest and most basic of human matters—procreation, kinship, marital intimacy—and our unwillingness to pay disrespect to human embryos as a powerful statement of our societal commitment to the value of human life generally that we come to the important questions: What practices, what acceptable harms, are ultimately consistent with such a commitment? What research goals are we willing to sacrifice to sustain it? If we believe that there is some risk on both sides, are we endangering respect for the sanctity of human life more immediately in permitting the creation of embryos for research or in slowing the pace at which we address the needs and wants of existing human beings?[10]

For Steinbock this last question is easily decided in favor of advancing the goals of research. As we have seen, she takes it as obvious that we have an interest in opposing frivolous or crassly commercial uses of human embryos, but equally obvious that symbolic commitments to human life ought to give way when embryo research makes it possible "to save many lives and ameliorate many conditions which make life miserable." With a speed reminiscent of John Robertson's treatment of symbolic issues in the defense of reproductive liberty,[11] Steinbock gives the "vital interests of real persons" trump over all other moral considerations. Indeed, so obvious is the importance of embryo research vis-à-vis symbolic commitments to the sanctity of life or the integrity of reproduction to Steinbock that it seems to require no proof. That is, she merely assumes rather than argues for the importance of the information to be gained through embryo research: Possible goals of embryo research include "developing more adequate contraception, determining causes of infertility, investigating the development and potential transformation of moles into malignant tumors, evaluating the effects of teratogens on the early embryo and understanding normal and abnormal cell growth and differentiation." Embryo research "may be particularly valuable for understanding, preventing, and treating cancers, and for studying and treating genetic disease" (p. 204). Given the present state of embryo research and the limits of Steinbock's own professional competence, a certain humility in expressing anticipated benefits is appropriate. Still, because the force of her position depends on convincing us that the human interests to be served by embryo research are compelling enough to override widespread moral and religious anxieties about the production of research embryos, one expects more evidence than she offers.

This very objection was raised by several critics in response to the report of the HERP. Central to the panel's defense of federal funding for embryo research is the claim that withholding public funds or banning the fertilization of oocytes for research purposes impedes research of "great scientific and therapeutic value."[12] As Daniel Callahan points out, however, the report gives us simply a list of research possibilities rather than a substantive argument for proceeding at this time. Although it contains an extensive discussion of the moral status of the preimplantation embryo, there is no discussion of what he calls "the moral status of the proposed research." Although the panel rigorously acknowledges the need to balance the respect owed the preimplantation embryo against the imperatives of research, the report is "utterly silent on how research claims and possibilities should be evaluated for their moral weight and benefit" or what criteria are necessary to establish proportionality.[13] Despite invoking the history of embryo research in the private sector and in countries where federal support exists, the HERP report makes no mention of results achieved or benefits gained.[14]

Sheldon Krimsky and Ruth Hubbard[15] contend that the panel conflates "scientific interest" and "human benefit." There is no question that research into the processes of fertilization, early cell division, implantation, and embryonic development is of immediate scientific interest and that it holds some therapeutic promise (e.g., for improving the safety and efficacy of assisted reproduction). Why assume, however, that advancing the state of procreative technology should be a research priority or that overcoming infertility should lay a serious claim on medical resources and public funds? Why even assume that better technology is the best way to address infertility? Embryo research holds promise for improving techniques in preimplantation genetic diagnosis and developing more adequate methods of contraception. Yet why think that the ability to identify susceptibility to a range of genetic disorders is obviously and transparently beneficial or that introducing more effective artificial contraception obviously serves "vital human interests"?

Of course, a case can be made for the place of medically assisted reproduction in the allocation of health care resources and for research aimed at improving outcomes in reproductive medicine, just as a case can be made for developing safe and effective methods for understanding and addressing genetic disorders or preventing unplanned pregnancies. The claim to be seeking a balance between respect for the human embryo as a potential form of life and the imperatives of research, however, risks being disingenuous, where the importance of the research in question is merely taken for granted and where no serious attention is given to the existence of genuine conflicts between competing and qualitatively different interests. It may be that embryo research will allow us to "save lives and prevent misery." We might come to agree that saving lives and preventing the sorts of misery that can be prevented through embryo research are worth overriding religious and moral reticence about the manipulation and destruction of embryonic life. We might even come to agree that they are important enough to warrant suspending current limits on the use of embryos for research, for example, suspending limits on research after the appearance of the primitive streak. Any argument that treats these conclusions as self-evident, however, begs the question.

Thus, one objection we can raise to the argument in favor of permitting research embryos advanced by Steinbock and reflected in the report of the HERP concerns the sincerity of the commitment to respect for the human embryo and the adequacy of the criteria used in weighing competing values. In addition, Steinbock's distinction between moral status and moral value is problematic. She takes it as obvious that we should find the creation of human embryos for crassly commercial purposes or for use in frivolous research distasteful. Equally distasteful is the prospect of human embryos generated merely to have an ample supply of research material.

It is not at all clear, however, why this should be obvious, particularly why we should find the latter so obviously distasteful. On her own account, there is nothing intrinsically valuable or obligating about the human embryo. Without interests, she argues, a being "can have no claim to our moral attention and concern" (p. 68). Rather, we choose to confer value on the embryo just as we choose to value trees, national flags, and fine art. Although we can and sometimes do choose to value and therefore protect trees as works of nature, however, more often we do not, and trees in an arboretum have a distinctly different value than trees in an area slated for commercial development. National flags are both objects of reverence and articles of clothing depending on fashion trends, and what will count as fine art depends on the sensibilities of a given culture's elites. If we do not recognize the human embryo as potential life, as laying some claim on us morally that distinguishes it from a tree, as having a significance independent of our bestowal, what prevents us from producing as many embryos as we need for research just as we grow trees for furniture or auction art for charity? As a potential human being, the embryo or presentient fetus "is a powerful symbol of human life" argues Steinbock. "This is enough of a reason not to treat it as a mere commodity or convenient tool for research" (p. 167). Yet is not the embryo or presentient fetus "a powerful symbol of human life" precisely when it is recognized as having a transcendent value, a moral standing that, even if not equivalent to full personhood, distinguishes it from things and non-human forms of life?

The questions raised earlier point to a still deeper but related objection to the interest view. There is no doubt that the moral status of the preimplantation embryo is a fundamental issue in the assessment of embryo research. A narrow focus on the question of whether the preimplantation embryo ought to be shown the same respect as an infant or a child, whether or not the preimplantation embryo has interests that could be violated in the course of research, however, neglects critical questions about the setting, as well as the character and conduct, of embryo research. As Mary Mahowald[16] argues, moral status language abstracts the question of how we ought to treat human embryos from "the social context in which decisions about disposition of embryos, zygotes or gametes are made."

One consequence is that, for the most part, the debate about acceptable limits for embryo research ignores the question of who is really likely to benefit from embryo research. Improving success rates for medically assisted reproduction serves those who have access to specialized infertility treatments. Developing better methods for preimplantation genetic testing benefits those who are able to take advantage of opportunities for preimplantation diagnosis. Discovering safer and more effective contraception is useful to those who are able to choose from the full range of available methods. The high cost of specialized fertility services in the United States makes medically assisted reproduction and preimplantation screening genuine options only for those who have the financial resources. Despite the higher incidence of primary infertility among young African Americans with low income, the typical infertility patient is white, middle to upper income, and over 30 years of age.[17] In developing countries around the world, one-third or more of all couples lack access to reliable methods of contraception already available elsewhere. According to a recent report of the United Nations Population Fund, lack of access to desired methods of contraception results in 75 million unwanted pregnancies a year. Many women turn to unsafe abortion as their only option, resulting in more than 70,000 deaths a year.[18] Even a cursory look at the history of international population policy suggests that the existence or even the availability of contraceptives is much less important in the success or failure of family planning programs than cultural, political, and economic factors. It is not unreasonable to ask: Whose interests or what interests are at stake in funding embryo research? Whose lives are we really interested in saving, whose misery in preventing? What role will scientific or medical advancements actually play in the amelioration of those human miseries that concern us?

It might be argued that the potential clinical applications of embryo research are broader than I have indicated, that research into cell growth and differentiation holds promise for understanding how to prevent and treat cancer and other diseases that occur across populations—the prevention and treatment of which are in everyone's interest. It might also be argued that it is not unjust for infertility patients to benefit from the immediate clinical applications of embryo research if they also bear the primary burden as research subjects. Fair enough. But there is nothing in the argument from moral status that requires us even to ask whether embryo research or the creation of embryos for research is just or responsible under existing social, cultural, economic, or political conditions. In much the same way as appeals to moral status in the abortion debate have the effect of isolating decisions about continuing or ending pregnancy from the physical and social contexts that mediate and constrain the experience of pregnancy, appeals to the moral status of the preimplantation embryo isolate judgments about how far we can go in research from the institutional and social conditions under which scientific goals are defined and resources allocated.

The deep context: medically assisted reproduction

There is a more immediate and even more important "social context" that is obscured in arguments from moral status. It should seem obvious that we cannot separate the business of embryo research from its setting in the practice of medically assisted reproduction. It almost goes without saying, as Krimsky and Hubbard[19] observe, that without the medicalization of infertility and the public acceptance of IVF as a proper scientific and medical response, there would be no way to justify the collection of eggs and their fertilization outside a woman's body. Societal acceptance of IVF constitutes the essential port of entry into all forms of human embryo research.

In vitro fertilization is the "port of entry" for human embryo research in both a practical and a conceptual sense. The most immediate applications of embryo research are in reproductive medicine and the clinical treatment of infertility. Current methods for recruiting and harvesting ova and techniques for effecting fertilization outside the body were developed for IVF programs. In the short term, women undergoing assisted reproduction are likely to be the major source of research ova.[20] More important, the mainstreaming of IVF as a treatment for infertility signified a radical shift in personal, social, and scientific relationships to reproduction. As Lee Silver[21] argues, the birth of the first IVF baby represented a "singular moment in human evolution," a moment in which it became possible "in a very literal sense . . . to hold the future of our species in our own hands." Although developed for the treatment of infertility, IVF undeniably opens up possibilities for reproductive and genetic manipulations far beyond assisted reproduction. By "bringing the embryo out of the darkness of the womb and into the light of day," IVF allows for and makes acceptable the manipulation of the embryo on the cellular level, the transfer of embryos from "one maternal venue to another," and the ability to access and alter genetic material.[22]

Yet, the debate over the limits of embryo research prescinds unselfconsciously from judgments about goals and methods in reproductive technology. In this sense, the debate is "disembodied." It is as if eggs did not come from within particular women or embryos were not formed from the gametes of particular individuals. That is not to say that issues of informed consent or worries about harms to donors do not arise. Rather, the problem is that the question of how we ought to treat the preimplantation embryo is abstracted from the larger question of what we are doing when we intervene in the process of reproduction. More important, the problem of determining the scope of embryo research is addressed as though it had no relation to the rationale for introducing IVF into the clinical setting.

It is precisely when we resituate embryo research within the practice of medically assisted reproduction that we see why the creation of embryos for research purposes is troubling. By "re-embodying" the debate, we raise up what the moral status or interest view neglects: the intrinsically physical, social, and relational character of procreation; the ambiguity attached to our expanding power to alter the conditions under which fertilization and gestation occur; and the relationship between the expansion of reproductive technologies and the social meanings of sexuality, procreation, and parenthood. It is only against the backdrop of a technological capacity that has the potential to be alienating as well as generative, destructive as well as creative, that we can fairly weigh the cost of severing the act of initiating human embryonic life from intentions and commitments to care for and sustain it.

Elsewhere I have joined with feminists and others in arguing for caution in the development and clinical application of reproductive technologies.[23] There is no doubt that advances in reproductive medicine expand treatment options for couples struggling with infertility and provide new possibilities for biological reproduction. The ability to intervene in the process of reproduction gives new hope for overcoming both female and male factor infertility as well as for preventing and treating genetic diseases. Worldwide, IVF has already resulted in more than 150,000 live births, most of which would not have been possible without medical assistance. Just as the introduction of effective oral contraceptives gave women greater freedom in determining when they would reproduce, the advent of collaborative reproduction opens unprecedented possibilities for deciding how we will reproduce.

Yet medically assisted reproduction is not without risks. Drug regimes used to provide multiple ova for therapies such as IVF, GIFT, and ZIFT[24] pose both long-term and short-term threats to women's health, including the immediate risk of hyperstimulation and the possibility of slightly increased risk of ovarian and breast cancer. Although studies show no increased incidence of birth defects associated with the use of reproductive technology, the long-range effects of the drugs used to initiate and sustain assisted pregnancies on the reproductive capacities of offspring are still unknown. Women conceiving through IVF and IVF-related therapies experience higher rates of ectopic pregnancy, miscarriage, and multiple gestation.

Perhaps more important and more relevant for our purposes are the emotional, relational, and social costs. Specialized treatment for infertility can be invasive, intrusive, emotionally draining, and financially exhausting. The turn to reproductive technologies can provide new avenues of possibility; it can also draw patients deeper into the repeated cycles of hope and despair that characterize the experience of infertility. The appearance of highly sophisticated therapies "ups the ante" for the infertile, creating the new burden of "not trying hard enough." Often, patients cannot even begin to resolve the crisis of involuntary childlessness until they have sought every possible treatment and exhausted all medical options.

In addition, the advent of procreative technologies furthers the medicalization of infertility, constraining options for resolving the crisis of involuntary childlessness (e.g., adoption) and drawing attention away from the medical and social causes of infertility. While expanding possibilities for biological parenting, assisted reproduction also severs connections long thought important between sexuality, procreation, and parenthood. To many, new ways of configuring the family are welcome; still, doubts linger about the extent to which primary biological and genetic relationships can be refashioned without ultimately harming children.

Perhaps most troubling for feminists is the capacity of procreative technologies to "disembody" reproduction. As Margaret Farley[25] observes, "for many feminists the sundering of the power and process of reproduction from the bodies of women constitutes a loss of major proportions." Women's previous experience with reproductive technologies suggests that women's own agency is likely to be submerged in the network of multiple experts needed to achieve IVF. Far from this accomplishing a liberation from childbearing responsibilities, it can entail "further alienation of our life processes."

For feminists such as Patricia Spallone and Gena Corea, the submersion of women's agency to the "experts" has frightening social and political implications. "Scientist-controlled, technological reproduction offers solutions," argues Spallone, but in ways that ultimately disempower women and at the cost of forcing women to hand over their very "life power" to the (primarily male) medical establishment. "Women's struggle for sexual, reproductive, economic and social autonomy," she warns, "is undermined by the proliferation of a kind of reproduction which necessitates interference from the state and its institutions, especially medical science professionals."[26]

Still, I believe that reproductive technologies can be used justly and responsibly and without "making women redundant," as feminists rightly fear. Along with Christian ethicist Lisa Sowle Cahill, I take the view that the human ideal for procreation and parenthood is biological and relational partnership: a couple "committed to one another, as well as to the child-to-be, and who initiate their parental project with a loving sexual act."[27] It is a view that I would defend ultimately on theological grounds, although I believe it is defensible on non-theological grounds. The question posed by reproductive technologies concerns what exceptions to the ideal are justifiable. If the union of sexual intimacy, procreation, and parenthood cannot always be realized—indeed, if sometimes it ought not be—what possibilities for procreation and parenthood are consistent with a commitment to the value of biological and relational partnership?

Also with Cahill, I support the view that reproductive interventions are defensible to the degree that they maintain "the crucial biological relations that undergird the personal and social relations of spousehood, parenthood and childhood."[28] In vitro fertilization using gametes from within a marriage is more easily defended from this position, therefore, than IVF using donor gametes; in the former, procreation remains a shared biological endeavor, growing out of a sexual and marital relationship. That the sexual act "in which these physical relations are united and by which they are symbolized" is not realized can be justified, as Cahill argues, "by achievement of higher values: shared parenthood as part of the partnership of a couple committed to one another . . . and by the ability to maintain the important biological values. . . ."[29]

Reproductive interventions are defensible also insofar as they respect the well-being of offspring as well as the needs and rights of adult parties. They are defensible insofar as they honor individual women's agency in creating, sustaining, and bringing forth life. They are defensible to the extent that their use meets the norms of justice, that is, that they are used in a way that is socially responsible and in a way that respects obligations to offspring through the relationship of procreation. Reproductive technologies open the opportunity of biological parenting to those for whom it would be impossible, but not without a price; the technologies are both justified and properly constrained by the goal to which they aspire: the bringing forth of new life in loving and nurturing relationship.

It is in light of this account of the goals of reproductive technologies that it becomes possible to say what is troubling about the creation of embryos for research purposes. Although it is reasonable to argue that we do not harm very early embryos by bringing them into existence merely to use them for experimental purposes, to initiate human life in the absence of intentions to care for and sustain it is nonetheless an assault on the character of procreation. It is an extension of the power to remove conception from the body, to manipulate the basic material of reproduction, that moves outside the most compelling justifications for developing and exercising it. As I have argued, reproductive interventions can serve the goods of intimacy, generativity, and commitment to nurture, but interventions carry with them the risk of "further alienation from our life processes" and loss of regard for the embodied and relational character of reproduction. To initiate human embryonic life with the intention of bringing it to fruition is consistent with the best reasons for "paying the price" of intervening in biological reproduction. This remains so even if the well-being of procreators or potential offspring dictates that implantation not be attempted or if embryos that would otherwise be destroyed are later donated for research. To initiate human embryonic life in the absence of intentions to care for and nurture it is, however, inconsistent with the goals I have argued justify and ought to constrain reproductive interventions.

In excluding as oocyte donors women who are not scheduled to undergo a surgical procedure, the Human Embryo Research Panel itself recognized a distinction between the intention to initiate a pregnancy and the pursuit of research goals, however important. The panel argued that "women who are not scheduled to undergo a surgical procedure are not a permissible source of oocytes for research at this time, even if they wish to volunteer to donate their oocytes":

The Panel is concerned about the risks that current methods of oocyte retrieval pose to the health of donors. In order to obtain a number of fertilizable oocytes, hormonal stimulation and an invasive procedure are now required. Because alternative sources of oocytes are available, the Panel believes that such risks to donor cannot be justified. The Panel, however, is willing to allow such volunteers to donate oocytes if the intent is to transfer the resulting embryo for the purpose of establishing a pregnancy. . . . Absent the goal of establishing a pregnancy for an infertile couple, however, the lack of direct therapeutic benefit to the donor and the dangers of commercial exploitation do not justify exposing women to such risks.[30]

Although I have drawn the risks involved differently from the panel, it seems to me that we agree on at least this much: The goal of bringing about a pregnancy provides a rationale for accepting a degree of risk, for allowing certain kinds of harms to occur, that other goals do not.

Someone might argue that creating embryos for research does not undermine the relational and embodied significance of procreation as long as research embryos are not transferred for implantation. To sever the initiation of human life from intentions to care for and sustain it is only problematic, someone might say, if children are brought into the world within instrumental rather than nurturing relationships. Fertilizing oocytes for research is not the same as procreating; it does not violate the moral character of procreation to create embryos that will never develop into human personhood. To be sure, to bring a child to life in the absence of anyone committed to his or her well-being or merely for the use of others would be indefensible in light of the position I have defended. Yet initiating human embryonic life with the sole intention of obtaining research material is the appropriation of the power of procreation divorced from the context in which it finds its meaning and focus, whether or not the embryo is brought to personhood. I have argued that it is precisely the intention to create life for the purposes of establishing a parental relationship that provides the primary justification for intervening in the procreative process; it is therefore also the intention to create embryonic life for research purposes that is problematic.

Of course, the very meaning of *procreation* is no longer clear. Is the activation of eggs to begin development without fertilization, as in parthenogenesis, a "procreative act"? Is human cloning by nuclear transfer "procreation" or merely "replication"? The question of what ought to count as "reproduction" or "procreation" in the face of expanding possibilities is far too complex to answer here. We have only begun to debate the meanings of sexuality, reproduction, and parenthood under the radically different circumstances introduced by IVF. Yet, if cloning by nuclear transfer or parthenogenesis or fertilizing ova for research purposes are not properly called *procreative* acts, it is fair to ask whether they should be held to the moral standard for procreation I have invoked.[31]

Even if only a preliminary response can be given, it should be obvious why, in this account, cloning by nuclear transfer would violate the moral character of reproduction. I have defended a view of the significance of reproduction that underscores the integrity of its relational and biological dimensions. In addition to the risks of commercial exploitation that attend human cloning by nuclear transfer, it introduces the initiation of human life through a single progenitor. From a biological sense, cloning fails to honor the ideal of embodied partnership that I defended earlier.[32]

Parthenogenesis is a more difficult case. As described in the report of the Human Embryo Research Panel, ova that are activated to begin cleavage and development without fertilization lack the genes necessary to develop as viable human embryos. Unlike the research embryo, the parthenote intrinsically lacks the potentiality for development. Thus, it is reasonable to argue that the concerns about the conditions under which it is moral to initiate human life that I have raised with respect to the research embryo would not apply in the same way to parthenogenesis, just as it is reasonable to argue that concerns about the morality of human cloning would not apply directly to the use of cloning in initiating nonreproductive cell lines.[33] Throughout this chapter, however, my primary interest has been with justifications for intervening in the normal or "natural" process of reproduction. Rather than taking the removal of eggs from women's bodies and fertilization in vitro as routine or morally neutral and asking only "What are we permitted to do with gametes or embryos now that we have them?" I have insisted that we must continue to ask "Why are we doing this in the first place?" Taking seriously the risks to women's health and reproductive agency posed by reproductive technologies as well as the potential to undermine important connections between sexuality, procreation and parenthood, I have maintained that the intention to bring forth offspring in responsible and loving relationships provides the most compelling justification.

Finally, it might be argued that the creation of research embryos is not incompatible with the rationale for reproductive interventions if the research in question seeks to advance the goal of biological parenthood. If the availability of research embryos has the potential to improve the safety and efficacy of IVF, are not the goals of research in such a case consonant with the good of reproduction? On the face of it, this objection seems persuasive. If the achievement of biological parenthood drives our willingness to accept the risks of assisted reproduction, why not do anything necessary to advance that cause? It is not, however, only the ends of reproduction that are important in this analysis, but also the means. It is not only opening possibilities for biological parenting that is morally important, but also opening possibilities that are responsible to the goods at stake, that is, the embodied and relational character of procreation. It is only when we resist the temptation to split ends from means, when we reject the assumption that an end state can be clearly demarcated from the processes that lead up to it, that we see why creating research embryos is incompatible with commitments to maintaining the relational significance of procreation and why it remains so even when the research in question serves the overall goal.

Conclusion

In her statement of dissent, panel member Patricia King[34] stated that "fertilization marks a significant point in the process of human development, and the prospect of disconnecting fertilization from the rest of the procreative process in which there is an intent to produce a child is profoundly unsettling." I have tried to suggest here why, indeed, we might find the prospect of severing fertilization from the rest of the procreative process, or, more accurately, from the rest of the parenting project, profoundly unsettling. In the end, King was persuaded that the benefits to be gained through embryo research outweighed the anxieties, although she approved the use of research embryos only where the information needed could not be gained in any other way. Assessing the risks and benefits somewhat differently than King did, I remain unsettled.

Disagreements over the use of research embryos have centered, on the one hand, on conflicting assessments of the moral status of the preimplantation embryo and, on the other hand, on differing judgments about how to weigh moral anxieties over the treatment of human embryos against the social importance of the research.

I have argued that a narrow focus on moral status abstracts the question of acceptable limits to embryo research from its larger setting. Beyond the question of whether embryos can be harmed is the deeper question of how we justify interventions into the procreative process. Severing fertilization from reproduction, in the full sense, is problematic precisely because it stands outside of the goods and values that medically assisted reproduction most directly and appropriately serves. The risks to be weighed, therefore, involve not only the "interests" of the preimplantation embryo, but also societal interests in women's health and in the integrity of sexuality, reproduction, and parenthood.

I have left an important issue unaddressed. The argument I have offered rests on a particular account of the intrinsic relationship between sexuality, procreation, and parenthood, an account with which many in this society may disagree and one with important theological influences. It is not unfair to ask what weight such arguments should have in public and policy-oriented debates. Should arguments for banning the use of research embryos be accepted that depend on what may constitute a minority position on the goals of medically assisted reproduction?

The limits of this essay make an adequate answer impossible, although it does seem to me that there is an important place in public debate for perspectives that challenge the dominant research ethos, particularly when it concerns issues of such human importance as the limits of research and the nature of reproduction. Here, however, I share Lisa Sowle Cahill's conclusion: The important thing is not how to prevent embryo research or cloning from occurring. Indeed, given the vast commercial potential in reproductive and genetic technologies, I am not optimistic that it will be possible even to contain them well, let alone prevent them from being introduced. What is important is how to open up public discussion to values beyond unexamined scientific progress or self-determination.[35] For now, the important thing is to expand the range of what is taken to be morally important in the debate over the creation of embryos for research or the introduction of human cloning, to resituate the question of what it means to respect human embryos in our ongoing reflection about the meaning of intervention into human reproduction.

4

Casuistry, Virtue, and the Slippery Slope: Major Problems with Producing Human Embryonic Life for Research Purposes

JAMES KEENAN, S.J.

Contemporary proponents of producing human embryos for research purposes fail in three ways to make their case: They do not provide a standard to legitimate the new endeavors on which they want society to embark; they contradict by their recommended practices the legitimating attitude that they invoke; and they offer no grounds for public confidence that we can effectively safeguard against likely abuses. These three issues are treated respectively under the topics of casuistry, virtue, and the slippery slope.

In addressing these claims, I hope I am not considered an obstructionist in the current discussion. While I am opposed to producing human embryonic life for research purposes, I have not seen any reasons offered to think otherwise. I am stunned that proponents for this innovation have proffered neither ethical arguments for their proposals nor ethical standards for their protocols. My challenge to these proponents is not that they necessarily should abandon their position, but rather that they should offer some warrants for it. As I hope the reader will discover, I offer the proponents some specific direction about methods of ethical argumentation that may be suitable for their purposes. It is on that note that I conclude.

Casuistry

As participants on the National Commission for the Protection of Human Subjects of Biomedical and Behavioral Research (1975–1978), Albert Jonsen and Stephen Toulmin discovered that their commission was able to agree on acceptable forms of experimentation only through the use of cases. They discovered that whenever an individual member suggested a particular moral principle as the validating ground for the commission's conclusions, disagreement arose. When a member invoked a case analogous to the one being considered, the committee was able to achieve consensus from a variety of positions. A case, not a principle, became the locus of moral certitude for the pluralistic committee. This insight led to Jonsen and Toulmin's investigation of the history of moral reasoning, and the result was a compelling and sustained defense of casuistry.[1]

In this section I argue that casuistry affords a key method for addressing the moral legitimacy of the production of human embryos for research purposes; but before that, I want to make two extended, but preliminary comments. The first surveys recent literature on embryonic research; the second describes the recent studies on high casuistry that have appeared in the wake of Jonsen and Toulmin's study. These two steps serve to support my claim for the relevance of casuistry for the topic at hand.

International Comments on the Research of Human Embryos

A recent collection of essays by predominantly European scholars, edited by Donald Evans, studied the human embryo and the type of legal and moral guidelines that do or ought to direct research with human gametes and embryos.[2] Although this collection does not primarily address the issue of producing embryos solely for research, and although it is focused on the use of embryos for research in Europe, it is instructive for considering embryo research in the United States because it highlights the inability of national communities to rely on principles to achieve consensus on the broader topic of embryonic research. Indeed, what Arlene Klotzko says about the British Human Fertilisation and Embryology [HFE] Act (1990) seems to be true of national policies in Hungary, Spain, Germany, France, and Poland. She writes:

The HFE Act creates a highly elaborated framework governing the morally conscientious practice of embryo research. It is virtually a law without norms—or at least a law with very few. Instead the HFE Authority is created and empowered as a pragmatic means of facilitating medical advances. There is no real attempt at a principled approach to the vindication of patient rights.[3]

None of the national policies described in the Evans collection is grounded on a principled foundation.

Although the lack of a rationale explaining embryo research policy is curious, Evans's volume helps us to see why a foundation of principles is lacking and how we might profitably proceed in the absence of principles. First, many authors discuss at length the impossibility of ever achieving any certitude on the exact nature of the human embryo.[4] They claim that religious, cultural, philosophical, national, and personal biases so frame individual positions that when talking about the embryo we cannot expect ever to agree to a moral determination of its nature. Second, the editor suggests that the "nature" of the embryo does not really set the agenda in our current debates; rather, our willingness to manipulate the embryo determines our understanding of the nature of the human embryo. Evans writes: "it might well be that it is by discovering what I am prepared to do with the preembryo that I determine what I consider its status to be as opposed to trying to get clear about the matter in order to decide what I shall do."[5]

Maurizio Mori also wants to steer us away from talking about the particular nature of the embryo per se and to focus instead on the interaction we have with human reproduction. The issue is not so much what the embryo is, but rather what we are doing with human reproduction.[6] If the question is phrased in this way, then the issue is who we become when we do the research we are doing. This of course does not marginalize the embryo from the debate but rather acknowledges our role in the entire process. Thus, although we may be at a stalemate on the notion of potentiality in the embryo,[7] we may be able to recognize our place in the entire process of embryonic research and development.[8]

Finally, the authors argue that we need to see the present set of stalemates as occasions for finding alternatives to the usual method of moral argument, that is, the simple application of a principle to a situation.[9] This search for alternatives, argues the Danish philosopher Knut Ruyter, ought to lead us to consider the possibilities that the analogical logic of casuistry offers.[10]

Recent Research into High Casuistry

Casuistry emerges as a method of moral reasoning whenever extraordinary, new issues materialize. The development of high casuistry during the sixteenth century makes this clear. An example helps to illustrate the pattern. Although maritime insurance had been considered a form of usury since 1237, European explorations in the New World and trade with the East led Europeans to question this older moral guideline. By the beginning of the sixteenth century, the prohibition against underwriting expeditions appeared to be unworkable. Therefore, merchants petitioned faculty members of the University of Paris to render new decisions on maritime insurance. The faculty responded by arguing that the case of an insurer guaranteeing the arrival of the worth of a cargo was like the case of the captain of a ship who secures the arrival of the cargo. The merchants' question became a case, then, and was placed against another case that described already validated moral activity. By showing congruency between the two, the faculty provided new ways of circumscribing the decretal against insurance, distinguishing insurance from usury, and proposing ethical grounds to legitimate the insurance.[11] Casuistry was thus used to liberate institutions from normative determinations that did not keep pace with other developments.[12] With this freedom, however, came the need for new expressions of moral guidance, and casuistry also provided those bankers, merchants, missionaries, explorers, and princes bent on expansionism a new inductive method of moral logic to navigate the unfamiliar waters before them.

Consider an example more to the point, a classic case dealing with abortion: a pregnant woman flees from a charging bull, even as her flight prompts a spontaneous abortion. The case was first presented by Peter of Navarre (d. 1594), who illustrated the position of Antonius de Corduba (1485–1578) that a woman had a "right to protect her life even at the cost of causing an abortion."[13] Gabriel Vasquez (1551–1604) later employed the same case precisely to deny Corduba's position: The woman's flight was an attempt to save both her life and her fetus'; therefore her flight may result in the fetus' death, but she may not have an abortion to save her own life.[14] Ioannes Azor (d. 1603) used the case (changing the bull to a ranging fire) to argue that a woman could intend to protect her life and use certain means that are not of necessity aimed at abortion.[15] Thomas Sanchez (1550–1610) expanded on the case when considering whether a pregnant woman can take a drug with doubtful effects when she and her fetus are both doomed to death and no other drugs are available. He added the fleeing woman who can escape the bull only by jumping from a cliff.[16]

The inductive method of comparing cases employed by these writers is called *taxonomy* by Jonsen and Toulmin and is typical of high casuistry. High casuistry thus involves the analogous comparison of the new case against one or more cases that already enjoy successful resolution. This comparison helps bring to light the morally relevant circumstances that become decisive in determining the outcome of any case. Moreover, in the absence of relevant principles, the cases already successfully resolved become the standards against which to measure the circumstances of the new case. These standard cases Jonsen and Toulmin call *paradigms*.[17] Two such paradigms were the cases of the captain of the ship and a woman saving her life.

This taxonomic use of casuistry differs considerably from the standard understanding of casuistry that was current from the seventeenth century until recently. In that *geometric* casuistry, existing principles were simply deductively applied to cases and the case was solved. In geometric casuistry a principle and not the case is the standard; a case is thus measured against a principle rather than compared with other cases. One clear example of geometric casuistry is the application of the principle of double effect. It is important to remember, however, that even that principle developed from high casuistry. From a constellation of several similar paradigm cases, the central factors of congruency among them were eventually articulated into the four conditions of the principle.[18] Other methodological principles, like cooperation, toleration, and lesser evil, also emerged out of the taxonomies of high casuistry. Like double effect, they also replaced the paradigms themselves as the standards for attaining moral objectivity.

Geometric casuistry operates, then, when principles are firmly in place. In periods of great certainty, principles tend to supply ample and adequate understanding of the moral point of view that society has on a subject. The geometric method or the basic deductive application of a principle to a case is then the prevalent moral logic in times of certainty; the taxonomic or the basic inductive method is prevalent in times of experimentation and newness.

In the face of antiquated principles, sixteenth-century ethicists attentive to the newness of contemporary projects turned for guidance to cases, circumstances, new distinctions, and analogous logic. Those times are similar to our own; ethicists and historians revisiting this material are struck by the resemblances: new questions, new meetings between people of diverse religious and cultural backgrounds, weak principles, a time bent on expansionism, and, most importantly, a world where the advances in other fields outpace those in ethics.[19]

Bringing Casuistry into the Debate About Producing Human Embryos

When we read the literature concerning the production of human embryos for research purposes, we see the evident similarity between the sixteenth-century merchants and the contemporary proponents of embryonic research. Among both proponents and opponents of the research there is a general recognition that relevant principles (Kantian categorical imperative, double effect, and the slippery slope) are woefully inadequate. In fact, the proponents of producing human embryos for research (hereinafter known as simply, "the proponents,") generally make their case negatively by arguing against principles that would restrict embryo research rather than positively for principles that would justify the research. For instance, Bonnie Steinbock,[20] Dena Davis,[21] and David Heyd[22] each attack any attempt to apply the categorical imperative to the treatment of human embryos. They basically adopt Steinbock's argument that these entities are not yet human persons and do not have interests, although they may have value.[23] They conclude that the imperative cannot be applied to these non-interested entities.

Likewise, Carol Tauer and Bonnie Steinbock critique those who, by invoking the principle of double effect, argue that only research on spare embryos is permissible because the intention of their production was not originally to experiment on them and destroy them. Steinbock, for instance, claims that the production of the other human embryos is for a good purpose as well.[24] Dismissing any intrinsic value to the embryos, she invokes basic consequentialism to vindicate her argument, not realizing that the principle that her opponents employ is precisely founded on non-consequentialist claims.[25] Tauer takes Steinbock's analogy and expands it, suggesting that one who invokes it could also justify deception: "[I]f clinicians are interested in research they may even choose to fertilize a large number of oocytes in the hope that some will be 'left over' for research."[26] Whereas the purpose of Steinbock's critique is to undo the dividing line between research embryos that are spares from those that are intentionally produced for research, Tauer is more interested in revealing a slippery, self-serving casuistry behind those who invoke the principle to work on spares.

Steinbock and Tauer's engagement with the principle highlights two important insights. First, both are right to reject the claims of those who invoke the principle: Double effect does not apply to the case of the spares; the more appropriate principle could be the principle of lesser evil. Second, neither advances any ground for whether producing embryonic life for research purposes is ethical. However, Tauer differs from Steinbock in this: She acknowledges that when we erase the dividing line, we are not necessarily on moral ground. As Tauer points out, research on embryos secured either way may be right or wrong. Her claim is simply that how embryos are produced is not morally significant.

Finally, Davis,[27] Steinbock, and Tauer all take aim at the slippery slope argument. Again Steinbock is influential: She argues that its supporters "assume, without justification, that it is impossible to set limits and create restrictions that will prevent predicted dire consequences."[28] I agree with these critics, having argued elsewhere that the slippery slope has no final claims in closing debates.[29]

The proponents demonstrate, then, the futility of existing moral principles to serve as barriers that could morally distinguish experimenting with spares from producing embryos for experimentation. Like those forward-looking ethicists of the sixteenth century, they show that we are in newly ambiguous territory and that the guidance provided by existing principles is not helpful. Having made that point, however, they do not imitate their forbearers in the next step of high casuistry, that is, providing a paradigm, first to legitimate their claims and second to serve as a reliable action guide. This is remarkable, because in failing to provide a paradigm they provide no grounds for their argument nor a standard of moral rightness by which we can maintain a measure of moral objectivity in dealing with this at least morally ambiguous activity. Moreover, if the proponents did provide some analogous paradigm cases, they would shift the debate dramatically.

As in the sixteenth century, the turn from principles to cases simultaneously turns debate from the nature of the moral object to a description of human agency. The Paris faculty did not discuss the nature of usury; they presented a captain of a ship securing a cargo's arrival. Spanish casuists did not discuss abortion, but whether a pregnant woman's options were like those of the woman fleeing for her life. Casuists shifted the debates away from that tendency in ethics to discuss a moral object metaphysically toward a moral description of human practical activity. If the proponents were to turn to paradigms, they could follow Mori's suggestion and talk, not about the nature of the embryo but rather about what it is that we humans are doing when we produce human embryos for research purposes only.

The proponents, however, simply prove that some of their opponents' arguments are wrong. This method of argumentation is called *retortion*. Retortion is a valid form of argument and sufficient when one is replying to a proponent attempting to introduce a new, morally dubious practice. Retortion is not sufficient, however, when one introduces change. When new practices are being introduced, which are at best morally problematic, proponents must provide a moral foundation for their practices and moral standards to guide society's engagement of those practices. Thomas Kuhn made this clear in his important work where he argued that for proponents to replace a paradigm, they must not only demonstrate the lack of validity of the existing paradigm, they also must both validate their paradigm and present its operational structure.[30]

That their argument is solely one of retortion can be seen by the three stages of their argument. First, they note that, faced with spares, it is better to put them to the good purpose of research than to simply discard them. For example, Tauer recounts what others claim: "[T]here are other alternatives for the surplus embryos besides entering them into a research protocol. But if they otherwise would have been discarded or left in storage indefinitely, then to study them in research might be regarded as the least bad of the available choices."[31]

Second, they oppose any claims for distinguishing embryos that are spares from embryos that are produced for research purposes. They highlight the "difficulties in defending a rational ethical distinction between what one can do to spare embryos" and "what one can do to embryos created for the sole purpose of research."[32]

Third, they claim, therefore, that if it is permissible to experiment on spare embryos, then there are no reasons for not opposing producing embryos for research. The argument rests on this double-negative construction. Davis writes: "In sum, none of the arguments most commonly used against embryo research can support the distinction between what one can do to spare embryos and what one can do to embryos made for research. In terms of how embryos may ethically be used, it appears to make no ethical difference where embryos come from."[33]

Davis is not alone; John Robertson claims that "if embryos are too undeveloped physically to be harmed, it should not matter whether researchers use embryos left over from IVF or embryos created solely for research."[34] Likewise, Carol Tauer argues, "If it is not wrong to use a preimplantation embryo in research, then how can it be wrong to intend this use at the time of fertilization?"[35]

Curiously, then, the standard for the rightness of producing new embryos depends (according to the proponents) on the practice of experimenting on spare embryos. None of the proponents, however, establishes this practice as a moral or ethical standard. Like Davis, every proponent seems to point to the morally ambiguous situation we find ourselves in having left-over, unimplanted embryos. To give them good purpose, we submit them to experimentation instead of simply discarding them. The moral treatment of these spare embryos is determined then by default: Not knowing what to do with these spare embryos, we use them for research rather than simply discarding them. This is a good example of the principle of the lesser evil. If that principle, however, justifies the use of spare embryos, how can it justify the production of embryos for research? Do any of the proponents really believe that that principle applies to the production of embryos?

Other proponents could disagree with Tauer's line about the implicit need to validate the experimental use of spare embryos. They might argue that because the embryos are without interests, our treatment of them does not need to be considered morally and that discarding or experimenting on them is morally insignificant. Then, in a manner of speaking, by retortion, the proponents have backed themselves into a corner where there is no ethical standard, neither principle nor paradigm case, that provides a moral measure of the rightness or wrongness of our activities, whether with spare embryos or with produced embryos. This is known as pure moral relativism.

This is clearly present in the Human Embryo Research Panel report. The report acknowledges that opponents would allow that "research on embryos remaining from infertility treatments (or preimplantation diagnosis) may be justified as a byproduct of the otherwise well-intentioned act of trying to conceive a healthy child, whereas the express fertilization of oocytes for research purposes lacks even this minimal justification." On the other hand, proponents "who would permit the fertilization of oocytes expressly for research often argue that the resulting embryos have equivalent moral status to embryos remaining from fertility treatment, and thus they should be acceptable for research under similar guidelines."[36]

Of this debate, the report simply states, "These arguments are metaphysically complex and controverted, and the Panel did not come to any conclusion about their validity or weight."[37]

This conclusion is stunning because the report proceeds immediately to name six ways that research on embryos would be helpful and then recommends research on embryos, both spares and those specifically produced for research.[38] Without providing grounds for its position and without determining any moral standard (neither principle nor case) for what the action of producing a human embryo is like, the report simply presumes that the action is morally acceptable on the basis of the importance of research. This decision should disturb anyone familiar with the numerous examples in this century of unethical experimentation on subjects whose status was never ascertained but was justified in the name of the importance of research.[39] As Daniel Callahan has recently objected, "simply projecting possible good consequences of research hardly constitutes such a defense. . . ."[40]

Some proponents could again say that they have made, à la Steinbock, a decision on the moral status of the subjects. Here they might say that they have declared that, lacking interests, the embryo is not a human person. This may be true; my own Roman Catholic tradition denies that claim. Were we to grant the proponents' assertion that we cannot determine what the human embryo is, we still need to know what it is that we humans are doing when we produce human embryos for research purposes only. The proponents, however, do not address that question; they only address the claims of their opponents and leave us with no moral grounds for their innovation or any standards for their innovative protocols. We are thus still morally adrift.[41]

Opponents to the NIH Research Panel agree with this critique: There is no methodological framework or any particular principles or paradigm cases for weighing or measuring the morality of the proposal to produce embryos. For instance, the Ramsey Colloquium objects that there is only one guiding principle: "the principle that research involving preimplantation embryos is acceptable public policy only if the research is acceptable public policy."[42] Daniel Callahan[43] likewise writes:

How are we to go about establishing some kind of proportionality between the claims of research (which the report at one point calls a "duty") and that of the "moral weight" of the embryo? Some astonishment is in order at this point. Though the report sets up a clear moral tension between those goods, it is utterly silent on how research claims and possibilities should be evaluated for their moral weight and benefit. It is no less silent on how, even with that information in hand, a moral calculus is to be constructed to do the necessary balancing.

In fact, a panel member, R. Alta Charo, commented: "in the end, the Panel's actual policy choices were highly consequentialist,"[44] and acknowledged that "what is missing from the Panel's report is any theory explaining why the presence of a collection of factors, each inadequate in itself, would yield a compelling argument for a particular moral status to be assigned at any particular stage."[45]

These persons complain then that proponents offer no calculus for mediating the claims of research against the claims of the embryo. While agreeing with the opponents, I suggest that the calculus is missing because of a more fundamental flaw in the proponents' arguments. That flaw is their failure to provide any positive foundational argument (even an analogous one that a paradigm case provides) for determining the moral nature of our activity. Omitting that case, they have no standard.

Virtue

If the proponents were to offer a case, it could bear an analogous relationship not with what an embryo is, but more with what we are doing when we produce human embryos for research. To this proposal some proponents might remark that, in lieu of either a case or a principle, they offered a virtue, "respect" for the human embryo. The panel, after all, proposed that respect was owed to the human embryo. John Robertson too endorses this proposal:

Identifying the symbolic component in embryo research (and other biological controversies) is essential to sharpen debate and give competing considerations their due. Labeling an ethical concern as "symbolic" is not to denigrate it, but rather to situate it accurately vis-à-vis the interests with which it conflicts. A key point is that symbols do not make moral claims on us in the same way that persons and living entities with interests do. Because symbolic meanings are so personal and variable, subordinating them to research goals usually violates no moral duties.[46]

Curiously, the proponents advance the applicability of the concept of respect only to our experimentation on embryos, not to our production of them. Again, the proponents sidetrack any discussion about the moral nature of our activity of producing embryos for research purposes. Thus Robertson[47] describes what is at stake in this respect by noting that the entire issue is "about what cost in foregone knowledge should be tolerated to demonstrate the respect for human life that limiting embryo research symbolizes." For Robertson, respect, then, is the price we pay for research. He does not consider that respect might generate positive guidelines. Rather, respect functions negatively: We should not treat embryos in a "demeaning" way, for example, for testing the safety of cosmetics. Robertson is not alone; the panel and Davis argue in the same way.[48]

This method of argumentation is similar to that which we saw before. Rather than proposing a constructive foundation, guidelines are established negatively, on three levels. First, the proponents claim that since before 14 days, embryos are not human persons with interests, they cannot be treated by principles as human ends. Because we should not treat them as ends, we should by default at least treat them respectfully. Second, because this respect is not of persons, this virtuous stance requires no specific "duties." Third, this respect means not treating preimplantation human embryos in demeaning ways.

The proponents introduce "respect" as the only marker for how we should treat the embryos; they leave us with an extraordinarily fluid concept without any measurable claim on us. Not surprisingly, opponents object. Courtney Campbell is "troubled by doubt as to whether the philosophical value the panel has attributed to the preimplantation human embryo will have any moral significance within the research process."[49] He adds, "My concern was to examine how the moral respect the panel confers on the embryo will be meaningful in the context of scientific research."[50] Callahan's views are even stronger:

[I]t is better and more honestly done by simply stripping preimplantation embryos of any value at all. If we look under the rhetoric of respect, that seems to me the actual meaning of what the panel has done. At best, the kind of respect it would accord embryos is to them as a class, not as individual embryos. Those embryos that stand in the way of research are to be sacrificed—as nice a case of the ends justifying the means as can be found.[51]

As a virtue ethicist and a casuist, I find that the proponents, having discredited casuistry by their insufficient argumentation, likewise undermine the attempts of virtue ethicists who claim that virtues give concrete guidance. The proponents claim that respect means not demeaning human embryos. They describe what we should not do; but, if virtue inclines us toward the good, then respect must tell us what we should do, not simply what we should not do.

My complaint is all the more important when we consider how it is that we presently treat human embryonic life. Dena Davis provides an illustration from a typical IVF narrative:

[A] woman is made to hyperovulate, some eight or ten ova are fertilized, and perhaps half of the resulting embryos are transferred to the womb; if pregnancy is achieved, those embryos are often "selectively reduced" to twins; and, meanwhile, the remaining embryos are frozen in case the couple needs to try again. If unused, the spare embryos are eventually destroyed or donated to research.[52]

When we understand that "embryonic reduction" is a euphemism for selective abortion, we realize that the IVF protocol today now includes not only the wastage of preimplanted spare embryos but also the probable destruction of some fetal life.

The very topic of spare embryos highlights not only the way technology has out-paced ethics, but also how our "respect" for embryonic life is hardly adequately engaged. As The *New York Times* correspondent Gina Kolata writes: "Tens of thousands of embryos are steadily accumulating in tanks of liquid nitrogen across the country, an eerie consequence of the recent success of in vitro fertilization. . . . [T]he ranks of frozen embryos raise a host of legal, emotional, and ethical questions."[53]

What does this say about the way we are respecting the human embryo or the way we are ethically exercising our agency in human reproduction? In fact, there is so little regard for embryonic life that that becomes an argument for permitting the production of human embryos for experimentation purposes! The HERP report admits: "a complete prohibition in this area is likely to be difficult—if not impossible to enforce. . . . In the words of the Australian Senate Select Committee, "any intelligent administrator of any IVF program can, by minor changes in his ordinary clinical ways of going about things, change the number of embryos that are fertilized."[54]

What then is the culture of respect for the human embryo today? Ambiguous at best. What is particularly troublesome about the proponents' position is, then, that they do not use the concept of respect in any way to stave off the growing disregard for embryonic life. On the contrary, ironically, the concept of respect gives them the latitude to produce embryos for research and then destruction. In effect they argue that if we grant them the right to open the door to the production of human embryos for research purposes, they will use "respect" as the "wedge" to restrict the experimentation to non-demeaning purposes. In effect, by "respect," they will be producing and destroying more embryos than they have yet done so.

Proponents might respond that I am unfair; after all, a limit has been imposed by this concept. So Ronald Green responded to Campbell and Callahan: "we concluded that symbolic, biological and other matters make it wise to accord a measure of respect to the preimplantation embryo and we expressed this respect in the specific limits we recommend be imposed on research."[55]

But Green has not demonstrated how we positively measure that respect against the claims of research.[56] Moreover, he does not apply respect for embryos to any other existing practice. Either the proponents are introducing something new, or the proponents are legitimating the status quo. If new, then what positive ground is being won with regard to the treatment of embryos?

For instance, why would respect for embryonic life not prompt the panel members to critically examine the practice by IVF administrators who produce more spare embryos than are necessary and who do this solely to generate embryos for research? Where is the censure of "embryonic reduction"? Why is there not some inclination by the proponents to suggest that IVF protocols try to reduce the dependency on multiple embryos for implantation? In short, is there any way that the proponents by introducing the virtue of respect improve our cultural sense of value for what we do with the embryo?

The emptiness of the symbolic nature of respect is picked up again by panel member Charo: "Labeling peoples' interests as symbolic does denigrate their ethical concerns, because it fails to distinguish in a principled way among extremely important, important, and unimportant symbolic values."[57]

Relying on an Orwellian concept of respect, the proponents do not present credible grounds for their position.

Slippery slope

Invoking the slippery slope argument to foreclose discussion is often a sign of intransigence. One can look on the slippery slope, however, not to forecast the future, but to express concern about the present. When a slippery slope argument is used to close debate it is nothing but an authoritarian tool; but it can legitimately suggest that necessary standards need to be in place before the public can be confident in a proponent's proposal.[58] Thus, another member of the Human Embryo Research Panel invokes the slope as a concern about the proponents' point of view. Patricia King[59] writes, "I do not believe that this society has developed the conceptual frameworks necessary to guide us down this slope." The report noted her concern but refused to endorse it.

In light of the present debate on human embryos one can certainly ask these proponents what standards are in place to guarantee (humanly speaking) an effective set of moral guidelines to maneuver in this new field. Thus far, the proponents have failed terribly: They have rejected the claims of principles invoked by their opponents and proffered none in their stead; they have not offered any concrete standard in terms of the paradigm cases that the National Commission for the Protection of Human Subjects discovered and employed; they have proposed a weak notion of the virtue that undermines what the virtue ought to promote; and, they have claimed that invoking the slippery slope argument is "without justification." In a word, they have proved nothing more than that some of their opponents are not right. This failure occurs in a culture more accustomed now to the proliferation and destruction of human embryos than any before.

If the proponents want to advance their case, then they will need to provide both moral grounds to legitimate it and moral standards to guide us. This foundation does not necessarily have to be rooted in principles. I have suggested that invoking paradigm cases might provide a better reference point for legitimating their claims. Of course, they could turn to virtues, but then they would have to define virtues that lead us rather than simply restrain us. By either case, the proponents would do better, because each method, casuistry and virtue ethics, aims to evaluate not moral objects, but rather human activity.

In the international discussion about whether to produce embryos for research, the topic of human agency is comically absent. Like the question of spare embryos, the attention is singularly focused on the embryos and never on what we are doing. We overlook our agency: It is as if our questions are about whether to research on something that someone anonymously delivered to the lab.

As Maurizio Mori suggests, we need to critically examine of what moment there is to the production of human embryos for research purposes. A good set of analogous cases could help us to understand what this activity means and whether it is moral. Those cases could be crafted around virtues, for virtues help us to understand who it is that we are becoming by our own human agency. Thus the real cases that we need to look at are about ourselves and not primarily the embryos. For, in fact, it is we, not the embryos, who are on the slippery slope.

The proponents do little to assuage our anxiety about being on that slippery slope. By their language, they seem unaware of the concerns of much of society. For instance, when David Heyd refers to the activity as "the creation" of human embryos for experimentation, he proffers a poor descriptive, both ethically and strategically speaking, for what we are doing when we are producing human embryos. Ethically, it suggests that we are something that we are not: creators. Strategically, it suggests that we are usurping the place of God when we are producing human embryos for research purposes. Indeed, in explaining the White House's swift rejection of producing embryos for research, Charo wrote that senior White House staffers decided that "creating embryos for research exceeded the public's (and their) tolerance for exotic research."[60]

Conclusion

Good casuistry, like good virtue ethics, is persuasive. As I have hopefully demonstrated in this essay, the proponents have not been persuasive. Clearly, panel members were persuaded into believing that producing human embryos for research purposes is ethically right. They have not, however, communicated the grounds for being persuaded, and that has been their task. As Kuhn noted, innovators must be persuasive on two fronts: on the legitimacy of their claims and on the reliability of the operational structure or protocols of the innovation.

Unlike the panel members, I am not at all confident in the moral understanding of ourselves or of our activity as we engage the human embryo. I have only hinted at what I perceive to be the largely unexplored moral terrain of what it is we are doing when we manipulate the human embryo, but I have also demonstrated the poverty of moral argumentation proposed by those who purport to lead us into newer territories. They do not instill trust. On the contrary, they make us alarmed that we have followed them in the first place.

The same problem arises, I think, when we hear interests in human cloning. Here, too, we hear claims of "why not?" or "what's wrong with this?" In these claims we hear nothing but retortion used as the operating method of moral argumentation. Likewise, we watch an endless debate about the nature of the human embryo and see the innovators use this impasse to circumvent the more important question of who we are as we clone, as we genetically engineer the embryo, or as we produce embryos for research.[61]

I propose to the innovators that they enter into serious argument with those of us less optimistic and more concerned, nay alarmed. First, I invite them to admit that when human beings manipulate human embryos they/we are doing something with our very selves. A discussion appealing to a relational anthropology could help us achieve better understanding of who we are as a species as we manipulate human embryos.[62] Second, I suggest that the innovators admit that the topic of manipulation is problematic and that they cannot simply invoke old standards for guidance in very new terrain. Third, for this very reason, they should abandon arguments from retortion as insufficient: Retortion only claims that existing distinctions and standards are not valid. If they are not valid to prohibit innovation, they are not valid to legitimate it. Fourth, as we try to come to some self-understanding about ourselves in this (broadly conceived) manipulation, I invite the innovators to articulate and explore some virtues that could shore us up and guide us reflectively as we enter into the admittedly problematic field of manipulation. Certainly, we are now only on the verge of crossing the boundary into the new land of embryonic manipulation, and certainly, we can expect that we shall not simply have a brief foray there. Rather, I suspect, that for better or worse, some researchers shall set up tents there, and because of that we should ask what long-standing ethical dispositions should be developed for this work.

Here I think of a variety of essays in medical ethics that invoke the virtues of prudence, justice, humility, and wisdom.[63] Fifth, I propose that the innovators study casuistry. Clearly, taxonomic casuistry provided some moral compass for the expansionist tendencies of the late fifteenth and early sixteenth century Europeans. The innovators would do well, then, to consider the importance of cases, analogies, paradigms, and inductive reasoning. Here, I am not suggesting that this study would give them full license. Casuistry has helped to see which forms of embryonic manipulation are morally valid and which are not.[64]

At the dawn of work in embryonic manipulation, innovators would do well exploring, then, the two fields of virtue ethics and casuistry. Whereas weaving these two fields might remind some of reckless cross-breeding, I believe that such attempts are neither novel nor fruitless. John Noonan[65] remarks often in his historical studies of development in moral doctrine that the two reliable moral guides in times of innovation have always been the cultivation of truly virtuous dispositions and the development of rationally compelling, inductive moral logic.

5

Every Cell Is Sacred: Logical Consequences of the Argument from Potential in the Age of Cloning

R. ALTA CHARO

In Monty Python's *The Meaning of Life* there is a song that pokes fun at the Catholic Church's opposition to contraception and, by extension, at the classic argument from potential that any entity which has the potential to become a baby must be treated as sacredly as babies. The song, entitled "Every Sperm Is Sacred,"[1] goes:

Every sperm is sacred.
Every sperm is great.
If a sperm is wasted,
God gets quite irate.

One can only imagine what Monty Python will do with the advent of human cloning. Suddenly, many formulations of the argument from potential lead to the conclusion that not only is every embryo or fertilized egg to be treated as sacred, but so should every nucleus-bearing cell in our bodies.

The logical conclusion of such an analysis is, of course, absurd. It would mean that every avoidable discard of a live cell from our bodies would be sinful. Cell-recovery technology would need to be built into our showers, our clothes, and every other aspect of our daily lives. It is no wonder that no one will apply the argument from potential this way.

That does not mean, however, it is not worth our time to explore the way in which the argument from potential interacts with the new insights gained from cloning technology. With the insights that this combination provides, the analytical aspects of the argument from potential grow even weaker, forcing us to articulate better the real reasons for opposition to things such as research on human embryos. Better articulation, in turn, leads to some possible compromises in that debate, compromises that just might provide an avenue for permitting embryo research to go forward while at the same time demonstrating some degree of respect and deference to those troubled by cavalier destruction of the possible future children represented by those embryos. To do this, however, it is best to start in the beginning.

Consider somatic cell nuclear transfer cloning. Somatic cells, which make up most of our bodies, contain within them a full set of genetic material representing the genes needed to code for every aspect of an animal's body.[2] Until the 1980s, however, scientists believed that the process of specialization placed all genes in a state akin to a permanent vegetative state (PVS), except those needed to code for the specialized function. In other words, unnecessary genes became permanently unusable. Researchers at the Roslin Institute in Scotland, however, demonstrated that by starving the cell into a state amenable to reproduction, and then combining it with the cytoplasm of an enucleated egg cell, the genes previously thought to be in PVS could be awakened and coaxed into performing as if the cell were an ordinary fertilized egg, that is, to divide and develop into a fetus, baby, and thence adult sheep.[3] In other words, the previously dormant genes were not in PVS, merely in a reversible coma.

The prospect of using nuclear transfer cloning in humans to actualize the potential of every nucleus-bearing differentiated somatic cell raises the question: What distinction is there between ordinary cells and those entities, such as fertilized eggs or embryos, for which the argument from potential is used to justify deferential treatment?

For those opposing embryo research, the most widely shared analysis of the moral status of the embryo focuses on the notion that a fertilized egg is a genetically unique, complete cell with the potential to become a baby. Thus, it is argued, it is wrong to interfere with that potential by destroying the cell via destructive embryo research. In essence, the moment—or, at least, the process—of fertilization becomes the key dividing line between unprotected and protected forms of human life.[4] Due in large part to its genetic completeness and uniqueness, many hold that the fertilized egg has now become a member of the moral community of humanity.[5]

Of course, it is well understood that each aspect of this argument is subject to criticism. For example, the genetic "uniqueness" criterion is used to assert that the fertilized egg now exists in a one-to-one correspondence with a future baby, that is, that the embryo now represents a single individual. This assertion is especially important for those who seek to identify the moment at which the "soul" enters the body,[6] but it also resonates strongly with those who merely seek to identify the moment at which the embryo shares a key characteristic with the rest of those who claim unambiguous moral status.

Reproductive biology, however, reveals that a single fertilized egg can twin (thus creating two babies from one "unique" embryo) and, perhaps even more conceptually complicating, that two different embryos can merge to form a single baby whose body is a mosaic of the two different genetic patterns embedded in the two original embryos. Thus, genetic uniqueness does not entirely correspond with human individuality.[7]

A classic response to this, however, focuses on the combination of genetic uniqueness and completeness to represent a form of potential. In other words, the unique, complete embryo now represents a potential baby. Basically, the argument from potentiality is an argument for treating the acorn with respect because it could become an oak.

The first form of objection to this argument is empirical; even under optimal conditions within a woman's womb, nearly 60% of all fertilized eggs fail to implant or complete their development, with their loss either unnoticed during a menstrual cycle or, in later stages, marked by a miscarriage.[8] Thus, as members of a British medical society studying embryo manipulation observed: "[I]t is morally unconvincing to claim absolute inviolability for an organism with which nature itself is so prodigal."[9] Of course, however, the fact that few embryos survive under optimal conditions is not necessarily an excuse for affirmatively destroying even more of them.

A more significant objection to the argument from potentiality concerns its reliance on treating acorns in many respects as if they were already oaks. Assume, for the sake of simplicity, that unambiguous moral status is achieved by being born. Does the potential to be born entitle an entity to be treated as if it had already been born?[10] As philosopher Joel Feinberg pointed out, when Roosevelt, Carter, and Reagan were boys, they were potential presidents, but that did not confer upon them the prerogatives of office until that potential was actualized upon election and inauguration.[11] More seriously, Michael Tooley notes that the very reason we treat already born babies as sacred is that they are capable, however primitively, of forming preferences, a necessary condition for having interests that are entitled to be respected. Because embryos lack the capacity to form preferences,[12] they perforce have no interest one way or the other in their own continued survival, thus obviating the need to protect their viability.[13]

A response to Tooley's argument can be found in the writings of phenomenological personalists, who stress the unity of the personality and the body.[14] Rather than a Cartesian-style dualism, in which the personality is some sort of extra quality that is added to the body, such that a body may be treated as inconsequential before the entrance or emergence of the personality, phenomenologicalists view the body itself as the subject of consciousness. Thus, an early form of the body, such as embryo, is merely one stage of many in the life cycle of the personality. The fact that the embryo has no consciousness to form preferences and thus have interests is a mistaken form of reductionist argumentation; because the person is *always* in a state of evolution toward perfection of its potential, no stage can be severed from another, and a wrong committed at any stage of the body's development is a wrong committed to the personality at every state of its development.[15]

This argument, in turn, however, depends on viewing the embryo as an entity with the potential to be a baby. It is on this point that one finds interesting intersections with arguments concerning embryo research and cloning.

The idea of a genetically complete or relatively complete entity with the "potential" to be born as a distinct baby has been criticized as an over-broad basis for the argument from potential. Peter Singer and Deane Wells, for example, have argued that a single sperm and single egg in a petri dish represent a complete, unique human genome that, if contact and fertilization is left unimpeded, will continue to divide into an embryo, and thence a baby. Thus, they conclude that the argument from potential ought to encompass this situation and not rely so heavily on the moment of fertilization.[16] As philosopher Jonathan Glover[17] has put it, "if it is the cake you are interested in, it is equally a pity if the ingredients were thrown away before being mixed or afterwards."

In his re-examination of the argument from potential, Massimo Reichlin attempts to refute this argument. He explains that the sperm and egg are not the same ontological entity as the embryo (and baby) until they are joined. It is this moment, or process, of joining that marks the moment when the biological being that is the baby has begun. The only way to argue that this is the commencement of that being, however, is by reference to the argument that this "being" is one that is contiguous with all forms of its body at times during which it has the requisite "potential" to be a baby, in essence circling around to the phenomenological argument.

To distinguish the sort of potential possessed by a fertilized egg from that possessed by a sperm and egg in a petri dish, Reichlin distinguishes between "active" and "passive" potential. Passive potential, he notes, is that which would permit the being to develop if subject to external actions that help bring out certain traits that are present, albeit not central to its essence. Thus, a tree is a potential table in this passive sense, as it could be turned into a table by an external agent. It cannot become a table without external assistance, however, and if it is never turned into a table, its essential "tree-ness" is not affected.

Active potentials, in contrast, are those that are intrinsic to the entity itself, that is, "those inherent to the very nature of the being. . . . all those things which it will be of itself if nothing external hinders it . . . a tendency which is dependent on its very nature."[18] Because it is the essence of the entity to become something, it is not in need of external assistance to ensure its transformation. A child will grow larger because that is its essential trait. It does not take an external agent to make it grow larger, although it does need certain things to make that process continue unimpeded, for example food and water.

By this notion, however, an interesting observation can be made about embryos. A fertilized egg or early embryo in a petri dish most certainly has an intrinsic tendency to continue growing and dividing. Without the provision of an artificial culture medium, however, it will never grow and divide more than about 1 week. If the provision of such a medium is considered a form of external assistance akin to that at issue in passive potentiality, then the fertilized egg is a potential week-old embryo, not a potential baby.[19] Because it is not a potential baby, it need not be treated with a degree of respect that forestalls destructive research. By this line of reasoning, abortion might still be prohibited because it interferes with the natural development of a fetus, but destructive research on an in vitro embryo would not be prohibited, as it interferes with nothing more than the potential development of an embryo; no potential baby is at stake.

This argument, as is well known, holds no sway among opponents of embryo research. Opposition to embryo research is sufficiently widespread to have rendered the National Institutes of Health (NIH) wary of funding this kind of work, even after regulatory obstacles were removed. Instead, the NIH requested guidance from an expert panel. The panel's report, which recommended limited embryo research when sound scientific questions were presented,[20] generated a congressional backlash that resulted in legislative restrictions on the uses of federal funds for any research that puts human embryos at risk of destruction.[21]

Thus, it would seem that proponents of the argument from potential make no distinction between embryos in vitro and embryos in vivo. This implies that whatever external assistance is needed to ensure development of in vitro embryos into babies is consistent with the type of assistance encompassed by the idea of "active" potential.

It is here that the question of cloning gets intriguing, as one might well ask why the assistance needed to get a skin cell to generate a baby is any different from the assistance needed to get an in vitro embryo to develop into a baby. Both need a culture medium. For skin cells, that medium is found partly in the cytoplasm of an enucleated egg, but a medium it is nonetheless. The skin cell needs an electric shock. Again, however, it is unclear why electricity, as opposed to the warmth of the incubator used in ordinary management of an in vitro embryo, is of ontological significance.

The real response probably lies in an argument about the "implicit nature" of a fertilized egg versus that of a skin cell.[22] It can be argued that the "implicit nature" of an embryo is to divide and grow into a baby, whereas the implicit nature of a skin cell is to divide into more skin cells. Of course, however, it has been shown that the implicit nature of an in vitro embryo is merely to divide;

absent extensive external assistance, a baby is not its natural endpoint, only a mass of nonviable cells.

In addition, the "implicit nature" of a skin cell is also to divide and grow. With the discovery that the genes coding for non-skin functions are merely dormant rather than dead comes the observation that the nature of skin cells and that of embryonic cells are not terribly different. This observation is made more acute by noting that the transformation of cells from embryonic to fetal to adult is one marked by a gradual decline in the functioning of their nonspecialized genes; the distinction between these stages of cell life is not clean but blurred. Furthermore, when current research on somatic cell nuclear transfer cloning unlocks the secrets to the role of the egg's cytoplasm in regulating the expression of genes that code for development of an entire organism, the next step in cloning will be to eliminate the need for fusion with an enucleated egg; all the material needed to regulate gene expression is present in the cytoplasm of the skin cell as well, and turning that expression on by manipulation of the skin cell alone will be the final step in eliminating all pertinent difference between embryonic cells and adult cells.

The observation that cloning further undermines the logical integrity of the argument from potential opens up new possibilities for exploring the nature of opposition to embryo research and, perhaps, holds some promise for finding some compromises.

The NIH's Human Embryo Research Panel took note of a technology called *blastomere separation*, also known as *embryo splitting*, by which a single embryo can be multiplied. The technique involves separating one or more cells from an embryo. These separated cells can then themselves be cultured so that they divide into embryos. The result is the creation of an identical twin embryo.

One possible compromise in the area of embryo research depends on the use of this technique. Imagine a single fertilized egg that is called "Johnny." As Johnny divides and grows into an embryo, there is a request to use this material for embryo research. One possibility is to detach a cell from Johnny's embryonic body. The embryo "Johnny" is then permitted to continue dividing and is eventually transferred to a womb for development into the baby "Johnny." The detached cell, meanwhile, is cultured to grow into an embryo that can be used for research.

Opposition to the destruction of developing life arises from many instincts, not just those associated with variations on the argument from potential. One of those instincts is the idea that it is wrong for humans to have unlimited power to alter the future. Those familiar with science fiction, such as *Star Trek*, will recognize a persistent theme about the nature of the future, to wit, that it consists of possible timelines akin to a series of railroad tracks stretching off into the distance. Once a human life has commenced developing, some view us as having been committed to a particular track, for example, a track into the future in which Johnny is born. To destroy Johnny as an embryo is to wrench the train onto a different track. This degree of control is viewed with alarm by some who worry about the hubris it implies.

By permitting Johnny to be born, however, and working only on a single cell detached from Johnny's body, there is no deviation from the track that was determined at the moment of Johnny's emergence as a developing form of human life. It is akin to taking a cell from Johnny's body long after he was born and using that cell in an experiment, something that is done all the time when we work on human tissue taken from surgical waste.

Of course, some argue that at the moment a cell is detached from the embryo known as "Johnny" a new and separate individual, called "Jimmy," has emerged. In essence, this separation has shifted the train to a track in which identical twin boys Johnny and Jimmy are born. Any action that prevents them from coming to fruition is wrong, just as cutting off the original lifeline of Johnny was wrong.

With the advent of nuclear transfer cloning, however, comes the prospect of a technique that can reliably permit the generation of Johnny, Jimmy, Joey, and tens or hundreds more identical embryos. For those whose opposition to embryo research arises from this discomfort with control of the future, it is possible that at some point it will be difficult to believe that we must be committed to a future with hundreds of genetically identical boys. Although it might not seem that the quantitative difference in the number of identical embryos ought to make a qualitative difference in how one regards them, it is quite possible that it would. Indeed, this is precisely the fear that underlay much of the opposition to using cloning to generate multiple genetic copies of babies; people worried that in a world in which there were a hundred genetically identical people it would be hard to regard each one with the same respect and sentiment as one would regard those people if they were singletons, or at most quintuplets or sextuplets. Thus, instinct tells us that with larger numbers comes the possibility of declining regard.

The compromise for embryo research, then, might well be to insist that no unique embryo be destroyed; each unique combination of genetic material representing a possible future baby must be given a chance at development toward that outcome. Cells from these embryos could be removed, however, and cultured and used for research. Every Johnny would be given a chance to develop to birth, and no new, unique Johnny would be abandoned. Johnny's cells could, however, be used for the myriad research applications that have been documented elsewhere, applications that hold promise for understanding cancer, ameliorating infertility, and preventing developmental abnormalities.[23]

This solution will not satisfy those who premise their opposition to embryo research strictly on the argument from potential. To those who oppose embryo research because of a genuine attachment to the idea that a fertilized egg or embryo represents a singular predecessor to a knowable future individual, however, cloning offers the following challenge: Must every one of those future individuals necessarily come into being? If so, then how does one ignore the loss of other future individuals represented in nearly every other cell in the body?

Conclusion

Although somatic cell nuclear transfer cloning does involve the use of an enucleated egg to re-initiate the gene expression that codes for development of a complete organism, it also mirrors the processes of cell division and development experienced by a fertilized egg in all ways relevant to the argument from potential. Thus, it challenges those who would oppose research on embryos to better articulate the precise nature of their opposition, particularly in light of the substantial scientific gains to be made from such research. Furthermore, cloning also re-opens discussion of a compromise in the debate over embryo research, offering the prospect of protecting the future that has commenced in the form of an embryo while also permitting important scientific research to go on using copies of that embryo. A fresh debate over this and other possible ways to proceed with embryo research would be welcome.

II

DEBATES SURROUNDING CLONING AND EMBRYO RESEARCH

6

Cloning Human Beings: An Assessment of the Ethical Issues Pro and Con

DAN W. BROCK

The world of science and the public at large were both shocked and fascinated by the announcement in the journal *Nature* by Ian Wilmut and his colleagues that they had successfully cloned a sheep from a single cell of an adult sheep.[1] Scientists were in part surprised because many had believed that after the very early stage of embryo development at which differentiation of cell function begins to take place it would not be possible to achieve cloning of an adult mammal by nuclear transfer. In this process the nucleus from the cell of an adult mammal is inserted into an ennucleated ovum, and the resulting embryo develops following the complete genetic code of the mammal from which the inserted nucleus was obtained. Some scientists and much of the public were troubled or apparently even horrified, however, at the prospect that if adult mammals such as sheep could be cloned, then cloning of adult humans by the same process would likely be possible as well. Of course, the process is far from perfected, even with sheep; it took 276 failures by Wilmut and his colleagues to produce Dolly, their one success, and whether the process can be successfully replicated in other mammals, much less in humans, is not now known. Those who were horrified at the prospect of human cloning were not, however, reassured by the fact that the science with humans is not yet there, for it looked to them now perilously close.

The response of most scientific and political leaders to the prospect of human cloning, indeed of Dr. Wilmut as well, was immediate and strong condemnation.

In the United States, President Clinton immediately banned federal financing of human cloning research and asked privately funded scientists to halt such work until the newly formed National Bioethics Advisory Commission could review the "troubling" ethical and legal implications. The Director-General of the World Health Organization characterized human cloning as "ethically unacceptable as it would violate some of the basic principles which govern medically assisted reproduction. These include respect for the dignity of the human being and the protection of the security of human genetic material."[2] Around the world similar immediate condemnation was heard as human cloning was called a violation of human rights and human dignity. Even before Wilmut's announcement, human cloning had been made illegal in nearly all countries in Europe and had been condemned by the Council of Europe.[3]

A few more cautious voices were heard both suggesting some possible benefits from the use of human cloning in limited circumstances and questioning its too quick prohibition, but they were a clear minority. In the popular media, nightmare scenarios of laboratory mistakes resulting in monsters, the cloning of armies of Hitlers, the exploitative use of cloning for totalitarian ends as in Huxley's *Brave New World*, and the murderous replicants in the film *Bladerunner* all fed the public controversy and uneasiness. A striking feature of these early responses was that their strength and intensity seemed far to outrun the arguments and reasons offered in support of them—they seemed often to be "gut level" emotional reactions rather than considered reflections on the issues. Such reactions should not be simply dismissed both because they may point us to important considerations otherwise missed and not easily articulated and because they often have a major impact on public policy. The formation of public policy should not, however, ignore the moral reasons and arguments that bear on the practice of human cloning—these must be articulated in order to understand and inform people's more immediate emotional responses. This chapter is an effort to articulate, and to evaluate critically, the main moral considerations and arguments for and against human cloning.

Although many people's religious beliefs inform their views on human cloning, and it is often difficult to separate religious from secular positions, I shall restrict myself to arguments and reasons that can be given a clear secular formulation and will ignore explicitly religious positions and arguments pro or con. I shall also be concerned principally with cloning by nuclear transfer, which permits cloning of an adult, not cloning by embryo splitting, although some of the issues apply to both.[4]

I begin by noting that on each side of the issue there are two distinct kinds of moral arguments brought forward. On the one hand, some opponents claim that human cloning would violate fundamental moral or human rights, while some proponents argue that its prohibition would violate such rights. On the other hand, both opponents and proponents also cite the likely harms and benefits, both to individuals and to society, of the practice. While moral and even human rights need not be understood as absolute, they do place moral restrictions on permissible actions that an appeal to a mere balance of benefits over harms cannot justify overriding. For example, the rights of human subjects in research must be respected even if the result is that some potentially beneficial research is more difficult or cannot be done, and the right of free expression prohibits the silencing of unpopular or even abhorrent views; in Ronald Dworkin's striking formulation, rights trump utility.[5]

I shall take up both the moral rights implicated in human cloning and the more likely significant benefits and harms of cloning because none of the rights as applied to human cloning is sufficiently uncontroversial and strong to settle decisively the morality of the practice one way or the other. Because of their strong moral force, however, the assessment of the moral rights putatively at stake is especially important. A further complexity here is that it is sometimes controversial whether a particular consideration is merely a matter of benefits and harms or is instead a matter of moral or human rights. I shall begin with the arguments in support of permitting human cloning, although with no implication that it is the stronger or weaker position.

Moral arguments in support of human cloning

A. Is There a Moral Right To Use Human Cloning?

What moral right might protect at least some access to the use of human cloning? Some commentators have argued that a commitment to individual liberty, as defended by J. S. Mill, requires that individuals be left free to use human cloning if they so choose and if their doing so does not cause significant harms to others, but liberty is too broad in scope to be an uncontroversial moral right.[6] Human cloning is a means of reproduction (in the most literal sense), and so the most plausible moral right at stake in its use is a right to reproductive freedom or procreative liberty.[7]

Reproductive freedom includes not only the familiar right to choose not to reproduce, for example, by means of contraception or abortion, but also the right to reproduce. The right to reproductive freedom is properly understood to include as well the use of various artificial reproductive technologies, such as in vitro fertilization (IVF), oocyte donation, and so forth. The reproductive right relevant to human cloning is a negative right, that is, a right to use assisted reproductive technologies without interference by the government or others when made available by a willing provider. The choice of an assisted means of reproduction, such as surrogacy, can be defended as included within reproductive freedom even when it is not the only means for individuals to reproduce, just as the choice among different means of preventing conception is protected by reproductive freedom. The case for permitting the use of a particular means of reproduction is strongest, however, when that means is necessary for particular individuals to be able to procreate at all. Sometimes human cloning could be the only means for individuals to procreate while retaining a biological tie to the child created, but in other cases different means of procreating would also be possible.

It could be argued that human cloning is not covered by the right to reproductive freedom because, whereas current assisted reproductive technologies and practices covered by that right are remedies for inabilities to reproduce sexually, human cloning is an entirely new means of reproduction; indeed, its critics see it as more a means of manufacturing humans than of reproduction. Human cloning is a means of reproduction different from sexual reproduction, but it is a means that can serve individuals' interests in reproducing. If it is not covered by the moral right to reproductive freedom, I believe that must be not because it is a new means of reproducing but instead because it has other objectionable moral features, such as eroding human dignity or uniqueness; I shall evaluate these other ethical objections to it later.

When individuals have alternative means of procreating, human cloning typically would be chosen because it replicates a particular individual's genome. The reproductive interest in question, then, is not simply reproduction itself but a more specific interest in choosing what kind of children to have. The right to reproductive freedom is usually understood to cover at least some choice about the kind of children one will have; for example, genetic testing of an embryo or fetus for genetic disease or abnormality, together with abortion of an affected embryo or fetus, is now used to avoid having a child with that disease or abnormality. Genetic testing of prospective parents before conception to determine the risk of transmitting a genetic disease is also intended to avoid having children with particular diseases. Prospective parents' moral interest in self-determination, which is one of the grounds of a moral right to reproductive freedom, includes the choice about whether to have a child with a condition that is likely to place severe burdens on them and to cause severe burdens to the child itself.

The more a reproductive choice is not simply the determination of oneself and one's own life but the determination of the nature of another, as in the case of human cloning, the more moral weight the interests of that other person, that is, the cloned child, should have in decisions that determine its nature.[8] Even then, however, parents are typically taken properly to have substantial, but not unlimited, discretion in shaping the persons their children will become, for example, through education and other childrearing decisions. Even if not part of reproductive freedom, the right to raise one's children as one sees fit, within limits mostly determined by the interests of the children, is also a right to determine within limits what kinds of persons one's children will become. This right in-

cludes not just preventing certain diseases or harms to children but also select-
ing and shaping desirable features and traits in one's children. The use of human
cloning is one way to exercise that right.

It is worth pointing out that current public and legal policies permit prospective parents to conceive, or to carry a conception to term, when there is a significant risk, or even certainty, that the child will suffer from a serious genetic
disease. Even when others think the risk or presence of genetic disease makes it
morally wrong to conceive, or to carry a fetus to term, the parents' right to reproductive freedom permits them to do so. Most possible harms to a cloned child
that I shall consider below are less serious than the genetic harms with which
parents can now permit their offspring to be conceived or born.

I conclude that there is good reason to accept that a right to reproductive freedom presumptively includes both a right to select the means of reproduction and
a right to determine what kind of children to have by use of human cloning. The
particular reproductive interest of determining what kind of children to have is
less weighty, however, than other reproductive interests and choices whose im-
pacts fall more directly and exclusively on the parents rather than the child.
Accepting a moral right to reproductive freedom that includes the use of human
cloning does not settle the moral issue about human cloning. Because there may
be other moral rights in conflict with this right or serious enough harms from
human cloning to override the right to use it, however, this right can be thought
of as establishing a serious moral presumption supporting access to human
cloning.

There is a different moral right that might be thought to be at stake in the dispute about human cloning—the right to freedom of scientific inquiry and research
in the acquisition of knowledge. If there is such a right, it would presumably be
violated by a legal prohibition of research on human cloning, although the government could still permissibly decide not to spend public funds to support such
research. Leaving aside for the moment human subject ethical concerns, research
on human cloning might provide valuable scientific medical knowledge beyond
simply knowledge about how to carry out human cloning. Whether or not there
is a moral right to freedom of scientific inquiry, for example, as part of a right
to free expression, prohibiting and stopping scientific research and inquiry is a
serious matter and precedent that should only be undertaken when necessary to
prevent grave violations of human rights or to protect fundamental interests. Even
for opponents of human cloning, however, the fundamental moral issue is not acquiring the knowledge that would make it possible, but using that knowledge to
do human cloning. Because it is possible to prohibit human cloning itself, without prohibiting all research on it, it is not necessary to limit the freedom of scientific inquiry in order to prevent human cloning from taking place. This means
as well, however, that a right to freedom of scientific inquiry could only protect
research on human cloning, not its use. For this reason, I believe the fundamen-

tal moral right that provides presumptive moral support for permitting the use of human cloning is the right to reproductive freedom, not the right to freedom of scientific inquiry. My discussion in what follows principally concerns the moral issues in the use of human cloning, not those restricted to research on it.

B. What Individual or Social Benefits Might Human Cloning Produce?

Largely Individual Benefits

The literature on human cloning by nuclear transfer, as well as the literature on embryo splitting when it is relevant to the nuclear transfer case, contain a few examples of circumstances in which individuals might have good reasons to want to use human cloning. A survey of that literature strongly suggests, however, that human cloning is not the unique answer to any great or pressing human need and that its benefits would at most be limited. What are the principal benefits of human cloning that might give persons good reasons to want to use it?

1. Human cloning would be a new means to relieve the infertility some persons now experience. Human cloning would allow women who have no ova or men who have no sperm to produce an offspring that is biologically related.[9] Embryos might also be cloned, either by nuclear transfer or embryo splitting, in order to increase the number of embryos for implantation and improve the chances of successful conception.[10] While the moral right to reproductive freedom creates a presumption that individuals should be free to choose the means of reproduction that best serves their interests and desires, the benefits from human cloning to relieve infertility are greater the more persons there are who cannot overcome their infertility by any other means acceptable to them. I do not know of data on this point, but they should be possible to obtain or gather from national associations concerned with infertility.

It is not enough to point to the large number of children throughout the world possibly available for adoption as a solution to infertility unless we are prepared to discount as illegitimate the strong desire many persons, fertile and infertile, have for the experience of pregnancy and for having and raising a child biologically related to them. Although not important to all infertile (or fertile) individuals, it is important to many and is respected and met through other forms of assisted reproduction that maintain a biological connection when that is possible; there seems no good reason to refuse to respect and respond to it when human cloning would be the best or only means of overcoming individuals' infertility.

2. Human cloning would enable couples in which one party risks transmitting a serious hereditary disease, a serious risk of disease, or an otherwise harmful condition to an offspring to reproduce without doing so.[11] Of course, by using donor sperm or egg donation, such hereditary risks can generally be avoided now without the use of human cloning. These procedures may be unacceptable to

some couples, however, or at least considered less desirable than human cloning because they introduce a third party's genes into their reproduction instead of giving their offspring only the genes of one of them. Thus, in some cases human cloning would be a means of preventing genetically transmitted harms to offspring. Here, too, there are no data on the likely number of persons who would wish to use human cloning for this purpose instead of either using other available means of avoiding the risk of genetic transmission of the harmful condition or accepting the risk of transmitting the harmful condition.

3. Human cloning of a later twin would enable a person to obtain needed organs or tissues for transplantation.[12] Human cloning would solve the problem of finding a transplant donor who is an acceptable organ or tissue match and would eliminate, or drastically reduce, the risk of transplant rejection by the host. The availability of human cloning for this purpose would amount to a form of insurance policy to enable treatment of certain kinds of medical needs. Of course, sometimes the medical need would be too urgent to permit waiting for the cloning, gestation, and development of the later twin necessary before tissues or organs for transplant could be obtained. In other cases, the need for an organ that the later twin would himself or herself need to maintain life, such as a heart or a liver, would preclude cloning and then taking the organ from the later twin.

Such a practice has been criticized on the ground that it treats the later twin not as a person valued and loved for his or her own sake, as an end in itself in Kantian terms, but simply as a means for benefiting another. This criticism assumes, however, that only this one motive would determine the relation of the person to his or her later twin. The well-known case some years ago in California of the Ayalas, who conceived in the hopes of obtaining a source for a bone marrow transplant for their teenage daughter suffering from leukemia, illustrates the mistake in this assumption. They argued that whether or not the child they conceived turned out to be a possible donor for their daughter, they would value and love the child for itself and treat it as they would treat any other member of their family. That one reason it was wanted was as a means to saving their daughter's life did not preclude its also being loved and valued for its own sake; in Kantian terms, it was treated as a possible means to saving their daughter, but not solely as a means, which is what the Kantian view proscribes.

Indeed, when people have children, whether by sexual means or with the aid of assisted reproductive technologies, their motives and reasons for doing so are typically many and complex and include reasons less laudable than obtaining life-saving medical treatment, such as having a companion like a doll to play with, enabling one to live on one's own, qualifying for public or government benefit programs, and so forth. Although these other motives for having children sometimes may not bode well for the child's upbringing and future, public policy does not assess prospective parents' motives and reasons for procreating as a condition of their doing so.

One commentator has proposed human cloning for obtaining even life-saving organs.[13] After cell differentiation, some of the brain cells of the embryo or fetus would be removed so that it could then be grown as a brain-dead body for spare parts for its earlier twin. This body clone would be like an anencephalic newborn or presentient fetus, neither of which arguably can be harmed because of their lack of capacity for consciousness. Most people would likely find this practice appalling and immoral, in part because here the cloned later twin's capacity for conscious life is destroyed solely as a means for the benefit of another. Yet if one pushes what is already science fiction quite a bit further in the direction of science fantasy and imagines the ability to clone and grow in an artificial environment only the particular life-saving organ a person needed for transplantation, then it is far from clear that it would be morally impermissible to do so.

4. Human cloning would enable individuals to clone someone who had special meaning to them, such as a child who had died.[14] There is no denying that if human cloning were available some individuals would want to use it in order to clone someone who had special meaning to them, such as a child who had died, but that desire usually would be based on a deep confusion. Cloning such a child would not replace the child the parents had loved and lost, but rather would create a new and different child with the same genes. The child they loved and lost was a unique individual who had been shaped by his or her environment and choices, not just his or her genes, and more importantly who had experienced a particular relationship with them. Even if the later cloned child could not only have the same genes but also be subjected to the same environment, which of course is in fact impossible, it would remain a different child from the one the parents had loved and lost because it would share a different history with them.[15] Cloning the lost child might help the parents accept and move on from their loss, but another already existing sibling or another new child who was not a clone might do this equally well; indeed, it might do so better because the appearance of the cloned later twin would be a constant reminder of the child they had lost. Nevertheless, if human cloning enabled some individuals to clone a person who had special meaning to them and doing so gave them deep satisfaction, that would be a benefit to them even if their reasons for wanting to do so, and the satisfaction they in turn received, were based on a confusion.

Largely Social Benefits

5. Human cloning would enable the duplication of individuals of great talent, genius, character, or other exemplary qualities. The first four reasons for human cloning considered above all looked at benefits to specific individuals, usually parents, from being able to reproduce by means of human cloning. This reason looks at benefits to the broader society from being able to replicate extraordinary individuals—a Mozart, Einstein, Gandhi, or Schweitzer.[16] Much of the appeal of

this reason, like much thinking both in support of and in opposition to human cloning, rests on a confused and mistaken assumption of genetic determinism, that is, that one's genes fully determine what one will become, do, and accomplish. What made Mozart, Einstein, Gandhi, and Schweitzer the extraordinary individuals they were was the confluence of their particular genetic endowments with the environments in which they were raised and lived and the particular historical moments they in different ways seized. Cloning them would produce individuals with the same genetic inheritance (nuclear transfer does not even produce 100% genetic identity, although for the sake of exploring the moral issues I have followed the common assumption that it does), but neither by cloning nor by any other means would it be possible to replicate their environments or the historical contexts in which they lived and their greatness flourished. We do not know, either in general or about any particular individual, the degree or specific respects in which their greatness depended on their "nature" or their "nurture," but we do know in all cases that it depended on an interaction of them both. Thus, human cloning could never replicate the extraordinary accomplishments for which we admire individuals like Mozart, Einstein, Gandhi, and Schweitzer.

If we make a rough distinction between the extraordinary capabilities of a Mozart or an Einstein and how they used those capabilities in the particular environments and historical settings in which they lived, it would also be a mistake to assume that human cloning could at least replicate their extraordinary capabilities, if not the accomplishments they achieved with them. Their capabilities too were the product of their inherited genes and their environments, not of their genes alone, and so it would be a mistake to think that cloning them would produce individuals with the same capabilities, even if they would exercise those capabilities at different times and in different ways. In the case of Gandhi and Schweitzer, whose extraordinary greatness lies more in their moral character and commitments, we understand even less well the extent to which their moral character and greatness was produced by their genes.

None of this is to deny that Mozart's and Einstein's extraordinary musical and intellectual capabilities, nor even Gandhi's and Schweitzer's extraordinary moral greatness, were produced in part by their unique genetic inheritances. Cloning them might well produce individuals with exceptional capacities, but we simply do not know how close their clones would be in capacities or accomplishments to the great individuals from whom they were cloned. Even so, the hope for exceptional, even if less and different, accomplishment from cloning such extraordinary individuals might be a reasonable ground for doing so.

I have used examples here of individuals whose greatness is widely appreciated and largely uncontroversial, but if we move away from such cases we encounter the problem of whose standards of greatness would be used to select individuals to be cloned for the benefit of society or humankind at large. This problem inevitably connects with the important issue of who would control access to and use of the technology of human cloning, because those who controlled its use would be in a position to impose their standards of exceptional individuals to be cloned. This issue is especially worrisome if particular groups or segments of society, or if a government, controlled the technology, for we would then risk its use for the benefit of those groups, segments of society, or governments under the cover of benefiting society or even humankind at large.

6. Human cloning and research on human cloning might make possible important advances in scientific knowledge, for example, about human development.[17] Although important potential advances in scientific or medical knowledge from human cloning or human cloning research have frequently been cited in some media responses to Dolly's cloning, there are at least three reasons why these possible benefits are highly uncertain. First, there is always considerable uncertainty about the nature and importance of the new scientific or medical knowledge that a dramatic new technology like human cloning will lead to; the road to that new knowledge is never mapped in advance and takes many unexpected turns. Second, we also do not know what new knowledge from human cloning or human cloning research could also be gained by other methods and research that do not have the problematic moral features of human cloning to which its opponents object. Third, what human cloning research would be compatible with ethical and legal requirements for the use of human subjects in research is complex, controversial, and largely unexplored. For example, in what contexts and from whom would it be necessary, and how would it be possible, to secure the informed consent of parties involved in human cloning? No human cloning should ever take place without the consent of the person cloned and the woman receiving a cloned embryo, if they are different. We could never, however, obtain the consent of the cloned later twin to being cloned, so research on human cloning that produces a cloned individual might be barred by ethical and legal regulations for the use of human subjects in research.[18]

Moreover, creating human clones solely for the purpose of research would be to use them solely for the benefit of others without their consent, and thus unethical. Of course, once human cloning was established to be safe and effective, then new scientific knowledge might be obtained from its use for legitimate, nonresearch reasons. How human subject regulations would apply to research on human cloning needs much more exploration than I can give it here in order to help clarify how significant and likely the potential gains are in scientific and medical knowledge from human cloning research and human cloning.

Although there is considerable uncertainty about most of the possible individual and social benefits of human cloning that I have discussed, and although no doubt it may have other benefits or uses that we cannot yet envisage, I believe it is reasonable to conclude that human cloning at this time does not seem to promise great or unique benefits to meet great human needs. Nevertheless, a case can be made that scientific freedom supports permitting research on human cloning to go forward and that freedom to use human cloning is protected by the important moral right to reproductive freedom. We must therefore assess what moral rights might be violated, or harms produced, by research on or use of human cloning.

Moral arguments against human cloning

A. Would The Use of Human Cloning Violate Important Moral Rights?

Many of the immediate condemnations of any possible human cloning following Wilmut's cloning of an adult sheep claimed that it would violate moral or human rights, but it was usually not specified precisely, or often even at all, what the rights were that would be violated. I shall consider two possible candidates for such a right: a right to have a unique identity and a right to ignorance about one's future or to an open future. The former right is cited by many commentators, but I believe even if any such right exists, it is not violated by human cloning. The latter right has only been explicitly defended to my knowledge by two commentators and in the context of human cloning only by Hans Jonas; it supports a more promising, even if in my view ultimately unsuccessful, argument that human cloning would violate an important moral or human right.

Is there a moral or human right to a unique identity, and if so would it be violated by human cloning? For human cloning to violate a right to a unique identity, the relevant sense of identity would have to be genetic identity, that is, a right to a unique unrepeated genome. This would be violated by human cloning, but is there any such right? It might be thought there could not be such a right because it would be violated in all cases of identical twins, yet no one claims in such cases that the moral or human rights of each of the twins have been violated. Even the use of fertility drugs, which increases the probability of having twins, is not intended to produce twins. This consideration is not, however, conclusive.[19] It is commonly held that only deliberate human actions can violate others' rights but that outcomes that would constitute a rights violation if done by human action are not a rights violation if a result of natural causes; if Arthur deliberately strikes Barry on the head so hard as to cause his death he violates Barry's right not to be killed, but if lightening strikes Cheryl, causing her death, then we would not say that her right not to be killed has been violated. The case of twins does not show there could not be a right to a unique genetic identity.

What is the sense of identity that might plausibly be what each person has a right to have uniquely, that constitutes the special uniqueness of each individual?[20] Even with the same genes, two individuals, for example, homozygous twins, are numerically distinct and not identical, so what is intended must be the various properties and characteristics that make each individual qualitatively unique and different from others. Does having the same genome as another person undermine that unique qualitative identity? It does only according to the crudest genetic determinism, a genetic determinism according to which an individual's genes completely and decisively determine everything else about the individual, all his or her other non-genetic features and properties, together with the entire history or biography that will constitute his or her life. There is no reason whatever to believe this kind of genetic determinism exists, and I do not think that anyone does. Even with the same genes, as we know from the case of genetically identical twins, while there may be many important similarities in the twins' psychological and personal characteristics, differences in these develop over time together with differences in their life histories, personal relationships, and life choices. This is true of identical twins raised together, and the differences are still greater in the case of identical twins raised apart; sharing an identical genome does not prevent twins from each developing a distinct and unique personal identity of their own.

We need not pursue what the basis or argument in support of a moral or human right to a unique identity might be—such a right is not found among typical accounts and enumerations of moral or human rights—because even if we grant that there is such a right, sharing a genome with another individual as a result of human cloning would not violate it. The idea of the uniqueness, or unique identity, of each person historically predates the development of modern genetics and the knowledge that, except in the case of homozygous twins, each individual has a unique genome. A unique genome thus could not be the ground of this long-standing belief in the unique human identity of each person.

I turn now to whether human cloning would violate what Hans Jonas called a right to ignorance or what Joel Feinberg called a right to an open future.[21] Jonas argued that human cloning in which there is a substantial time gap between the beginning of the lives of the earlier and later twin is fundamentally different from the simultaneous beginning of the lives of homozygous twins that occurs in nature. Although contemporaneous twins begin their lives with the same genetic inheritance, they also begin their lives or biographies at the same time, and thus in ignorance of what the other who shares the same genome will by his or her choices make of his or her life. To whatever extent one's genome determines one's future, each begins ignorant of what that determination will be and thus remains as free to choose a future, to construct a particular future from among open alternatives, as are individuals who do not have a twin. Ignorance of the effect of one's genome on one's future is necessary, Jonas holds, for the spontaneous, free, and authentic construction of a life and self.

A later twin created by human cloning, Jonas argues, knows, or at least believes he or she knows, too much about himself or herself. For there is already in the world another person, one's earlier twin, who from the same genetic starting point has made the life choices that are still in the later twin's future. It will seem that one's life has already been lived and played out by another, that one's fate is already determined, and thus the later twin will lose the spontaneity of authentically creating and becoming his or her own self. One will lose the sense of human possibility in freely creating one's own future. It is tyrannical, Jonas claims, for the earlier twin to try to determine another's fate in this way. Moreover, even if it is a mistake to believe the crude genetic determinism according to which one's genes determine one's fate, what is important for one's experience of freedom and ability to create a life for oneself is whether one thinks one's future is open and undetermined and thus still to be determined by one's own choices.

One might try to interpret Jonas' objection so as not to assume either genetic determinism or a belief in it. A later twin might grant that he is not determined to follow in his earlier twin's footsteps, but that nevertheless the earlier twin's life would always haunt him, standing as an undue influence on his life and shaping it in ways to which others' lives are not vulnerable. The force of the objection still, however, seems to rest on a false assumption that having the same genome as his earlier twin unduly restricts his freedom to choose a different life than the earlier twin chose. A family environment also importantly shapes children's development, but there is no force to the claim of a younger sibling that the existence of an older sibling raised in the same family is an undue influence on his freedom to make a life for himself in that environment. Indeed, the younger twin or sibling might gain the benefit of being able to learn from the older twin's or sibling's mistakes.

In a different context, and without applying it to human cloning, Joel Feinberg has argued for a child's right to an open future. This requires that others raising a child not so close off the future possibilities that the child would otherwise have as to eliminate a reasonable range of opportunities for the child to choose autonomously and construct his or her own life. One way this right to an open future would be violated is to deny even a basic education to a child, and another way might be to create it as a later twin so that it will believe its future has already been set for it by the choices made and the life lived by its earlier twin.

A central difficulty in evaluating the implications for human cloning of a right either to ignorance or to an open future is whether the right is violated merely because the later twin may be likely to believe that its future is already determined, even if that belief is clearly false and supported only by the crudest genetic determinism. I believe that if the twin's future in reality remains open and his to freely choose, then someone's acting in a way that unintentionally leads him to believe that his future is closed and determined has not violated his right to ignorance or to an open future. Likewise, suppose I drive down the twin's street in my new car that is just like his, knowing that when he sees me he is likely to believe that I have stolen his car and therefore to abandon his driving plans for the day. I have not violated his property right to his car even though he may feel the same loss of opportunity to drive that day as if I had in fact stolen his car. In each case he is mistaken that his open future or car has been taken from him, and thus no right of his to them has been violated. If we know that the twin will believe that his open future has been taken from him as a result of being cloned, even though in reality it has not, then we know that cloning will cause him psychological distress, but not that it will violate his right. Thus, I believe Jonas's right to ignorance, and our employment of Feinberg's analogous right of a child to an open future, turns out not to be violated by human cloning, although they do point to psychological harm that a later twin may be likely to experience, and that I will take up later.

The upshot of our consideration of a moral or human right either to a unique identity or to ignorance and an open future is that neither would be violated by human cloning. Perhaps there are other possible rights that would make good the charge that human cloning is a violation of moral or human rights, but I am unsure what they might be. I turn now to consideration of the harms that human cloning might produce.

B. What Individual or Social Harms Might Human Cloning Produce?

There are many possible individual or social harms that have been posited by one or another commentator, and I shall only try to cover the more plausible and significant of them.

Largely Individual Harms

Harm 1. Human cloning would produce psychological distress and harm in the later twin. This is perhaps the most serious individual harm that opponents of human cloning foresee, and we have just seen that even if human cloning is no violation of rights, it may nevertheless cause psychological distress or harm. No doubt knowing the path in life taken by one's earlier twin may in many cases have several bad psychological effects.[22] The later twin may feel, even if mistakenly, that his or her fate has already been substantially laid out and so have difficulty freely and spontaneously taking responsibility for and making his or her own fate and life. The later twin's experience or sense of autonomy and freedom may be substantially diminished, even if in actual fact they are diminished much less than it seems to him or her. Together with this might be a diminished sense of one's own uniqueness and individuality, even if once again these are in fact diminished little or not at all by having an earlier twin with the same genome. If the later twin is the clone of a particularly exemplary individual, perhaps with some special capabilities and accomplishments, he or she may experience excessive pressure to reach the very high standards of ability and accomplishment of the earlier twin.[23] All of these psychological effects may take a heavy toll on the later twin and be serious burdens under which he or she would live.

One commentator has also cited special psychological harms to the first, or first few, human clones from the great publicity that would attend their creation.[24] Although public interest in the first clones would no doubt be enormous, medical confidentiality should protect their identity. Even if their identity became public knowledge, this would be a temporary effect only on the first few clones, and the experience of Louise Brown, the first child conceived by IVF, suggests this publicity could be managed to limit its harmful effects.

Although psychological harms of these kinds from human cloning are certainly possible, and perhaps even likely, they do remain at this point only speculative because we have no experience with human cloning and the creation of earlier and later twins. With naturally occurring identical twins, while they sometimes struggle to achieve their own identity, a struggle shared by many people without a twin, there is typically a very strong emotional bond between the twins, and such twins are, if anything, generally psychologically stronger and better adjusted than non-twins.[25] Scenarios are even possible in which being a later twin confers a psychological benefit on the twin; for example, having been deliberately cloned with the specific genes the later twin has might make the later twin feel especially wanted for the kind of person he or she is. Nevertheless, if experience with human cloning confirmed that serious and unavoidable psychological harms typically occurred to the later twin, that would be a serious moral reason to avoid the practice.

In the discussion of potential psychological harms to a later twin, I have been assuming that one later twin is cloned from an already existing adult individual. Cloning by means of embryo splitting, as carried out and reported by Hall and colleagues at George Washington University in 1993, has limits on the number of genetically identical twins that can be cloned.[26] Nuclear transfer, however, has no limits to the number of genetically identical individuals who might be cloned. Intuitively, many of the psychological burdens and harms noted earlier seem more likely and serious for a clone who is only one of many identical later twins from one original source so that the clone might run into another identical twin around every street corner. This prospect could be a good reason to place sharp limits on the number of twins that could be cloned from any one source.

There is one argument that has been used by several commentators to undermine the apparent significance of potential psychological harms to a later twin.[27] The point derives from a general problem, called the non-identity problem, posed by the philosopher Derek Parfit and not originally directed to human cloning.[28] Here is the argument. Even if all the psychological burdens and pressures from human cloning discussed could not be avoided for any later twin, they are not harms to the twin and thus not reasons not to clone the twin. This is because the only way for the twin to avoid the harms is never to be cloned or to exist at all. Yet no one claims that these burdens and stresses, hard though they might be, are so bad as to make the twin's life, all things considered, not worth living— that is, to be worse than no life at all. Thus the later twin is not harmed by being given a life with these burdens and stresses because the alternative of never existing at all is arguably worse—he or she loses a worthwhile life—but certainly not better for the twin. Furthermore, if the later twin is not harmed by having been created with these unavoidable burdens and stresses, then how could he or she be wronged by having been created with them? If the later twin is not wronged, then why is any wrong being done by human cloning? This argument has considerable potential import, for if it is sound it will undermine the apparent moral importance of any bad consequence of human cloning to the later twin that is not so serious as to make the twin's life all things considered not worth living.

Parfit originally posed the non-identity problem, but he does not accept the above argument as sound. Instead, he believes that if one could have a different child without these psychological burdens (e.g., by using a different method of reproduction that did not result in a later twin), there is as strong a moral reason to do so as there would be not to cause similar burdens to an already existing child; I have defended this position regarding the general case of genetically transmitted handicaps or disabilities.[29]

The theoretical philosophical problem is to formulate the moral principle that implies this conclusion and that also has acceptable implications in other cases involving bringing people into existence, such as issues about population policy. The issues are too detailed and complex to pursue here, and the non-identity problem remains controversial and not fully resolved, but suffice it to say that what is necessary is a principle that permits comparison of the later twin with these psychological burdens and a different person who could have been created instead by a different method and thus without such burdens.

Choosing to create the later twin with serious psychological burdens instead of a different person who would be free of them, without a weighty overriding reason for choosing the former, would be morally irresponsible or wrong, even if doing so does not harm or wrong the later twin who could only exist with the burdens. At the least, the argument for disregarding the psychological burdens to the later twin because he or she could not exist without them is controversial and, in my view, mistaken; unavoidable psychological burdens to later twins are reasons against human cloning. Such psychological harms, as I shall continue to call them, do remain speculative, but they should not be disregarded because of the non-identity problem.

Harm 2. Human cloning procedures would carry unacceptable risks to the clone. One version of this objection to human cloning concerns the research necessary to perfect the procedure, and the other version concerns the later risks from its use. Wilmut's group had 276 failures before their success with Dolly, indicating that the procedure is far from perfected even with sheep. Further research on the procedure with animals is clearly necessary before it would be ethical to use the procedure on humans. Even assuming that cloning's safety and effectiveness is established with animals, however, research would need to be done to establish its safety and effectiveness for humans. Could this research be done ethically?[30] There would be little or no risk to the donor of the cell nucleus to be transferred, and his or her informed consent could and must always be obtained. There might be greater risks for the woman to whom a cloned embryo is transferred, but these should be comparable with those associated with IVF procedures, and the woman's informed consent too could and must be obtained.

What of the risks to the cloned embryo itself? Judging by the experience of Wilmut's group in their work on cloning a sheep, the principal risk to the embryos cloned was their failure to successfully implant, grow, and develop. Comparable risks to cloned human embryos would apparently be their death or destruction long before most people or the law consider them to be persons with moral or legal protections of life. Moreover, artificial reproductive technologies now in use, such as IVF, have a known risk that some embryos will be destroyed or will not successfully implant and will die. It is premature to make a confident assessment of what the risks to human subjects would be of establishing the safety and effectiveness of human cloning procedures, but there are no unavoidable risks apparent at this time that would make the necessary research clearly ethically impermissible.

Could human cloning procedures meet ethical standards of safety and efficacy? Risks to an ovum donor (if any), a nucleus donor, and a woman who receives the embryo for implantation would likely be ethically acceptable with the informed consent of the involved parties. What of the risks to the human clone, however, if the procedure in some way goes wrong, or unanticipated harms come to the clone? For example, Harold Varmus, former director of the National Institutes of Health, has raised the concern that a cell many years old from which a person is cloned could have accumulated genetic mutations during its years in another adult that could give the resulting clone a predisposition to cancer or other diseases of aging.[31] Moreover, it is impossible to obtain the informed consent of the clone to his or her own creation, but, of course, no one else is able to give informed consent for their creation either.

I believe it is too soon to say whether unavoidable risks to the clone would make human cloning unethical. At a minimum, further research on cloning animals, as well as research to better define the potential risks to humans, is needed. For the reasons given earlier, we should not set aside risks to the clone on the grounds that the clone would not be harmed by them because its only alternative is not to exist at all; I have suggested that this is a bad argument. We should not, however, insist on a standard that requires risks to be lower than those we accept in sexual reproduction or in other forms of assisted reproduction. It is not possible now to know when, if ever, human cloning will satisfy an appropriate standard limiting risks to the clone.

Largely Social Harms

Harm 3. Human cloning would lessen the worth of individuals and diminish respect for human life. Unelaborated claims to this effect in the media were common after the announcement of the cloning of Dolly. Ruth Macklin has explored and criticized the claim that human cloning would diminish the value we place on, and our respect for, human life because it would lead to persons being viewed as replaceable.[32] As I argued earlier concerning a right to a unique identity, only according to a confused and indefensible notion of human identity is a person's identity determined solely by his or her genes. Instead, an individual's identity is determined by the interaction of his or her genes over time with his or her environment, including the choices the individual makes and the important relations he or she forms with other persons. This means in turn that no individual could be fully replaced by a later clone possessing the same genes.

Ordinary people recognize this clearly. For example, parents of a 12-year-old child dying of a fatal disease would consider it insensitive and ludicrous if someone told them they should not grieve for their coming loss because it is possible to replace him by cloning him; it is their child who is dying whom they love and value, and that child and his importance to them could never be replaced by a cloned later twin. Even if they would also come to love and value a later twin as much as their child who is dying, that would be to love and value that different child who could never replace the child they lost. Ordinary people are typically quite clear about the importance of the relations they have to distinct, historically situated individuals with whom over time they have shared experiences and their lives and whose loss to them would therefore be irreplaceable.

A different version of this worry is that human cloning would result in persons' worth or value seeming diminished because we would now see humans as able to be manufactured or "hand-made." This demystification of the creation of human life would reduce our appreciation and awe of it and of its natural creation. It would be a mistake, however, to conclude that a human being created by human cloning is of less value or is less worthy of respect than one created by sexual reproduction. It is the nature of a being, not how it is created, that is the source of its value and makes it worthy of respect. Moreover, for many people, gaining a scientific understanding of the extraordinary complexity of human reproduction and development increases, instead of decreases, their awe of the process and its product.

A more subtle route by which the value we place on each individual human life might be diminished could come from the use of human cloning with the aim of creating a child with a particular genome, either the genome of another individual especially meaningful to those doing the cloning or an individual with exceptional talents, abilities, and accomplishments. The child might then be valued only for its genome, or at least for its genome's expected phenotypic expression, and no longer be recognized as having the intrinsic equal moral value of all persons, simply as persons. For the moral value and respect due all persons to come to be seen as resting only on the instrumental value of individuals, or of individuals' particular qualities, to others would be to fundamentally change the moral status accorded to persons. Everyone would lose their moral standing as full and equal members of the moral community, replaced by the different instrumental value each of us has to others.

Such a change in the equal moral value and worth accorded to persons should be avoided at all costs, but it is far from clear that such a change would take place from permitting human cloning. Parents, for example, are quite capable of distinguishing their children's intrinsic value, just as individual persons, from their instrumental value based on their particular qualities or properties. The equal moral value and respect due all persons just as persons is not incompatible with the different instrumental values of people's particular qualities or properties; Einstein and an untalented physics graduate student have vastly different values as scientists, but they share and are entitled to equal moral value and respect as persons. It would be a mistake and a confusion to conflate the two kinds of value and respect. Making a large number of clones from one original person might be more likely to foster this mistake and confusion in the public, and if so that would be a further reason to limit the number of clones that could be made from one individual.

Harm 4. Human cloning would divert resources from other more important social and medical needs.[33] As we saw in considering the reasons for, and potential benefits from, human cloning, in only a limited number of uses would it uniquely meet important human needs. There is little doubt that in the United States, and certainly elsewhere, there are more pressing unmet human needs, both medical or health needs and other social or individual needs. This is a reason for not using public funds to support human cloning, at least if the funds actually are redirected to more important ends and needs. It is not a reason, however, either to prohibit other private individuals or institutions from using their own resources for research on human cloning or for human cloning itself or to prohibit human cloning or research on human cloning.

The other important point about resource use is that it is not now clear how expensive human cloning would ultimately be, for example, in comparison with other means of relieving infertility. The procedure itself is not scientifically or technologically extremely complex and might prove not to require a significant commitment of resources.

Harm 5. Human cloning might be used by commercial interests for financial gain. Both opponents and proponents of human cloning agree that cloned embryos should not be able to be bought and sold. In a science fiction frame of mind, one can imagine commercial interests offering genetically certified and guaranteed embryos for sale, perhaps offering a catalogue of different embryos cloned from individuals with a variety of talents, capacities, and other desirable properties. This would be a fundamental violation of the equal moral respect and dignity owed to all persons, treating them instead as objects to be differentially valued, bought, and sold in the marketplace. Even if embryos are not yet persons at the time they would be purchased or sold, they would be being valued, bought, and sold for the persons they will become. The moral consensus against any commercial market in embryos, cloned or otherwise, should be enforced by law whatever public policy ultimately is on human cloning. It has been argued that the law may already forbid markets in embryos on grounds that they would violate the thirteenth amendment prohibiting slavery and involuntary servitude.[34]

Harm 6. Human cloning might be used by governments or other groups for immoral and exploitative purposes. In *Brave New World*, Aldous Huxley imagined cloning individuals who have been engineered with limited abilities and conditioned to do, and to be happy doing, the menial work that society needed done.[35] Selection and control in the creation of people was exercised not in the interests of the persons created but in the interests of the society and at the expense of the persons created. Any use of human cloning for such purposes would exploit the clones solely as means for the benefit of others and would violate the equal moral respect and dignity they are owed as full moral persons. If human cloning is permitted to go forward, it should be with regulations that would clearly prohibit such immoral exploitation.

Fiction contains even more disturbing and bizarre uses of human cloning, such as Mengele's creation of many clones of Hitler in Ira Levin's *The Boys From Brazil*, Woody Allen's science fiction cinematic spoof *Sleeper* in which a dictator's only remaining part, his nose, must be destroyed to keep it from being cloned, and the contemporary science fiction film *Bladerunner*.[36] Nightmare scenarios like Huxley's or Levin's may be quite improbable, but their impact on public concern with technologies like human cloning should not be underestimated. Regulation of human cloning must assure the public that even such far-fetched abuses will not take place.

Harm 7. Human cloning used on a very widespread basis would have a disastrous effect on the human gene pool by reducing genetic diversity and our capacity to adapt to new conditions.[37] This is not a realistic concern because human cloning would not be used on a wide enough scale, substantially replacing sexual reproduction, to have the feared effect on the gene pool. The vast majority of humans seem quite satisfied with sexual means of reproduction; if anything, from the standpoint of worldwide population, we could do with a bit less enthusiasm for it. Early in the twentieth century, programs of eugenicists, like Herman Mueller's plan to impregnate thousands of women with the sperm of exceptional men, as well as the more recent establishment of sperm banks of Nobel laureates, have met with little or no public interest or success.[38] People prefer sexual means of reproduction, and they prefer to keep their own biological ties to their offspring.

Conclusion

Human cloning has until now received little serious and careful ethical attention because it was typically dismissed as science fiction, and it stirs deep but difficult-to-articulate uneasiness and even revulsion in many people. Any ethical assessment of human cloning at this point must be tentative and provisional. Fortunately, the science and technology of human cloning are not yet in hand, and so a public and professional debate is possible without the need for a hasty, precipitate policy response.

The ethical pros and cons of human cloning, as I see them at this time, are sufficiently balanced and uncertain that there is not an ethically decisive case either for or against permitting it or doing it. Access to human cloning can plausibly be brought within a moral right to reproductive freedom, but the circumstances in which its use would have significant benefits appear at this time to be few and infrequent. It is not a central component of a moral right to reproductive freedom and it serves no major or pressing individual or social needs. On the other hand, contrary to the pronouncements of many of its opponents, human cloning seems not to be a violation of moral or human rights. It does, however, risk some significant individual or social harms, although most are based on common public confusions about genetic determinism, human identity, and the effects of human cloning.

Because most moral reasons against doing human cloning remain speculative, they seem insufficient to warrant at this time a complete legal prohibition of either research on or later use of human cloning. Legitimate moral concerns about the use and effects of human cloning, however, underline the need for careful public oversight of research on its development, together with a wider public debate and review before cloning is used on human beings.

ACKNOWLEDGMENTS

I acknowledge with gratitude the invaluable help of my research assistant, Insoo Hyun, on this chapter. He not only made it possible to complete the paper on the NBAC's tight schedule, but also improved it with a number of insightful substantive suggestions.

7

Much Ado About Mutton: An Ethical Review of the Cloning Controversy

RONALD M. GREEN

I begin this discussion with the conviction that 10 or 20 years from now around the world a modest number of children (several hundred to several thousand) will be born each year as a result of somatic cell nuclear transfer (SCNT) cloning. I further assume that within the same period cloning will have come to be looked on as just one more available technique of assisted reproduction among the many in use: in vitro fertilization (IVF), egg and sperm donation, intracytoplasmic sperm injection, surrogacy. I hope to show why this outcome is both predictable and ethically acceptable.

Against this background, however, I also want to explore why, at a certain moment in the 1990s, the prospect of human cloning created so much controversy around the world and led many people to want it banned. My exploration of this question will not primarily be at the level of cultural analysis. Obviously, many identifiable cultural phenomena contributed to this emotional reaction—from popular fiction and films to broad anxieties generated by changing family patterns and rapid advances in the life sciences. These cultural factors lent energy to the controversy, and they merit study in their own right. Nevertheless, what I want to focus on are the patterns of moral reasoning that led so many people to oppose cloning. What the cloning controversy tells us, I think, is that there are ways of thinking about new biomedical technologies that tend to cast them in a very negative light. It is worthwhile to identify these patterns as we enter an era of accelerating advances in the life sciences.

I also want to show how some of these patterns of reasoning evidenced themselves in the report of the National Bioethics Advisory Committee (NBAC), *Cloning Human Beings*.[1] Issued at the outset of the cloning controversy, this report is in many ways a balanced document that seeks to calm fears and place the issue of cloning in an informed and reasoned context. At the same time, however, the NBAC's approach to the cloning issue reflects some of the patterns of reasoning that contributed during this period to widespread rejection of this innovative technology.

Justifying human cloning

I have said that I think cloning will eventually be an accepted—and morally acceptable—reproductive technology. Let me begin by indicating why I believe this is so in order to establish a framework against which we can measure the concerns of those holding a different view. The most likely use of cloning will be circumstances in which one or both members of a couple do not produce the gametes (eggs or sperm) needed for sexual reproduction but wish a child with some genetic relation to his or her parents. Couples in which the male partner has undergone bilateral orchiectomy (complete castration) or otherwise lacks viable sperm are one example. If such couples wish to have a genetic connection with their offspring, they can currently resort to sperm donation, with the result that the child will share half of his or her genetic material with the mother and none with the father. Because sperm donation introduces a third party into the relationship and raises complex questions about the child's future relation to his or her biological father, some couples in this position may reasonably prefer to have a cloned child who has all the genetic material of either the mother or the father. Somatic cell nuclear transfer cloning will make this possible. For similar reasons, lesbian couples will also find cloning an attractive alternative, permitting each member of the pair to bear a child with her partner's genotype. Sperm donation is an option here, but some lesbian couples do not wish to involve third parties in their reproductive lives.[2]

It has been said that cloning may prove attractive to couples each of whose members bears a serious recessive genetic disorder. I am not personally persuaded that this is true. The evolving technology of preimplantation genetic diagnosis (PGD) can provide such couples an alternative by permitting clinicians to create a number of embryos, test them to distinguish those that merely carry the disorder from those that will be affected by it, and then transfer only those embryos likely to be healthy. It is true, however, that the existence of multiple—and in some cases unknown—mutations may frustrate these efforts and render cloning a preferred approach for some people. In any case, some individuals who have experienced the birth of a child with a serious genetic disease may be assumed to wish to avoid the "lottery" of sexual reproduction altogether in the future.[3] Cloning is one way they can do this.

It may be objected here that all these scenarios privilege people's wish to have genetically related children. In a world of burgeoning populations where so many children are currently living in foster homes or orphanages, do we really want to encourage these questionable new forms of parenting? I could reply to these objections in many ways. Assisted reproductive technologies make little or no significant contribution to the growth in world population (which is largely occurring in underdeveloped countries where these technologies are not used).[4] More important, these objections do not apply exclusively to cloning. They arise in connection with any of the established reproductive technologies and are not usually considered a reason for prohibiting access to them. In any case, my aim here is not to evaluate all the arguments pro and con for permitting infertile people, lesbians, or others in similar circumstances to have children via cloning. I merely want to indicate that there are good reasons, not all of which will be equally compelling to everyone, why cloning may be both desirable and allowed. We currently have a wide array of assisted reproductive technologies (ARTs) to help couples with reproductive problems. Cloning, I believe, will soon be regarded as merely another one of them.

Cloning is also likely to be the principal instrument of future gene therapy. Many serious genetic disorders have their start during the period of embryonic and fetal development. If we are to prevent or correct them by gene therapy, we must intervene early. The technical challenge is to insert a corrected gene into every cell of a developing embryo, something that is very difficult using most viral or other gene vectors, which penetrate only one out of hundreds or thousands of cells. This problem can be overcome by means of cloning.[5] Researchers can introduce the vector into a large population of differentiated cells gathered from adult or embryo donors. They can test to identify those few cells where the gene becomes properly inserted into the nuclear DNA. Using the nucleus of such a cell, they can then perform a cloning procedure to produce an embryo that, as it grows, possesses the corrected gene in every cell of its body. With the Human Genome Project greatly expanding our knowledge of the genetic basis of diseases, there will be increasing numbers of people who will want to intervene at the genetic level early in life. Cloning may be widely used in this connection.

Questionable patterns of moral reasoning

From its start, the cloning issue has been approached with a series of concerns, questions, and standards for evaluation that made negative conclusions about it almost inevitable. In this part of my discussion, I want to itemize those approaches and compare them, as necessary, with less forbidding standards applied to other, widely accepted areas of biomedical practice and innovation.

Nightmare Scenarios

Perhaps the most obvious feature of the early cloning debate was the prevalence of nightmare scenarios with little or no basis in facts or technical possibilities. Fictional literature and popular films fed some of these scenarios[6]; others were based on an unreasonable and uninformed estimate of what cloning technology involves or the role of genes in human development.

One such vision may partly explain the immediate impulse to political (and even presidential) involvement in the cloning debate. It is the specter that cloning will be used by a tyrannical regime to mass-produce an army of superwarriors. Against a background of Nazi breeding experiments, popular films like *The Boys From Brazil*, and very prevalent fears of Saddam Hussein's development of biological weaponry, these visions were understandable, but not in any way justified. Lurking here was the serious misconception that cloning can make possible the industrial-scale manufacture of desired human genotypes, bypassing pregnancy and years of childrearing. In reality, if Saddam Hussein were to embark on this route as a means of conquest, his program would require the reproductive enslavement of tens of thousands of women, and he would have to wait 20 years to see the results of his efforts. In addition, if Hussein really were committed to this idea, he could accomplish the same end by means of old-fashioned sexual reproduction using selected male and female breeders or their gametes— as in the Nazi Lebensborn program more than half a century ago. Because genotype is not phenotype—a theme I will return to shortly—there is also a high likelihood that many of Saddam's cloned warriors would no more exhibit his desired traits than would selected sexually reproduced children or even a well-trained population of normal recruits. Like Ferdinand the bull, many of Hussein's cloned superwarriors might prefer to sit out the next Gulf war smelling the flowers. It is probably true that these particular nightmare scenarios did not have much impact on informed discussion about cloning. Nevertheless, at some level they undoubtedly lent some of the emotional energy to the cloning debates.

Another prevalent nightmare scenario during this period was the vision of sexual reproduction being replaced by new commercialized reproduction revolving around the sale of proven or desired genotypes. The vision of thousands of Cindy Crawfords, Brad Pitts, or Michael Jordans danced frighteningly before some critics' eyes. These concerns were fed by the prompt appearance of spurious websites offering cloned copies of celebrities (one even promised an instant Elvis). Unlike the fear of cloned warriors, the problem here was not misinformation. Commercialized mass reproduction like this is technically possible. Furthermore, because a clone can be produced from virtually any intact diploid body cell—

one derived from a blood spot or even a hair follicle—cloning poses novel problems in terms of reproductive privacy and the unconsented use of one's genome by other people. Were this reproductive scenario to come to pass, doctors, dentists, hairdressers, and others with access to celebrities' DNA might have to sign agreements not to use it for personal gain.

These worries about commercialized genotypes betray not technical ignorance but an interesting and, to some extent, self-contradictory assessment of human beings' reproductive desires. On the one hand, many who oppose cloning criticize what they regarded as an obsessive concern with the perpetuation of one's genotype. On the other hand, some of these critics also seem to believe that many parents will gladly forego sexual reproduction—and hence the perpetuation of their genotypes—in order to have a celebrity child. In fact, there is substantial evidence that people, even those suffering from infertility who must use donor gametes, basically want to have children like themselves. The "Noble Prize-Winners" sperm bank opened some years ago by Linus Pauling has done little business. Couples using donor gametes frequently select a sperm or egg donor with desirable qualities like evidence of advanced education or physical attractiveness. As Teri Royal, director of one of the nation's largest fertility registries, observes, however, these couples typically want a child whose intelligence is comparable with their own and with whom they'll be able to relate. "They're not looking for any Mensa applicant," she says.[7]

The fear that people will readily abandon normal parenting and reproductive patterns points to a deeper problem in the moral reasoning of many who strongly oppose human cloning: their fundamental mistrust of natural human inclinations. We often encounter new technological or social developments that seem to threaten widely accepted forms of sexual expression, parenting, or family relations. In responding to these perceived threats, it is always important to respect the power and persistence of normal human drives and to resist the impulse to overreact to new developments in repressive ways. After all, if heterosexual sexual expression and familial affection are important enough to fear their loss, they are also not likely to be massively abandoned when confronted by alternate modes of behavior. Those afraid that cloning might lead people to relinquish sexual reproduction commit the same error in reasoning as homophobic people who fear that tolerance of homosexuality will lead to a mass exodus from heterosexuality. Both fail to trust in the force of the values that they are seeking to defend.

Risk Concerns

The bulk of informed critical opinion about human cloning has been focused not on nightmare scenarios but on possible risks to the children born as a result of cloning procedures. These risks are either physical or psychological. Because human cloning has never been accomplished, many of these harms are speculative in nature. This is not itself a count against them, because caution is always in order when possibly significant risks are involved. Nevertheless, the highly speculative nature of these discussions points to a larger problem in this debate. As we will see, cloning critics have frequently invoked standards of caution and non-injury for this technology that have not been—and probably should not be—applied to other biomedical or reproductive innovations. In addition, the debate has frequently been framed as though the only questions of importance are those about risk to prospective children. Other interests and considerations, especially those of parents, are often omitted from consideration. The result is an evaluation process that has the tendency to lead toward negative conclusions because no substantial values are advanced on the other side.

There is an important lesson here. It is easy to exaggerate the risks of technological innovations. Quite apart from the ease of constructing catastrophic "worst case" scenarios when unknown risks are multiplied by unknown risks, change itself is often perceived as dangerous because it threatens known and established values. The benefits of technological innovations, however, are often less obvious because what is unknown cannot be assessed. Imagine the content of a report on that new invention, the automobile, written by a national technology commission in 1895. To speculative fears of the psychological damage resulting from high-speed travel might have been added real concerns about the massive displacement of horsebreeders, blacksmiths, and others. This is not to say that anticipatory technology assessment and policy analysis are inappropriate. Certainly we have had too little of it in connection with some risky technologies. The point is that one must be aware in making such assessments of the built-in forces that tend to lead to negative conclusions and resistance to change.

I will indicate some of the ways that these misleading patterns of reasoning evidence themselves in some assessments of cloning's risks. First, however, I must state emphatically that concern about the harmful effects of cloning on the children produced by this technology is completely appropriate. I need to do this because two positions sometimes advanced in this context hold otherwise. One is the view that no person can be harmed by cloning because it involves human embryos, which are not regarded as juridical human beings in United States law (and in many people's ethical views). What is at stake in the cloning debate, however, are not embryos but future born children. Even though they may not be in existence when a cloning procedure is begun, children produced by cloning can be adversely affected by it. It is well established in ethics and law that children who are born alive can recover damages for prenatal injury done to them. The same applies to harm done through cloning.

A second view denying the possibility of harming children through cloning is based on the writings of Derek Parfit, David Heyd, and others.[8] In the cloning debate, John Robertson has most frequently voiced it.[9] According to this view, judgments of harm always involve the comparison of an individual's condition *ex ante* (before the alleged injury was done) with the individual's condition *post ante* (following the alleged injury). Harm is done if someone is made worse off as a result of another's actions. Robertson acknowledges that cloning may cause some very serious physical and psychological injuries to children. Because none of these children would have been conceived without use of the cloning procedure, however, we cannot say that they have been made "worse off" by it. Sustaining this claim, says Robertson, would involve showing that the child's life is of such low quality that it would have been better off if it had never come into being at all. Because even individuals born with serious ailments and disabilities are usually glad to be alive, however, it cannot be said that a cloned child would have preferred never to live. Researchers, clinicians, or parents will clearly harm a child by cloning only in rare cases where the child's suffering is so great that most individuals with the same problems would rationally prefer to die.

Robertson buttresses his case by appealing to practices and attitudes that he believes evidence widespread moral support for this position. They include our reluctance to make negative judgments about couples with serious hereditary diseases who choose to have children and our unwillingness to lock up or punish women who risk their future child's health by engaging in forms of substance abuse during pregnancy. According to Robertson, the absence of negative judgments in these cases is a sign of our conviction that parents cannot wrong their children by bringing them into being even in degraded circumstances.

To respond fully to Robertson's arguments would require a separate discussion.[10] Let me briefly suggest, however, why I believe Robertson's view is wrong. Like other approaches to complex new issues, it proceeds from received moral concepts and takes them into uncharted areas where they no longer work very well. In this case, the received concept is "harm," understood in terms of the comparison of an individual's condition before an allegedly injurious activity occurs with the individual's condition after it. Because birth technologies typically involve individuals—children to be—who are not yet in existence at the time the reproductive technology is employed, and because we have no experience in applying this concept of harm to novel circumstances before an individual ever exists, however, this mode of reasoning is likely to mislead.

If the *ex ante/post ante* conception of harm were the only one available to us, we might have to live with it, but it is not. Harms can occur without someone being made worse off than they were before. This is because, at its base, our understanding of what constitutes a harm is the outcome of a complex social and ethical decision aimed at discouraging conduct whose consequences we find undesirable. Harms are those things we do not want people to commit. In most instances, the things that we want to discourage are those that tend clearly to degrade someone else's condition. Hence the prevalence of the *ex ante/post ante* mode of analysis. Sometimes as well, however, there are forms of conduct we are unwilling to tolerate that do not make people worse off in a strict sense. We nevertheless still designate this conduct as harmful—and say that people have been harmed by it—if the conduct has consequences to which we are averse.

Legal reasoning provides an interesting illustration of this point. In the area of misrepresentation law, courts have sometimes awarded the victims of fraudulent stock schemes damages for the loss of promised gains.[11] In terms of the *ex ante/post ante* approach, we cannot straightforwardly say that such persons have been made "worse off." Their net worth may even have increased as a result of the fraud, though not to the extent they had wished and been promised. Nevertheless, to discourage swindling, courts have not hesitated to regard the victims of such schemes as having been harmed. It is possible, of course, to try to fit these judgments into the *ex ante/post ante* framework by arguing that, as a result of the fraud, the victim has been made worse off than he or she reasonably expected to be. This expansion of the concept of harm to include the comparison of expected with actual outcomes, however, takes it beyond any simple *ex ante/post ante* model.[12] It also supports the claim that our more basic purpose in using the harm concept is to identify behaviors we wish to discourage.

Similarly, we have very good reasons for wanting to discourage practices leading to the conception of children who will have significant impairments. Even if it cannot be said with confidence that the resulting children are less happy than are children born without handicaps, bringing handicapped children to the level where they can thrive requires considerable social expense and effort. That many of these children must struggle through painful surgeries or other medical interventions is another reason for seeking to discourage practices leading to such births.[13] On the other hand, it is also true that we have no good reason to want to bring damaged children into being. No one is harmed if they are never conceived. This conclusion is supported by the fact that "no one" exists before conception whose interests in coming into being we need seriously entertain. It is also supported by our common sense attitudes and existing reproductive practices. Outside of special historical circumstances when a high birth rate is needed for the survival of existing cultures, people are not usually censured for failing to have children. Nor is anyone criticized for failing to have all the children that they could have. Taken together, these considerations make it reasonable to conclude that if somebody chooses to have a child, which they are not morally obligated to do, they should try to see that the child is born within the existing parameters of good health. Failing to do this is conceptualized as committing a harm to the child. This is true despite the fact that, within the framework of traditional notions of harm, it is hard to see how the child itself is made "worse off."

It is no objection to this understanding to say that we do not ordinarily blame people who carry genetic diseases when they choose to have children whom they know may inherit those diseases. This issue involves complex balancing judgments in which the final direction of our thinking depends on a host of considerations, including, in addition to the outcome for the child, such things as parents' rights and interests. We may believe that a child is harmed by knowingly being brought into existence, say, with cystic fibrosis. We may also, however, choose to reserve any criticisms of the child's parents because we believe that, on balance, it is wrong to intrude on their right of reproductive decision making. Similarly, we may conclude that policies of incarcerating substance-abusing pregnant women are unwise because they drive such women away from prenatal care.[14] This does not, however, mean that we do not regard the knowing infliction on an infant of cocaine addiction or AIDS as a harm.

Robertson's mistake in drawing conclusions based on our reluctance to make negative judgments lies in confusing global ethical conclusions with specific ethical components of those conclusions.[15] We can judge a total pattern of behavior as morally acceptable (having a child when one carries a genetic disease; treating rather than imprisoning pregnant women) while still regarding some aspects of it (the parents or women's behavior) as harmful.

The upshot of this reasoning is that, despite Robertson's or others' contentions, the instinct to assess cloning in terms of possible harms to the child is sound. This leaves unaddressed, however, the question of whether any of the speculative or real harms that have been mentioned are sufficiently grave to lead us to conclude that human cloning should not be attempted. In approaching this issue it is useful to distinguish between physical and psychological harms because the former are somewhat more concrete. What I want to suggest now is that, in most discussions of the ethics of cloning, no one has shown that harms in either of these areas are likely to be so great as to lead us to want to ban cloning research or its most likely clinical applications.

Physical Harms

Even if it were technically possible, it certainly would not have been reasonable to try to clone a human being in the period following the announcement of Dolly. A fundamental principle of human subjects research is that appropriate studies using animals, preferably of closely related species, should first be undertaken to determine the safety and efficacy of procedures before they are applied to human beings. No one has yet accomplished this for human cloning. Furthermore, initial human research will have to be done with embryos not intended for transfer, as was true in the case of IVF research in the 1960s and 1970s. (I will return to this point when I look more closely at the NBAC's report.) Only once animals evidencing no anomalies have been born and lived a normal life span and a series of viable and apparently healthy human embryos have been produced can researchers offer fully informed and freely consenting parents the opportunity to participate in further research by attempting a live birth.

A critical question is what the precise baseline of possible harm to the child should be. I have already rejected Robertson's suggestion that we can permit any degree of harm so long as it does not reach the point where most people would prefer to die. In contrast, I think that in terms of health we must strive to give a child a start in life roughly equivalent to others in its birth cohort.[16] This reflects our interest in discouraging behaviors leading to suffering on the child's part or creating significant additional burdens for the child's parents or society. As one possible measure of this, we can say that a child is harmed when he or she is deliberately or knowingly brought into being with health problems or disabilities serious enough to warrant a malpractice suit in the context of obstetrical or pediatric medicine.

When new reproductive technologies are involved, however, this does not necessarily mean a risk standard equivalent to that of normal conception and birth. As has been true with the introduction of IVF, assisted hatching, intracytoplasmic sperm injection, and other new reproductive technologies, a somewhat elevated risk level for the child above the baseline of unassisted reproduction might be permissible. The reason for this is not, as Robertson believes, because harm to the child is offset by the benefit to it of being born. No such benefit exists. Rather, it is the benefit to the child's otherwise infertile parents that justifies this small increment of risk. When one has experienced infertility, the desire to have a child is legitimate and pressing. In other areas, parents' wishes are commonly regarded as justifying modest increments of risk of harm to their children. (For example, even though the risks of birth defects are somewhat higher in such cases, we sympathize with couples who marry late and who try to start a family.) Because parents will bear many of the emotional and financial costs of a child's congenital problems, they should also have a right, within reasonable limits,[17] to accept these small increments of risk for their child.

Before leaving the matter of physical harms, I must note that risk assessments for cloning research should stay focused on risks to the child to be: not on gametes or embryos. During the initial debates surrounding cloning, commentators reported that 277 attempts had been made to clone Dolly. Many people naturally assumed that this would be a morally unacceptable loss rate if human subjects were involved. These numbers are, however, misleading. Most of this loss took place in the initial efforts to achieve cell division to the blastocyst stage following nuclear transfer.[18] These failures represent a massive loss of oocytes and somatic cell nuclei that, at least until there is some technical innovation in the source of ova,[19] will have to be remedied if human cloning is ever to be efficient and cost effective. The loss of oocytes and somatic cell nuclei does not, however, represent a moral problem. Neither egg cells nor body cells have a moral claim on us. The final number of blastocyst-stage embryos produced was 29, of which 13 were judged viable for transfer. One lamb, Dolly, resulted. If this were human research and the high loss rate did not indicate an elevated congenital risk for the resulting child, these numbers would pose no significant moral problem. A high ratio of transferred embryos to births is already common in current human IVF procedures. Only those who regard the early embryo as morally equivalent to a child will be troubled by this rate of loss.[20]

The stir about these numbers is important, however, because it highlights two recurring features of the cloning controversy. One is the poor quality of much press coverage and reporters' tendency to emphasize seemingly disturbing news. The other is the constant presence in these reproductive debates of emotional energy drawn from our abortion controversies. Properly understood, the ratio 276 to 1 points to nothing more than the rudimentary state of cloning technology. For some who view the early human embryo as sacrosanct, however, this ratio represents a potentially catastrophic loss of human life and confirms their fears that cloning will lead to the massive abuse of human beings. These worries may be legitimate, of course, but they should not be wrongly intensified by a particular—and I think erroneous—moral estimate of the early embryo.

Psychological Harms

In many discussions of cloning, the risk of physical damage captured less attention than a host of possible psychological harms for the child. Underlying these concerns is a novel feature of cloning, especially somatic cell cloning: the possibility of replicating in an infant the genotype of someone who is already alive or has lived before. The principal worry is that the cloned child would be exposed to acute, and ultimately oppressive, expectations for its development. A child brought into being with the genes of a successful parent, an outstanding athlete, or a prima ballerina might be harmed in several ways. Parental expectations may force the child into intensive programs of training or into career directions that do not correspond to the child's real interests. Failure to live up to the expectations established by the genotype donor might cause the child to experience reduced self-esteem. Parents might emotionally distance themselves from a cloned child they regarded as having failed to live up to his or her promise. Peter Singer, for example, asks whether parents of offspring produced by cloning "would be able to love their children with the uncritical love of parents who love their children for what they are."[21]

When the genotype donor has been selected because of his or her accomplishments, cloning would also seem to place the child in a no-win situation. The child's successes will be regarded as genetically inevitable while failures are likely to be attributed to an unwillingness to make the efforts needed to materialize his or her genetic promise. Finally, when intrafamilial cloning is involved (the cloning of a child who is the genetic replica of a parent), some fear that all these concerns may be compounded by problems of excessive intimacy and interdependency between parents and child.[22]

What are we to say about these scenarios of psychic damage? First, if true, they represent a level of harm to the child that warrants concern. The fact that these harms will not be immediately observable and that significant injury may not be evident until long after many cloned children are born makes it reasonable to ask whether cloning should be allowed in the first place. How likely, however, are these harms to occur? A major problem here, as many have noted, is that the reasoning rests on the fallacious premise that our genes strictly determine us: that genotype is phenotype. Although genes do influence many features of our physical, intellectual, and temperamental make-up, they are only one factor in the complex web of events that shape our life. Interactions with the environment from the moment of conception onward profoundly influence the expression of genes. In the words of Richard Lewontin:

The fallacy of genetic determinism is to suppose that the genes "make" the organism. It is a basic principle of developmental biology that organisms undergo a continuous development from conception to death, a development that is a unique consequence of the interaction of the genes in their cells, the temporal sequence of environments through which the organisms pass, and random cellular processes. . . . As a result, even the fingerprints of identical twins are not identical. Their temperaments, mental processes, abilities, life choices, disease histories, and deaths certainly differ, despite the determined efforts of many parents to enforce as great a similarity as possible.[23]

What does the faulty premise of genetic determinism mean for these arguments about speculative psychological harms? First of all, it suggests that in cases where parents are well informed of their limited ability to use cloning to determine a child's talents or disposition, many of the feared pressures and expectations will not exist. Parents may choose to use cloning to have a child more genetically related to one of them than would be true with other reproductive alternatives, but they will not bring to this the unreasonable expectation that the child will necessarily be very much like the genotype donor. This does not mean that parents may not harbor some wish that Mary will share her mother's passion (or ability) for ballet. Even the parents of sexually produced children, however, have such expectations and frequently do all they can to impose their wishes on children. (How many toddlers at alumni events have I seen wearing diminutive Dartmouth sweatshirts inscribed with their hoped-for graduation years?) If the parents of cloned children receive proper information, counseling, and support, their children may actually experience fewer pressures than many sexually reproduced children.

As a general rule, in seeking to prevent injury it is always ethically required to select the most efficacious and least restrictive means possible. Because cloning can benefit people, the aim is to permit people to use it while eliminating those aspects of it that lead directly to harm. This suggests that the proper mode of intervention is not to ban cloning but to reduce the ignorance and misinformation that can make it harmful. We can do this by requiring psychological workups and counseling for parents as a condition of their participation in cloning programs. Critics of cloning, in their haste to construct scenarios of possible harm, have often failed to consider the range of alternatives for minimizing damage.

Some bioethicists, while recognizing the error in strict genetic determinism, still fear that cloning is nevertheless a technology that may lead some parents to excessively intrude on their child's life. Dena S. Davis, for example, makes a distinction between what she calls logistical and duplicative cloning and singles out the latter for special criticism.[24] Logistical cloning involves the use of this technology to have a child with some degree of genetic relation to the parent when this would not otherwise be possible (as in the case of parents who lack gametes). Duplicative cloning has as its express aim a child with exactly the same genes as the selected genotype. It occurs when parents seek to have a child whom they hope will have a greater chance of being a prima ballerina or a sports star or will be a replica of a parent or deceased loved one. Davis believes that, however well informed such parents may be, duplicative cloning poses unavoidable dangers.

Borrowing a concept from Joel Feinberg, Davis asserts that every child has a "right to an open future," which includes the freedom needed to choose his or her own life purposes and goals. Parents have the corresponding obligation to preserve a child's nascent autonomy and to avoid forcing the child into a life based on their own preferences. Davis acknowledges that "this right to an open future" can be imperiled by attitudes and practices that parents bring to ordinary sexual reproduction. She believes, however, that duplicative cloning in particular is an invitation to harm:

True, everyone is born with a genetic inheritance, which enables some choices and not others, and, true, parents are often quite assertive in their drive to influence their children's life choices. But allowing parents to clone children for this purpose elevates the problem to a new level. . . . [P]arents who take expensive cumbersome steps to provide their child with a specific DNA in order to maximize the chances of success in a particular field, will, I suspect, find it almost impossible to accept if the child hates ballet or basketball, and chooses the life of an accountant or tympani player. Parents will be focused, from the child's first days, on such a narrow range of possibilities that the child's right to an open future, her chance to explore her own interests and options, will be radically limited.[25]

What can we say about this objection? First, to some extent Davis's fears may be well founded. Some parents, however well informed, may use cloning to exert undue pressures on their children, and they may be more likely to do this when duplicative cloning is involved. Nevertheless, even if we concede this, it is not an argument against cloning research or many of its likely clinical applications. Much cloning in the future will be logistical rather than duplicative, and it is not warranted to ban all attempts at cloning because one form has risks.

Beyond this, it is not clear that even those seeking duplicative cloning should be denied this opportunity as long as they are fully informed of the limits of such efforts. Davis is right to observe that such cloning may narrow or restrict the range of the child's future choices. Nevertheless, such occurrences are common in family life, and the idea that the child's "right to an open future" should always trump parental wishes is unreasonable. Throughout most of modern history, for example, whenever African-American, Jewish, or Native-American parents chose to have children, they imposed significant limitations on their child's "right to an open future." We do not conclude that these people ought not to have reproduced. Even today, parents make decisions about their own careers or their family's place of residence or religious affiliation that significantly limit their children's future choices, and we do not think it right to intrude in such matters.

The Amish, by denying their children more than an eighth grade education, greatly limit the children's abilities to become world-class scientists or scholars. U.S. law has accepted this as a price of parental religious freedom. Lawyers for the Amish have also successfully persuaded American courts that to require a high school education for these youngsters in the name of preserving their future autonomy would seriously jeopardize the children's ability to integrate themselves in the Amish community, a matter of parental discretion.

The point is that many parental interventions take place during the formative years when a child's most basic aptitudes and values are being formed and they thus effectively limit the child's range of future choices. To insist on the child's "right to open future" as a governing norm amounts to drastically limiting the freedom that parents have to raise their children as they wish. It also flies directly in the face of many currently allowable childrearing practices. Do parents who seek to use cloning to influence a daughter in the direction of becoming a prima ballerina compromise her future any more than parents who would enroll her for 12 years in a strict convent school in the hope that she will become a nun? If the latter is widely regarded as morally acceptable, why not the former? This is not to say that "the child's right to an open future" is not a valuable ideal toward which many will want to strive. In terms of the cloning debate, it may justify programs of counseling and support to steer parents away from abusive uses of duplicative cloning. It is by no means clear, however, that it justifies limiting or removing parents' ultimate freedom to make these reproductive decisions for themselves.

The National Bioethics Advisory Commission report

I want to conclude this ethical review of the cloning controversy by offering a brief critique of the National Bioethics Advisory Commission (NBAC) report and the NBAC's approach to the task it was given. Some of the larger problems that have troubled our approach to cloning are evident in the NBAC's work. Before doing this, however, I must offer two caveats. First, I am not an impartial critic. Having served during 1994 on the Human Embryo Research Panel (HERP), I have an investment in the way that the previous federal advisory group approached its job of addressing a very controversial issue in reproductive medicine. The NBAC chose to differ with the HERP approach on several matters, and my partisanship is evident. Second, I must acknowledge that the NBAC worked under

very difficult conditions. Newly created, operating with a partial staff and uncertain budget, its members were asked by President Clinton to produce a report
on a very complex bioethical issues in just 90 days' time. That the NBAC completed the report as requested and that, with its flaws, it is still a useful document is an important achievement.

Nevertheless, my first criticism is that the NBAC even chose to accept this assignment at all. At the outset, the NBAC's members made a strategic decision
that they would try, in a period of 90 days, to provide counsel that was likely to
lead to executive branch or legislative action on an issue of enormous complexity whose scientific and technical dimensions were not yet clear. Political scientist Andrea Bonnicksen asks a fair question: "What was the rush?"[26] No one reasonably believed that the announcement of Dolly would soon lead to efforts to
clone a human being. Why, then, accept this hurried time frame?

From my experience of the HERP, I understand that national commissions have
a built-in tendency to try to please those who create them.[27] The NBAC was
formed at the President's urging, and it is always difficult to turn down a presidential request. Nevertheless, with the 20/20 vision of hindsight, the NBAC might
have considered whether their first act should not have been to request more time
for study and deliberation. A time frame of one year for this issue, or the opportunity to periodically re-examine it over a longer period while continuing to
monitor and report on developments, would not have been unreasonable. The
larger lesson here, I think, is our tendency to overreact to bioethical innovations,
especially those related to reproductive medicine. At a moment when the President
and the public were responding to these developments in emotionally charged
ways, it was the duty of a national bioethics commission to restore some perspective to the debate. The NBAC chose to do this by trying to produce a balanced report as soon as possible. The effort to do this, however, may have added
fuel to the fire.

A second criticism relates to the high profile the NBAC gave to religious views
in the testimony and written reports it invited. Religious ethicists and religious
spokesmen certainly have a right to add their views to public debate on an issue
like this. Nothing within our tradition of separation of church and state requires
religious communities to silence themselves on matters they believe to be of public moral concern. In giving religious views a place in their process, some NBAC
members were also seeking to remedy what they regarded as a defect in the work
of the HERP. Viewing itself primarily as an expert commission, the HERP may
have underestimated its political role as a forum for airing diverse opinions and
as a place where the public could get a sense that their concerns were being
heeded. In several statements, Alta Charo, who served on both the HERP and the
NBAC, stated that in its approach to cloning the NBAC should correct the earlier panel's relative neglect of religious positions.[28]

Nevertheless, for a public panel to highlight religious views on an issue like
this also has its perils. As a religious ethicist, I believe that many religious tra-

ditions are poorly equipped to offer sound advice on reproductive technologies. Few religious spokespersons are up to date on the complex technical aspects of these debates, and religious traditions' conservativism is often most pronounced on issues related to sex and family. Because religions' ethical teachings on sexual ethics evolved over centuries within traditional cultural contexts, these traditions are often unable to respond rapidly to new possibilities made possible by technological change. Witness how long it has taken most religious communities to respond to the revolution represented by the advent of birth control and rapid population growth in our century (some have still not done so). The slow response to emergent biological understandings of homosexuality is another example.

Of course, because cloning touches on fundamental issues of family and personal identity it is good to have voices present that represent traditional perspectives. My point is not that those voices should not be heard. Rather, I want to alert us to the fact that whenever a dramatically new sexual or reproductive opportunity is developed religious spokespersons will figure predominantly among its critics. This is a special—and acute—case of the kind of opposition to change that increasingly occurs in life sciences research, especially in the area of human reproduction. A policy review process that foregrounds religious positions will tend to place these new technologies in a negative light.

My third criticism concerns the NBAC's willingness to recommend federal legislation prohibiting cloning. As numerous commentators have observed,[29] there has been surprisingly little of use to date of federal legislative power to prohibit research or clinical activities. Regulation results instead from a complex web of restraints. Human subjects regulations that govern federally funded research are one major component. Standards of care established by professional associations are another. Common law protections against medical malpractice work to discourage harmful research or clinical activities. Finally, voluntary moratoria by scientists themselves—the Asilomar initiative for recombinant DNA research is the leading example—may be used to slow research until pressing safety concerns are addressed. As a result of this loose-textured web of restraints, it is very had to entirely halt a promising line of research or the provision of greatly desired clinical services. Dedicated scientists who believe their research to be safe and important can refuse to cooperate with an ill-considered moratorium, and patients can vote with their feet and dollars by seeking services they want from private clinics here or abroad.

Fearing that this could happen with cloning, the NBAC called for a uniform federal ban on any attempt to clone a human being. The commission would permit human research as long as it was not intended to lead to the birth of a cloned child, and it also recommended a 3 to 5 year "sunset provision" in any legislation to allow reconsideration of the issue in the future.[30] These recommendations seem moderate, but they are actually quite radical. A federal ban, however circumscribed, shifts the emphasis from regulated support to outright prohibition.

Instead of inviting the best scientists to assume responsibility for the direction of the field in concert with the existing human subjects review process, a ban on cloning could lead the best researchers and institutions to avoid the field entirely.[31] This would leave cloning to irresponsible scientists at the margins of the profession (witness the emergence of Richard Seed). The argument that good preliminary research could still take place in this country as long as it did not aim at the birth of a child is undercut by the existing legal prohibitions of federal funding for embryo research. Deprived of federal support, researchers committed to perfecting human cloning may well find themselves attracted to more permissive jurisdictions overseas or may seek employment in offshore commercial enterprises offering cloning for a price. None of these outcomes enhances the possibility of good ethical oversight of this research.

The idea that Congress might act in the future to reconsider or lift a cloning ban is also naive. New reproductive technologies are caught up in our deep divisions over the abortion question and our polarized moral views on the status of the early embryo. In these debates, the legislative process is particularly vulnerable to pressure from militant minority groups. For nearly 20 years, federal funding for embryo research has been blocked by a coalition of "pro-life" groups. Similarly, once a federal law against human cloning is enacted, a small number of dedicated opponents can work to keep it in place. By urging a ban, the NBAC opened the door to this possibility.

My final criticism has to do with the NBAC's decision not to make any recommendations about the issue of human embryo research as it relates to cloning.[32] There were some very good reasons why the NBAC chose to bypass this issue. For one thing, its members rightly concluded that the most worrisome risks at this time have to do with the damage that cloning might do to any children born through this still undeveloped procedure. This meant that there was no reason to prohibit private cloning research using embryos as long as no effort was made to transfer these embryos to a womb. By not supporting a private sector ban on cloning research when no transfer was involved, the NBAC also refused to add its voice to those who would take advantage of the cloning controversy to further restrict embryo research in this country.

The real question, however, is why the NBAC failed to issue a more urgent appeal for federally funded research on cloning when no transfer was intended. I realize that I may seem detached from reality in suggesting that the NBAC should have done this. After all, the HERP had made a strong case for embryo research not long before, and Congress soundly rejected its recommendations. Why in the world would the NBAC want to get involved in this issue?

In answering this question, we must recall that the principal rationale behind the NBAC's call for a ban on human cloning were the unknown risks of this procedure for the child. If this ban were to be reconsidered in five years' time, as the NBAC recommended, we would thus need a body of experimental data offering a more precise idea of the risks full human cloning would entail. But how were we to learn about these risks? Research using human embryos not intended for transfer would be crucial, yet federal support for such research was prohibited. This means that the burden of providing the information needed for a critical review of the federal ban would fall on private research facilities that had few resources for such studies and that were largely exempt from human subjects regulations.

If the NBAC's members really believed that the most pressing questions around cloning concerned safety to the child, they would seem to have had an obligation to make clear the urgent need for federally funded research in this area. That they did not do tells me that they never really seriously considered the matter of immediate risks or how they might be assessed and reduced. Rather, the emphasis on these risks was a convenient way for the NBAC to ratify and continue the moratorium instituted by the President without having to resolve all the larger questions about cloning that had been raised.

The NBAC's approach here may be reasonable. I do not want to revisit the difficult choices the commission had to make to sustain its value and credibility. Nevertheless, the approach they took provides a vivid illustration of some of the dynamics whose presence in our ethical debates I have tried to signal. One is the sense of panic and the pressure toward prohibition that has accompanied this technology from the start. Our discussions about cloning have too often been an impulse toward prohibition in search of a rationale. Closely related to this is the tendency to posit risks without critical scrutiny of their likelihood or gravity. Highly speculative scenarios have been constructed with little examination of their logic, or, as in the case of the NBAC report, concrete risks have been alleged with no recommendations for how they might be measured or reduced. Finally, too little attention has been given to the other side of the issue: the reasons why cloning or cloning research might be advisable or the harms of prohibitions and research obstructions. Cloning critics have sometimes lived in a cost-free world where innovative research might be stopped by fiat with little price in terms of lost knowledge, undeveloped therapies, or damage to the research enterprise.

The immediate controversy around cloning has not been one of our better moments in the formation of public science policy. I have tried to signal some of the ways contributors to this debate have erred or exaggerated in their approach to the issues, and I have tried to highlight modes of reasoning that, although understandable, skew our discussions and block reasoned deliberation. By taking stock of the excesses in these debates, we can improve our response to cloning and other biomedical innovations in the future.

8

Born Again: Faith and Yearning in the Cloning Controversy

LAURIE ZOLOTH

Two pieces from the January 1, 2000, edition of the *New York Times* set the stage for this chapter. In the first, William Safire poses a question that he thinks might reasonably be asked in the twenty-first century. Given recent discussions about the possibility for tissue and organ regeneration through the use of human stem cells, it may soon not be "nutty" to ask the question, "Why die?" In a similar vein, Sheryl Gay Stolberg writes about likely biological advances in cloning, stem cell research, and gene therapy that are changing how we think about reproduction. She quotes Gregory Stock, the director of the Program in Medicine, Technology and Society at UCLA. According to Stock, "in the not-too-distant future, it will be looked at as kind of foolhardy to have a child by normal conception." Both Safire and Stolberg draw our attention to the mesmerizing quality of the future that reproductive technology appears to have opened. Ethicists, theologians, and moral philosophers find themselves in a public discourse marked by passionate interest in the immediate implications of this new science, in both the personal and the public sphere, and, not tangentially, the marketplace.[1] The cloning experiment's process was revealed only after the patients were obtained, and the details were given in the business section.

Consider the public debate about cloning. At the heart of the cloning controversy is the endless fascination that humans have in replication, both a narcissistic and a messianic impulse. Cloning the self intrigues precisely because it of-

132

fers an answer to the inevitability of alterity, estrangement, and death. As such, it reflects the deepest of yearnings: for redemption and resurrection into a better, purer, and transformed self, a self given a second chance at an embodied human journey.

The prospect of cloning a human being affords us the chance to reflect on the theological and ethical implications for personhood, citizenship, and social policy of such new reproductive technology. In this conversation, I want to offer the particularities of one non-inclusive claim within the Jewish tradition of bioethics, the curious corridor voice of feminist Jewish ethics. I want to speak this to you, as reader of this work, within the methods of traditional Jewish ethics: narratives, matters of detail, and disagreement. At stake in such reflection is the particularity of the theological contribution to the public discourse, a discourse that was, in the immediate aftermath of the announcement that cloning might be possible, immediately, universally, and joyfully seized upon by ethicists: a week of spectacular attention to our field, a sort of bioethicist WPA. What we knew, collectively, as observers, experts, and commentators was that this news was spiritually central to our shaken notions of modernity. Moreover, we agreed that it was high time to think through how this science deconstructs notions of love, intimacy, and the faithful union traditionally at the core of the human experience of being in a family. Could we not but shudder at Gregory Stock's vision of a future where normal conception was an aberration, where love, tenderness, and creation seem a sort of error?

Our first reflections were partial: In this chapter, I want to pull the discourse to a darker place. It is the job of the ethicist, perhaps especially the Jewish ethicist, to worry, to make trouble, especially about the meaning of the vulnerable self and the state. I want to suggest both that theologically trained bioethicists have unique contributions to make to the reflections on cloning and that we have as yet gotten it wrong in our replies. Although we are called by the media to be asked about theology, we need to raise questions more about the work of the love of each other, with the most serious and rigorous intent, and to remind, in our frail and stubborn creatureliness, of finality.

After the initial clamor about cloning, after we had all had the chance to be called by the press and see our friends on "Nightline," the scholarly response was to turn to the National Bioethics Advisory Commission (NBAC) to reflect and codify our positions. In doing this, Rabbi Elliott Dorff and Rabbi Moshe Tendler, two of our most gifted halachic authorities, articulated the Jewish position on this ethical dilemma. I am not going to raise objections to the halachic or theological reasoning of my colleagues in Jewish bioethics. As usual, Dorff and Tendler have provided us with a consistent, familiar, reliable account of the Jewish texts on healing that have led us to frame our view of reproductive technology. I think, however, that while they are on the right track of these texts, they are in the wrong country of discourse, a category mistake. So I want, in this chapter, to "walk off"

in another direction, remembering always that the root of the word *halachah* is
to walk a road. I want to argue that we need to be walking and thinking and arguing in the terrain of death and our staggering mesmerizing panic at our own
mortality.

Because we are afraid of death, we turn from what we must do to face it and
fill our souls with the yearning for ever-better rebirth (hence Americans and our
fetish of the new). Birth, in its messy, uncontrollable tumult, is the closest moment we ever have to facing our own death, of course. The Jewish rabbinic tradition requires women to re-enact this by the ritual immersion and the public
recitation of the prayer of rescue, both acknowledgments not only of the obvious risk involved in physical childbirth (a fact rather cheerily forgotten in all of
the cloning debates) but also of the fact that the birth of a child re-states the ending of the self. It is the entrance into the room of your life of the he-who-will-
hold-you-as-you-lie-dying.

In reflecting on this, I come, not to the texts of infertility or healing. I turn to
the book of Job, the book of loss, and to the persistent rabbinic phrase that occurs in the commentary on the book, variants on "Women brought death into the
world."[2] The plain meaning of the text is a reference to the Gan Edan story, but
the implication is more profound. It is women who bring birth into the world
and, by so doing, bring the aching inevitability of loss, the fragile infant whom
we will love and who will replace us, but who may die, and in so doing threaten
the very order of the air, the earth. With love, and relationality, comes this child
whose name may well be Cain, death in the world. It is a chance we take with
love and procreation left in the hands of women.

And yet: second chances. If the process can be controlled, made perfect, the
death taken out of it, the loss and the chance made safe by science, then it is a
"technique." We can debate it like we speak of tissue plasminogen activator and
streptokinase; we can even sell it, promising outcomes; ads can appear in
the Sunday paper. Our local in vitro fertilization clinic promises "a baby,
guaranteed."[3]

Missing persons

My contention, then, is that the cloning controversy reaches so deeply into the
popular imagination not because it is about birth, but because it is about the fear
of mortality that lurks always at the corners of birth and fecundity. Job, of course,
hearing about the death of his children, re-links this for us linguistically: "Naked
I was born out of my mother's womb, And naked shall I return there."[4]

Cloning is not about infertility, which can be more easily managed with other
means. It is surely not about children. Here is the clue. If we meant to talk about
children we would have to speak about the time it takes to explain spelling or
how best to wipe the table clean after the chalk is on it, or rocking the sick 4-
year-old to sleep after croup steals her breath. If cloning were about children, we

would need to be thinking about the 100,000 children in foster care in America and the way that race, illness, or oddity makes children unadoptable, untakeable. We would remember that every act is a public one and that each of those un-claimed children is ours. We might have to think aloud on "Nightline" about why we somehow cannot provide universal access to health care for the children we produce. Or why infant mortality, in those untechnical births of the poor, is higher in my city than in many developing countries. Or why we are mesmerized by the "way-coolness" of the scientific arts that assist impregnation, like intracytoplas-mic sperm injection (gendered the male act), and why we can barely fund infant nutrition (gendered the female act).

Cloning is about the imagined self reborn past death, into the future, a life lived in the imagined thenness, rather than the broken exilic nowness of the pre-sent. In fact, many of the moral parables of cloning begin with the case of the family whose only beloved child is dying. For Jews, this has played out in a po-tentiated, particular, post-Shoah narrative, cloning as a way to redeem the Holocaust, a kind of Passion and a resurrection of the lost dead.

In fact, Tendler and others justify a possible positive use of cloning for saving the genetic material of the last member of a Holocaust survivor family, which was the identical rationale that drove the first surrogacy case, Baby M. It is the yearning for the genetic, scientific fix for history itself.

The gender wars

It is the link between women and death and fecundity, however, that animates much of the cloning talk, a talk that is also about the profound ways that the gen-der wars have played out in modernity and the yearning for men to order and control how it is that women are closer to the mystery of reproduction of the self. At the heart of the controversy is a discussion in which the object of the gaze is on the body of the imagined child, through the woman, in which the woman be-comes a kind of device (replaceable if we could) for the production of, or rather the spacial housing for, the product of conception. Am I being too harsh? I think not—there was not one woman scientist involved in the presentation of the cloning event; the scientists were men, and the discourse and linguistic turn was deeply gendered as male. The implications of the act all revolved around the construc-tion of the embryo. The issues of motherhood—that is, what was the pregnancy like, or the birth, who was it exactly who nursed that clone, and who did the clone love, whose warm, breathing body did she turn to in the night—all were absent. What mattered was not the chanciness, vulnerability, or heart-stopping loss inherent, really, in all pregnancies, but the outcome, the product, hence the marketplace interest in the work.

The only woman who was mentioned by name, in fact, was Dolly Parton, in a casual sexist slur, and she only made it into the discourse because of the allu-sion to her breasts, in a sniggering, adolescent-boy nomenclature. The way that the name framed the discourse was significant—here we subliminally heard, every time the name was mentioned, the message that a woman's body, her breast, the very way that a woman uniquely and irreplaceably nurtures real human babies is a joke.

In a 1997 speech at the American Association of Bioethics,[5] bioethicists John Robertson and George Annas launched a hot debate entitled "Who Is the Mother?" Annas argued that the mother of the individual was the adult from whom it was cloned, but Robertson thought not, that it was the mother of the adult from whom it was cloned. Neither seemed to consider as a candidate the woman, still needed to carry the child to term, from whose actual body the child would be nurtured and would emerge, onto whose belly the child would be laid.

Jewish textual tradition is clear. We tend to forget in the disputes around matrilineal descent what a feminist stand it was to consider the mother as central to the being of the child rather than the property assertion of the father.

Power itself as suspect

Jewish tradition is also cautionary about the use of the specific body for the greater good. Several scholars have cited the Tower of Babel (Genesis 11:1–9) as the tale that warns us away from science. It is not the text that ought to alert us, however, it is the midrash. "When a person fell, the work went on, but when a brick fell, all wept."[6]

In making meaning of the texts, the rabbinic move was to point to the issue of justice, a critical reminder for us about the way that power and its uses, allies, and objects are at stake in the development of new technology that allows for transformative acts. Both towers to Heaven and massive shipbuilding projects take place against a society that is lost and that profits not a bit from the effort. In fact, it is the rabbinic penchant for critique that locates even Noah, master technocrat and ship's contractor, as complexly lacking in his total inability to struggle to fight for his community, to even ask the justice question, to think only of his family, the crew on his own boat. Power is often suspect in the rabbinic tradition, as opposed to study. Even if technology is mobilized, the body cannot be ignored and used for the project without rebuke. It is the nature of the exilic community to be uneasy about power, living as outsiders, tangentially, contingently (Genesis 2:15).

Can it be used, however, if it is really wonderful? Dorff and others traditionally point out the nature of the mandate to heal, but let me argue that technical manipulations of exactly this sort, even the redemptive and salvific acts, must be carried out in the midst of a redemptive community that bears both the responsibility and the meaning of each gesture of power. For an example, I have used the Golem texts in other work. As early as the Talmud, the rabbis took note of how very useful it would be to have a person whom they could make:

Rava said: If the righteous wished, they could create a world, for it is written, "Your inequities have been a barrier between you and your God." For Rava created a man and sent him to R. Zeira. The rabbi spoke to him but he did not answer. Then he said: "You are from the pietists: return to dust."[7]

Of course we can do this, they are saying confidently in the second century; there are some technical flaws, but still. The text is subversive, however. Your power is limited by justice. A man created, but not quite; a man not having the really Jewish thing intact, the ability to answer back, a recapitulation of Noah's failure to argue with God for his society, is the sign of something gone astray morally, an inequity that is the barrier.

Throughout the brutalizing medieval and early modern periods, the Golem tales flourish, and the yearning remains. Could we make an enhanced Jew, a Jew without death, a Jew who could save us? Cynthia Ozick's work in the Perlmutter novels is of course centered on this. The move always, however, ends in chaos. It is because it is a sophisticated kind of idolatry, more the making of the calf to keep us from death, than the creator. It fails because there need always to be three in the room of creation of a child, the rabbis remind us, a relationship of the other to the other and of each to Godself. It is, as Emmanuel Levinas reminds, likened to the three in every ethical gesture, the ethics that for Levinas is always, always before freedom.

The role of theological ethics

Is it too late for theological ethics? If we would strongly recommend against such a technology, what would be the effect of the theological voice on the deliberations of policy? How does a theological discourse on the nature of the right act or on human flourishing affect the power ideologies of commodification, autonomy, and rights such a science implies?

Here are notes toward an answer:

1. Robertson and others have argued that cloning, rather than being essentially different, is merely a continuation of advanced reproductive technology (ART). Because we now use this technology to offer all kinds of persons the "right" of reproduction, why stop now? This is arguing up the slippery slope. It is true enough that one cannot justify the technology by pre-existing technology, but it is worse still to justify it when the entire enterprise of ART is the oddest of mixes of unrestrained desire, the unfettered marketplace, and the seduction of experimental technology.

It is well past time to reflect rigorously on the entire process of "making" babies and of the problems of the marketplace as regulator of the process. It is true that cloning is not a deviation from the most basic assumptions of ART, which is the essential construction of infertility as a (dis)ease, an illness with a cure, a (dis)order of the mechanics or chemistry of the human self. In this formulation, the correct response is the one that we are accustomed to having to all disease: that a cure is necessary and lies firmly in the hands of the medical expert. We study earnestly the little diagrams of cells that tell you how they did it, the methodical details. Such a construction, however, is not simple. It needs specific overt and covert philosophical truth claims to support its direction. It justifies, of course, the establishment of a marketplace of competitive and complex expertise, an increasingly desperate and yearning public, and a central moral appeal to autonomous desire as a trumping concern in ethical reasoning. Every day the newspaper brings us new variety in the ways we can make babies. One day, on the front page of the *New York Times*: "For only 2,710 dollars you can buy a premade embryo, a pre-birth adoption." Another day, an ad offering $50,000 for the right sort of donor egg. And these are the "facts" that frame the narrative for us.

2. We say, as theologians, that it is not by might but by spirit that the world is held together, but we do not teach or act in such a way that we mean it. Part of the power of cloning derives from our own love, real love, of our own physical bodies, every little cell. Otherwise, why would noted theologians, me included, eat bran flakes and be found running at dawn, theologians who are concerned with their own bodies, panting down the street to save the flesh. This ironic stance is needed in the cloning debates. We need to speak of the goal of the agonistic human life: It is to move toward what the classic texts tell us is refinement of imperfection, not the *a priori* obliteration of imperfection. In this, we could serve to remind of something else: of the blinding power of human love, which sees and knows, right through the brokenness.

3. In a recent interview, Carl Djerassi noted: In a few years, in advanced countries, sexual activity, and the reproduction of healthy children will be entirely managed and distinct. This will just be what is possible, although it will come with a lot of ethical baggage.[8] We love that ethical baggage! Ethicists must be, in that scenario, customs inspectors at the border: rooting around and unpacking the baggage brought by the act of the scientists, unfolding the starched shirts, looking for the contraband, noting and recording carefully what is borne across our social borders in the name of a necessary, scientific voyage. Somewhere, for something, we have to summon up enough prophetic remembrance to say "no" like we mean it, to hold a partisan position without terror at our own toughness. Otherwise, why call oneself an ethicist?

The range of theological and philosophical commitments and communities that are represented in the field of bioethics offers an opportunity for a robust exchange of views from diverse epistemological stances. Much more work needs to be done. We need to reflect on the meaning not only of the performance gesture of cloning but also the act of the imagination that surrounds the act in the popular culture. In what way does the anticipation of this act in movies and literature frame our narrative of the actual event? There is more: What of the absurdity of the injustice of health care, the way that it is actually the poorest women of color, not the *New York Times* columnist who writes about it, who is far more likely to become infertile and then to have no access to even the most basic health care? What of the worry that Jews, persons of color, lesbians and gays, the deaf community, would never be reproduced and then would be instantly seen as defective merchandise?

Cloning long represented the "bright line" of reproductive technology. When bioethicists spoke of the dangers of earlier reproductive advances, we often noted with panic that the end of such work might be a cloned human person—only to be told calmly by scientists of the technological impossibility of this problem. Hence, cloning represents both the problem of our ability to set limits on a scientific discourse that is not our own and the most extreme example of the cascade of reproductive technology, a technology largely unregulated, undersupervised, and wildly lucrative for the practitioners. Speaking of cloning offers a new imperative for serious ethical reflection on the nature of the human moral gesture in science itself. Such speech is of central importance in a thoughtful consideration of not only cloning but also our collective human future.

Setting limits, however, standing at the borders of desire is what Jewish ethics is largely about—the term of art for this being "erecting a fence around the Torah." A commanded life does not allow for every single autonomous want to be sated, not that cheeseburger, not that lust, not that action on that day, not that harvest on *Shabbat* despite your hunger, not that answer to your need, and it does so without apology. All reproduction is a kind of hunger, the other hunger that compels the creaturely self to work and struggle in the world. The hunger of the infertile is ravenous, desperate, and frankly fed by the complexities of research, finances, and the special passion for creation from which it is difficult to turn.

4. Justice as equalness is not fully possible, not in the realm of death, not in the country of this debate, and it is in the arena of the family that we are intended to learn this. We need to make tangible that which is not seen in the cloning debate. What is transparent—in fact, what disappears from the discourse nearly entirely—is the actuality of the embodied relationship to the specified Other with a cause and concern and with creaturely imperfections just like our own. This is the deepest ethical danger—that in our progressively creative and procreative forward push, we will lope too easily into commodified, desiccated possession rather than love as the organizing principle of family formation.

If we focus on families, and the making, not of babies, but of relationships in the world created by complex negotiation among loving adults, then we have an ethical dilemma of a different nature. I talked about the enormity of love and anxiety that is mobilized by the erotic passions and the physical facticity of the newly born. At stake will be how it is to love like that, not the chosen one, not the close-as-can-be replica, but the surprising stranger who will live at your side. This creature that emerges from your creaturely self, a complete surprise (ask any parent, or any teenager, for that matter)—it is a stranger to whom you as parent would (and as ethicist Tom Murray reminds us, do) give your life. And it is a very hard stranger to love, coming yowling, needy, hungry, hands out, naked, speechless, not always the cutie-pie. It is where we learn to care, with love, for sweat, and feces, and urine and to love the other, and, hopefully, know that they will love us back when we become strangers in old age, our bodies vulnerable in exactly these animal ways. The act of parenting is the act of encounter with the other who is both not-you and of-you, your future and your responsibility, your obligation and your joy. In this way, we all learn to have the stranger, not the copy, live by our side as though out of our side.

Children are in large part about yearning. Like the women of the Bible, Sarah and Channah, teach us, the answer to the yearning is faith, and that has its costs— one loses one child in these stories. Channah's prayer is the first prayer, the rabbis remind us. But the answer is always unexpectedly freighted. The whole point of "making babies" is not the production, it is the careful rearing of persons, the promise to have bonds of love that extend far beyond the initial ask and answer of the marketplace.

5. Parenting, the creation of children into a relationship, has little in common with the search for perfection. The job of parenting is to prepare one's children to face death well and to do this by the stake of one's very life. Of course we hate to think about it, but I want to end as I began here, by speaking about the death of children. A story, with many details that I want you to face:

Several years ago, I was called to help at a difficult *taharah*. I was a member of the *Chevra Kadisha*—the holy friends—the volunteer Jewish burial society that ritually cleanses and dresses the bodies of the dead for a traditional burial. The small group of women were already at the funeral home, but they had gotten into trouble, and I left work and drove over. It was the afternoon before *Pesach*, 4 hours to the *seder*. The trouble was terrible trouble. The person who had died was a four-year-old girl, killed in a stupid senseless traffic accident as she ran joyfully toward her father. None of us had ever done the ritual cleansing of a child before, and no one had ever seen so very much blood. Everywhere we touched, the little baby body bled. Her hair was covered with blood, her fingernails. The work of the *Chevra* is to purify, but first we had to clean the tragedy off, and, not parenthetically, we had to save everything that was darkened with blood to bury with her. Then we said what Jews say at that moment, which are verses of the Song of Songs, and we put the earth brought in little bags from Jerusalem for this purpose on her eyes and her womb, her vagina, and we dressed her in the shrouds, and because they are only made for adult women, we had to roll up the sleeves. There are dozens of enacted details for the *mitzvah* to be proper. At that last moment, she was perfectly and transcendently beautiful, lost, and so dead.

Her mother came in to see her, and when she saw how the methodical work of the commanded act, the work of *mitzvah*, had given her dignity, and her sweet beauty back, she kissed her, and prayed, and promised her that she would see her when the Messiah came. Later, she turned firmly to us—I need you now to work to change the world, she said, to do *tikkun olam*, so that the Messiah will come soon, so I will see my M__ again—her faith blazing before me, the sheer fire of this, like the little flame we lit and left on the wood coffin in the coming darkness. We all had to leave and make Passover, the story that begins with the death of the babies of the Jews and ends with the free people. Ethics precedes freedom. In the years after, the mother kept in touch, urging me to study hard, to work for projects in her daughter's name; it is the way that Jews answer death, with the passionate search for justice. It is the not the body, it is a world reborn that her daughter needs.

I am not so certain. I understand the urge for second chances, the love of the particular little face. Whenever I hear people argue for cloning on the basis of the dead-child theory of meaning, I think of M__ and I remember how I wanted to hold her like Elisha holds the young child in the Biblical text, throw myself upon her, breath her back, knit her cells back into life.

It is at this very moment, like her mother, that we need to look at death in its terrible beautiful white face and think of justice. As the resolute, obligated, doubtful bearers of the stories of grace and loss, we need to worry, not about playing God, or the towers we can make, or of how we can outwit the nakedness that we are born into, but about the slow work of repair that falls to us, bewildered, freed slaves holding the Law in our hands, meaning, not in the narrow place, but on the vast plain of the possible, set free with much to do.

III

PUBLIC POLICY ISSUES

9

Responsibility and Regulation: Reproductive Technologies, Cloning, and Embryo Research

CAROL A. TAUER

In the United States, public policy prohibits federal funding of research involving in vitro fertilization or preimplantation human embryos.[1] At the same time, it sets no limitations on research conducted in the private sector or on private provision of reproductive technology services. In this chapter, I will show why this twofold policy is ethically problematic and will argue that public policy ought to choose between the following alternatives: *(1)* support research and provide regulation of both research and clinical use of reproductive technologies or *(2)* require that untested reproductive technologies and unregulated services be abandoned.

I will discuss the parallel between the current impasse in public policy and the impasse in moral debate on human embryo research, showing that the moral debate flounders because of different views as to where the burden of proof lies. Do those who defend embryo research have to show why it is morally justifiable, or do those who oppose it have to show why it is morally wrong?

In particular, I will point out how the disagreement on the burden of proof arises in the debate on the issue of bringing embryos into existence for purposes of research. Because the demand for a principled justification of this practice arises partly from the belief that it is an innovative type of research, I will review the history of the creation of embryos in research.

The background of the problem: cloning and embryo research

The cloning of Dolly from a mammary cell of an adult sheep and the announcement by Richard Seed of his intent to clone a human child from an adult somatic cell stimulated intense public discussion of the ethics of cloning. These discussions necessarily led to renewed consideration of the ethics of human embryo research. For example, some legislative cloning bills had an attachment prohibiting human embryo research, while others indicated that such a restriction was not implied by the bill's prohibition of cloning.[2] These connections are not gratuitous; the ethical issues raised by human cloning are closely related to concerns about human embryo research.

First and foremost, it would be impossible to do research that might lead to the eventual birth of a cloned human child without doing human embryo research. A human child necessarily has as his or her progenitor a human embryo regardless of how the embryo came into being, through natural intercourse, in vitro fertilization (IVF), or nuclear transfer (cloning).

With both cloning and embryo research, there are strong differences of opinion as to the moral status of the material under study. The question of the moral status of an oocyte whose nucleus has been replaced by that of a somatic or body cell is similar to the issue of the moral status of an oocyte fertilized by sperm. Not only is this question unresolved, but there is disagreement as to whether the moral status question is the crucial issue. Perhaps we should be guided instead by other morally relevant aspects of the situation: the meaning of parenting and procreation, the symbolism of creating human life that may not be intended to come to fruition, or the effects such practices have on us as moral agents.[3]

The potential benefits from cloning research as well as from much human embryo research are somewhat hypothetical and will require long-term investments to be realized. The type of cloning research advocated most strongly by researchers and clinicians is research to develop cell lines and tissues that would be therapeutically useful for transplantation. This therapeutic potential has also encouraged attempts to isolate stem cells and to develop stem cell lines from embryos resulting from IVF. Until recently it was not known whether successes with mice could be duplicated with human embryos. In November 1998, however, researchers supported by the Geron Corporation succeeded in developing human embryonic stem cells from blastocysts donated by couples in infertility treatment.[4] The potential therapeutic usefulness of these cells will depend on substantial investments in further research.

Neither cloning nor embryo research may legally be funded by federal agencies, in particular the National Institutes of Health (NIH). In the case of embryo research, the prohibition is of long standing, stemming from the 1979 requirement that any such research must be approved for public funding by the Ethics Advisory Board (EAB), a body that existed only briefly from 1978 to 1980.

Although that requirement has been removed from federal research regulations, it has been replaced by a congressional prohibition inserted into the yearly NIH appropriations bills since Fiscal Year 1996. The prohibition of federal funding for human cloning research resulted from an executive order issued by President Clinton a few days after the announcement of the birth of Dolly.

Yet there are no federal restrictions on either type of research when carried out in the private sector. Extensive experimentation on reproductive technologies, most involving human embryos, occurs in clinics that treat infertile couples. Commercial firms may see promise in research involving human cloning or embryonic stem cells and may decide to pursue this research, as Geron has. A scientist like Richard Seed may choose to investigate the possibility of human cloning with whatever resources he is able to gather. None of this privately funded and privately conducted research is prohibited or even regulated at the national level in the United States.

There are, nevertheless, some ethical distinctions between cloning and embryo research. Because there is a widespread consensus that it is morally unacceptable (at least at this time) to attempt to create a child cloned from a somatic cell, the end goal of birth cannot be invoked to justify cloning research. In fact, all cloning research including animal cloning might be considered questionable on grounds that it could prepare the way for the eventual cloning of a human child. On the other hand, the birth of a healthy child resulting from the use of IVF and related techniques is the explicit goal of much human embryo research. Making such techniques safer and more effective is precisely the reason the research is proposed and conducted. This goal, the eventual birth of a healthy child, may be considered one of the strongest moral arguments to justify human embryo research.

The paradox of public policy

The Human Embryo Research Panel (HERP) that was commissioned by the NIH in 1994 to make recommendations on the ethics of embryo research concluded that research was ethically acceptable under carefully defined conditions and qualifications. However, while the panel's recommendations were unanimously accepted by the Advisory Committee to the Director of NIH, they were never implemented because of the congressional prohibition of funding for embryo research.

It is unlikely that the U.S. Congress will change its policies on support for embryo research in the near future. Moreover, an executive order from President Clinton specifically prohibits federal funding of research that includes the fertilization of human oocytes.[5] Although the NIH has not vigorously contested the congressional or executive bans, in January 1999 lawyers for the NIH determined that congressional language did not cover research involving already established embryonic stem cell lines. This decision presumably allows the NIH to sponsor and fund research programs to explore the therapeutic potential of these cells.[6]

Although there has been much public interest in ethical issues raised by cloning, and more recently by embryonic stem cells, there has been little public debate on embryo research related to IVF. When the use of reproductive technologies results in ethical scandals such as eggs and embryos donated without knowledge or consent of the progenitors, or in legal morasses such as the status of a child born to a surrogate mother under a contract with a couple who utilized donated eggs and sperm, then there may be public astonishment as to how these things could happen. On such occasions there is often a flurry of newspaper editorials and letters from readers urging public policies that clarify and regulate appropriate uses of reproductive technologies.

Yet these technologies remain unregulated in the United States, with the exception of some individual state laws that are spotty and inconsistent with each other.[7] The absence of regulation also applies to research aimed at improving existing techniques and developing new ones. It may seem strange that a federal government so bent on outlawing any use of federal funds for research involving IVF is at the same time so uninterested in regulating these procedures and research on them in the private sector. This stance could stem from a libertarian view of private enterprise (but note the comprehensive regulation of prescription drugs and medical devices by the Food and Drug Administration [FDA]) or from a political calculation. On such a volatile and divisive issue, it may be pragmatically preferable to avoid substantive debate by simply prohibiting federal involvement while allowing *laissez faire* in the private sector. Cynthia Cohen suggests that "those in office would rather avoid the commotion that open discussion of the regulation of infertility practices would create."[8]

It should be noted that one of the arguments supporting federal funding of human embryo research is the need for some federal regulation of these practices. The HERP was concerned about the absence of generally accepted ethical standards, and it regarded federal funding, which necessarily involves regulations and guidelines, as a source for such ethical norms. Even though federal regulations apply only to institutions that accept federal funding or to testing of products before FDA approval, experience has shown that once federal regulations are in place, they set the ethical standard for all human subjects research. The concern about the underregulation of reproductive technologies and IVF research strengthens the case for federal involvement in these practices.

The moral debate, moral justification, and the burden of proof

The current status of public policy in the United States is well established: no public support or funding for embryo research but no interference with research or other practices in the private sector. Apart from the NIH's decision on stem cell lines, attempts to question this status quo seem likely to be fruitless. Public policy is at an impasse.

A similar impasse appears to hold in moral debate on the topic of embryo research, and here the disagreement may also be irresolvable. This disagreement reaches to basic issues in the logic of moral justification.

In the logic of moral justification, a crucial question often is, Where does the burden of proof lie? For example, in debates about how animals ought to be treated, one side may argue that as living, sentient beings with their own interests, animals ought not be used for our purposes (for food, clothing, sport, and so forth) unless there is a justifying reason such as no other source of life-sustaining food. Others take for granted that animals are not persons and were given to us to be used for our ends, perhaps citing Biblical texts supporting this view. It follows that our moral responsibility is limited to not causing them unnecessary pain and suffering. Some may argue that even though the animals themselves have little claim on us, it would be detrimental to our characters as moral agents if we treated them cruelly or wantonly; in fact, such practices might incline us to eventual callousness toward human beings.

Those who see an intrinsic and not simply instrumental value in animals place the burden of proof for using them on those who eat meat, hunt, use animals in research, and so forth. Those who regard animals as "fair game" for our needs put the burden of proof for *not* using them on those who claim that animals have rights and intrinsic value. According to the first view, you ought not use animals instrumentally unless you can show that you have adequate moral justification. According to the second view, you are free to make use of animals unless someone can demonstrate that the practice is morally wrong.

While I emphatically do not hold that the moral status of preimplantation human embryos is analogous to the moral status of animals, I propose that the debate on our ethical obligations regarding human embryos gives rise to analogous positions in the logic of moral justification.

Opponents of embryo research have criticized the HERP report by complaining that it contains no arguments other than consequentialist reasoning to justify embryo research.[9] Setting aside the issue of whether and when consequentialist arguments provide justification for a moral position, these critics place the burden of proof on defenders of embryo research. They begin with the supposition that such research is ethically highly problematic, perhaps *prima facie* impermissible, and that a strong justification is needed to overcome this supposition. But if consequentialist justifications are out of bounds (no prospect of good consequences may be sufficient to overcome the *prima facie* prohibition), then some justifying principle is needed. According to critic James Keenan, neither the HERP nor authors such as Bonnie Steinbock, Dena Davis, and I have provided such a principle.[10]

On the other hand, those who regard (some) embryo research as morally permissible may view the burden of proof as placed elsewhere. The HERP members concluded unanimously that the preimplantation embryo did not have the moral status of a full human subject, and thus it followed that it did not require all the protections due to such a subject. Embryo research was not *prima facie* impermissible. Although panel members differed in their individual approaches to determining what research was or was not acceptable, for some members the panel's position that the preimplantation embryo was not a human being or person[11] implied that embryo research was *prima facie* morally neutral (see below). One would have to show that certain kinds of research were unethical or immoral in order to argue that they should be prohibited. Moreover, this demonstration could not rely on the claim that research caused harm to or violated the rights of an entity that not only was not a human being or person but also was not even a sentient or differentiated organism.

There is a long tradition in moral philosophy and theology positing the concept of morally neutral acts. John Ladd explains: It is not the case that what is not morally good is morally evil; rather, most acts and practices are morally neutral. According to Ladd, the burden of proof is on the person who claims moral significance for anything, and without some evidence of moral rightness or wrongness, the thing is to be presumed morally neutral.[12] This view accords with a long tradition in Christian moral theology, where most acts and practices are characterized as morally indifferent. In that teaching, if an act or practice is neither morally wrong nor morally required, then one is at liberty to do what one wishes.[13]

If one starts from the position that research involving zygotes or preimplantation embryos is *prima facie* morally neutral, then one asks for reasons why it should either be morally prohibited or perhaps morally required. If one believes that such research is generally impermissible, however, or *prima facie* morally wrong, then one asks for principled arguments to justify research or to override the *prima facie* prohibition.

No one could defend a wide range of embryo research projects if he or she believed embryo research was *prima facie* immoral. Overcoming such a presumption would likely require an exceptional justification, perhaps a justification such as the survival of the human race. Defenders of embryo research are more likely to begin from the stance that the research in itself is morally neutral and that those who claim it is not must demonstrate its moral impermissibility.

This is the reason why much of the literature that supports embryo research is devoted to what Keenan calls retortion, or refuting opposing views. This literature reviews arguments purporting to show that embryo research is immoral; if these arguments can be refuted, then there is no reason for defenders of research to change their position. Of course there may be another argument just around the corner, but until it is articulated, it cannot be taken into account.

The Permissibility of Embryo Research

To opponents of embryo research, it may seem inconceivable that such research could be viewed as *prima facie* morally neutral. Whether it is or not depends largely on the moral status of the preimplantation embryo, which in turn depends on the ontological nature of this entity. Although some authors argue that the moral issues at stake are independent of the status of the embryo itself, I believe these issues are subsidiary ones. Issues such as the significance of procreation and parenthood, reverence and respect for developing human life, the effects of practices on us as moral agents and as a human community: these issues can only be raised after one has resolved the status of the embryo itself. If the embryo is a person or human being, it must be treated as one regardless of other consider-ations. If the embryo is not a person or human being, then subsidiary questions may be raised to determine what is ethically appropriate treatment.

Over the past half century, a plentiful literature has developed on the question of whether the conceptus is a full human being from the time of fertilization. While the issue is certainly still debatable, there is no question that a wide range of scholars have taken the position that it is not.[14] Thus, this is an intellectually credible position to take, one that is even considered legitimate by Catholic Church authorities.[15]

Beyond asserting that the early embryo is not a person or human being, most of the cited authors argue that for the first few days after fertilization (approxi-mately up to 14 days) the embryo is not even a human organism or a human in-dividual. Thus its destruction cannot be considered the killing of a human indi-vidual. Its discard or demise involves the loss of a collection of human cells, the sort of loss that is ordinarily considered morally neutral. The level of life of these cells has been compared with the life that persists in the cells of a human body after a person has been declared dead, genetically human life but not the life of a human being.

Although the status of the preimplantation embryo may not be that of a human being or human individual, however, there may be other reasons why we should not permit research that results in the destruction of embryos or the loss of their capacity for further development. In Mori's words, "It is possible that the em-bryo ought to be protected in a significant way, even if it is not a person."[16] On the assumption that the embryo is not a person, however, the burden of proof falls on those who nevertheless advocate significant protection for it.[17]

The Impasse in Moral Debate

Although I believe that the preimplantation embryo is neither a human individ-ual nor the sort of entity that demands significant protection, others hold that the preimplantation embryo is a human being or person, or may be a human being or person, and hence embryo research is *prima facie* prohibited. For these persons, the burden of proof is on the reverse side, and any research must have a moral justification that overrides the *prima facie* prohibition. The weight of this prohibition would appear to be so heavy that only an exceptional justification could override its claims.

There is no way that these two views can truly engage each other. Opponents of research require positive principled arguments to justify research, while defenders believe their task is to refute arguments that claim to show that research is immoral. This impasse in philosophical discussion is strikingly illustrated in debate on one specific issue: whether it is ethically permissible to bring embryos into existence for research purposes. Debate on this issue is crucial to the development of public policy, so it must be addressed before returning to consideration of public policy options.

Bringing embryos into existence for research purposes

The Moral Issues

Is it ever permissible to bring human embryos into existence for purposes of research? This question is frequently distinguished from the more general question of whether embryo research is permissible. Some writers oppose the creation of embryos for research purposes while they do not object to the use of embryos that remain after infertility treatment has been completed. These embryos, often called "surplus" or "spare" embryos, are contributed to research by couples who have achieved their reproductive goals or abandoned them. The use of surplus embryos in research is defended by the argument that they were initially created for a procreative purpose for which they are no longer needed, and hence they may now be used for another worthwhile purpose. The ethical basis for this argument may be the nature of the original intention (where procreation is regarded as a legitimate goal for IVF, but research is not) or the necessity to choose the "lesser evil" (assuming that the existence of surplus embryos forces us to choose among undesirable options: discard, indefinite frozen storage, or research use).

In my study, "Bringing Embryos into Existence for Research Purposes," I considered whether there are morally relevant differences between embryos fertilized for research and "surplus" embryos that are later designated for research.[18] Any such distinctions cannot flow from differences in the ontological and moral status of the embryos themselves, because these differences do not exist. Hence, the burden of proof lies on those who propose other morally relevant distinctions; the validity of these distinctions must be demonstrated. If proposed distinctions can be refuted, then there is no basis for claiming that research with surplus embryos is permissible, while developing embryos as part of a research protocol is prohibited.

Once again the debate may be stymied by disagreement as to where the burden of proof lies. In addition, much wariness about the practice of creating embryos for research stems from a mistaken assumption: the belief that deliberately fertilizing oocytes or creating embryos as part of a research protocol is a new idea.

A Historical View of Embryo Creation

At the time that the HERP announced its narrowly qualified acceptance of the creation of research embryos, many ethicists, politicians, and the press denounced these guidelines as opening the door to a practice for which our society was not ready. A member of the panel, Patricia King, lamented the lack of conceptual schemes to guide its reasoning,[19] and President Clinton indicated that the American public would not be willing to support such research.

The assumption of novelty continues to be prevalent. For example, in his discussion of the development of embryos for research, James Keenan frequently uses the terms "new" and "innovative" to characterize this practice. In his view, it is largely because the practice is so new and so different from any research done previously that its justification requires principled positive arguments, not merely refutations of opposing arguments.

This assumption is, however, clearly erroneous. In fact, the entire history of the research leading to the first successful IVF is the history of attempts to fertilize oocytes in the laboratory. Eventually these attempts succeeded, and the first IVF baby was born, followed by thousands of others in the ensuing decades.

The ethics literature contains scholarly discussions as to whether it is ethically permissible to make use of medical advances that result from unethical research. This discussion sometimes focuses on medical research conducted by the Nazis in concentration camps and institutions for retarded, mentally ill, and handicapped persons.[20] Yet I have never seen reference to reproductive technologies in this context. If the fertilization of embryos in research is a practice that is abhorrent to many or most people, then would it not be logical to question the continuing use of the results of such research? (Even the Catholic Church, which opposes the use of IVF and most other forms of assisted reproduction, does not invoke this argument to support its opposition.[21])

Note the following historical facts: Robert Edwards, who achieved the first successful human IVF pregnancy and birth in 1978, began to study fertilization in 1951, and by 1960 he was working with human eggs. Edwards's main practical problem was obtaining human eggs, as he had to persuade gynecologists to provide him with ovarian tissue removed during regular surgical procedures. He could then use his own sperm and that of other researchers to attempt to fertilize the maturing eggs.[22]

Although no embryos resulted for some time, this research surely was research on the creation of human embryos. There was no plan to transfer any embryos that might have resulted. The women whose ovaries contributed the eggs for this research were not infertile and probably did not know what their surgically removed tissue was being used for.[23]

The first successful laboratory fertilizations occurred in 1968, fully 10 years before the birth of Louise Brown, the first IVF baby. Edwards reports: "We fertilized many more eggs and were able to make detailed examinations of the successive stages of fertilization. We also took care to photograph everything because we would have to persuade colleagues of the truth of our discoveries."[24] The results of this work, undeniably the creation of embryos as part of a research protocol, were soon published in *Nature*.[25]

Still there was no plan to transfer these embryos to women. First the embryos had to be studied in order to ascertain whether they could be cultured to develop normally in the laboratory during the first few days after fertilization. The scientists did not know whether those that reached the blastocyst stage "had normal nuclei or chromosomes," so embryos had to be flattened on slides (destroyed) in order to determine this. Only when the researchers were convinced that the development of IVF embryos proceeded normally would they even attempt to transfer embryos to infertile women.

What is the point of my detailing this historical background? To illustrate concretely that it was only through years of attempted and actual fertilizations in the context of research that IVF and related techniques became possible. This sort of research is definitely not new. If it is research that society considers seriously immoral, then our widespread acceptance of procedures that are direct outcomes of this research ought to be questioned.

The work of the Ethics Advisory Board (EAB) in 1978 and 1979 also confirms that the development of embryos in research is not a new idea. The EAB, charged to examine the ethics of IVF and IVF research, specifically addressed the acceptability of federal funding for such research. Although discussions took many twists and turns, the final outcome was approval of federal funding as ethically acceptable.[26] The EAB's acceptance clearly extended to research that involves the creation of embryos, as the *Washington Post* reported in its account of the board's final meeting:

The board voted . . . that both basic research and the actual creation of so-called test-tube babies . . . are ethically acceptable, if the final goal is to produce children for [couples] who are otherwise unable to produce them. Also, said the board, research that merely joins sperm and ova to create laboratory embryos can be acceptable, even if the new embryo is then destroyed . . . if the aim is either to learn how to implant such embryos safely . . . , or to gain "important scientific information." [27]

The board used the rationale that it would be unethical to offer IVF as a clinical option unless research affirmed its safety and efficacy. Since IVF clearly was being offered and would increasingly be available, the board concluded that research to validate the procedure was ethically permissible and possibly required. Arguments from scientists claiming that it was irresponsible to offer untested therapies carried the day.

Although the EAB's rationale has both logical and ethical problems, their conclusion shows that 20 years ago, a national level ethics board judged the creation of research embryos to be ethically acceptable. The EAB applied this conclusion only to research to establish the safety and efficacy of IVF, however, and refrained from making a statement regarding research that had other types of goals.[28]

The alternatives: regulate or abandon

The Absence of Regulation

The preceding section shows that the practice of developing embryos in research and the arguments supporting its ethical acceptability are far from new. We have had several decades of experience of the results of this practice, and, at least in relation to the clinical outcomes (i.e., the menu of assisted reproductive technologies), attitudes throughout society appear fairly positive. Attitudes are even more positive among infertile couples who have benefited from these procedures and within support organizations for infertile couples such as RESOLVE.

None of these techniques for assisting infertile couples to have children would exist unless extensive research, including research involving the fertilization of oocytes, had been performed. American public policy tolerates a situation in which medical procedures are widely available as a result of research that public policy neither supports nor encourages and in which such medical procedures are neither regulated nor adequately scrutinized for safety and effectiveness. According to Cynthia Cohen, "Technological innovations and practice in reproductive medicine . . . are proceeding according to no validated information and no social consensus in the United States. . . . This lack of regulation of infertility procedures stands in contrast to the situation of much of mainstream medical practice in the United States."[29]

Although some needed regulation is unrelated to research, for example, clarification of legal custody and rearing rights in situations in which various parties claim to be the "real" parents, other missing regulations are directly related to research. There are two types: *(1)* the requirement that reproductive technologies be subjected to valid, peer-reviewed study, whether they are new or simply have never been adequately assessed; and *(2)* regulations that set standards for the ethical conduct of IVF and embryo research comparable with other ethical standards for human subjects research.

At the first meeting of the HERP in February 1994, embryologist Jonathan Van Blerkom addressed the panel. Describing the state of science in the area of IVF and embryo research, he presented a dismal picture. Because such research was mainly conducted as a corollary of clinical infertility treatment and in privately funded clinics, it lacked both the scientific and ethical controls that agencies like the NIH provided for other medical research. Without the elaborate scrutiny of peer review that federal granting processes involve, shoddy research practices had evolved, and little basic research was being conducted. As a result, IVF and related technologies continued to be inefficient (low success rate), unnecessarily costly, and often associated with health risks to women and prospective children.[30]

The EAB had suggested in 1979 that it was unethical to offer procedures like IVF without first doing the research necessary to validate these procedures. When the federal government failed to act on this proposal, it would have been logical for it to choose the implied alternative. If it is unethical for these procedures to be offered without research to ensure their safety and efficacy, and if as a society we choose not to support this research, then it would seem to follow that we ought not permit their use within the practice of medicine.

After two decades of worldwide availability of IVF, it may be too late to consider outlawing its use together with the many procreative variations it has spawned. So the other alternative is regulation. Cohen suggests that reproductive techniques call for even more attention than other types of medical treatment because they are distinctly different: "The major purpose of use of new reproductive technologies is to create human beings, and only incidentally to alleviate infertility. Because we place special value on the procreation and welfare of children . . . we are obliged to ensure that use of these techniques is carried out safely and efficaciously."[31] In fact, such obligations constitute an expression of respect for the process of bringing new human beings into existence.

The *status quo* cannot continue. The alternatives are abandoning the use of assisted reproductive technologies if our society is unwilling to conduct public discussion leading to regulation and oversight; or a coordinated public policy that includes both regulation of clinical procedures and support of research to validate new and already available procedures.

As we are just beginning discussion of cloning research, stem cell research, and their applications, we have an opportunity to avoid mistakes we have made regarding IVF and related technologies. From the very beginning we need public debate as to what scientific advances our society wishes to encourage and which it does not, realizing that this debate will necessarily lead to public policies on how research ought to be conducted and what goals are ethically acceptable. Experience has shown that transferring responsibility entirely to the private sector, while it may promote innovation and entrepreneurship, is inadequate as ethical and social policy.

The Ethical Imperative for Research

The low success rate for IVF is still of great concern. According to the latest available statistics, most attempts (oocyte retrieval cycles) do not produce a pregnancy, and even fewer produce a live birth. In 1997, 70.5% of ART (assisted reproductive technology) cycles did not result in pregnancy. (The ART cycles include two other procedures besides IVF, but they are grouped with IVF because their numbers are relatively small.) Only 14.8% of the cycles produced a single live birth, while 9.2% resulted in a multiple birth.[32]

Research is needed to improve the success rate and to inform clinicians as to how to avoid this enormous wastage of embryos. Studies suggest that chromosome errors, inherited or arising during maturation of the gametes or during fertilization, may be a major cause of embryonic mortality. Yet embryos that are chromosomally normal, the ones that clinicians would want to choose for transfer, cannot be distinguished morphologically (through microscopic examination) from those that are abnormal. According to geneticist Mary Seller, research is desperately needed to determine a reliable and noninvasive method for the identification of chromosomally normal embryos so that it is they that are transferred rather than the abnormal ones.[33]

Women whose eggs and embryos may be chromosomally defective or otherwise incapable of developing into fetuses are being subjected to strenuous and risky procedures that are highly unlikely to achieve pregnancy. In addition, because there are presently no reliable methods to assess developmental capacity, a number of embryos are usually transferred to the woman in hopes that at least one will implant and develop. This practice is one of the reasons for the huge increase in multiple gestation pregnancies in the last 20 years.

In 1997, multiple births constituted 38% of all births in women using assisted reproductive technologies, compared with about 2% of births in unassisted pregnancies. Between 1980 and 1997, the number of twin births in general rose 52%, and the number of triplet and higher births climbed 404%. This enormous increase is attributed to two interrelated factors: older age at childbearing and the extensive use of fertility-enhancing therapies, which are more likely to be sought by older women who have had difficulty conceiving.[34]

Triplet and higher multiple gestations are high-risk pregnancies by definition; for example, infant mortality rates are 12 times higher for triplet births than for single births.[35] The rise in multiple births has had a direct impact on the number of low-birth-weight and preterm infants, whose rates have increased during the 1990s despite the success of other measures to prevent such deliveries. Rates of low-birth-weight, very low-birth-weight, and infant mortality are 4 to 33 times higher for multiple births compared with single births.[36] A multiple gestation pregnancy is also much harder on the mother, often requiring lengthy confinement to bed and cesarean delivery.

To avoid these risks when a high (greater than twins) multiple gestation pregnancy has already been established, couples may be offered "selective reduction," where one or more fetuses are terminated for the sake of the well-being of the others. This process is deeply morally troubling. Moreover, the choice is emotionally excruciating for a couple who sought infertility treatment because they desperately wanted to have children.

The HERP advocated research that would allow fewer embryos to be transferred in each cycle in order to reduce the chances of multiple gestation pregnancies and births. Diagnostic tests and therapeutic procedures such as correction of polyspermy during early cell division could enable clinicians to select "developmentally competent" eggs for fertilization and embryos for transfer.

Research thus would not only improve successful outcomes (efficacy) but might even be imperative in order to prevent harms (safety). Clinicians may be causing harm in the course of providing purely elective procedures. Some argue that if reproductive technologies cause harm, then they should not be used, even though some children will not come to exist and some couples will not become parents.[37]

Many of these harms could be avoided, however, if the necessary research were done before a new procedure was offered clinically. Embryologist Alan Trounson describes a striking example:

I argued strongly that the risks of serious chromosomal abnormalities arising from the freezing of unfertilized eggs did not warrant the introduction of this technique into clinical IVF. The frozen–thawed human eggs should first be evaluated as pronuclear eggs or pre-embryos before the technique was considered for use clinically. Others did not agree and went ahead and introduced the technique into clinical IVF. . . . Many publications have subsequently identified genetic and developmental problems in the freezing of unfertilized eggs.[38]

In October 1997, Dr. Michael Tucker of Atlanta reported the first birth to an American woman using embryos fertilized from frozen eggs. Although countless previous efforts worldwide had ended in failure and the handful of purported successes were poorly documented cases, Tucker claimed his clinic's success was "not a fluke." One wonders whether the woman who agreed to this attempt understood the risks noted by Trounson, given her comment to the media: "They told me they had not had any success with it before, but I didn't care. I wanted to get pregnant."[39] Until January 25, 2000, the British Human Fertilisation and Embryology Authority banned the use of frozen eggs for infertility treatment. At that time the authority determined that research had proceeded far enough to allow the use of frozen eggs at one licensed infertility center, with the proviso that women be fully informed of the risks and of the poor chance of success.[40]

A second example cited by Trounson is the fertilization of eggs by injecting one sperm under the zona pellucida or shell of the ovum (the intracytoplasmic sperm injection [ICSI] procedure). Trounson argued that the clinical studies needed for safety had not been conducted, even though the process was already in wide use in Australia and the United States.[41] A retrospective study of this procedure published in 1996 concluded that "the evolution of pregnancies and occurrence of congenital malformations following treatment by ICSI were within the range observed with standard in vitro fertilization."[42] The safety data were collected only after many years of clinical use of the procedure, however, and they relied entirely on transferred embryos and their future development rather than on chromosomal studies before implantation. Other studies now suggest that there may be a "slight but significant" increase in sex chromosome abnormalities as a result of the ICSI procedure.[43]

A third example is zona removal ("assisted hatching") for fertilized eggs that have shown an inadequacy to achieve this naturally. The prospect of contamination of an unprotected fertilized egg through exposure to the various components added to the culture medium is real but unknown.[44]

Cloning as a New Reproductive Technique

The previous examples all involve reproductive techniques in actual use even though scientists raise questions as to the adequacy of preliminary testing. New approaches being considered include applications related to cloning or nuclear transfer. For example, researchers are attempting to transfer the genetic material (nucleus) from immature eggs of older women into enucleated eggs of younger women with the hope of avoiding the chromosomal defects that often occur in attempted pregnancies of older women.[45] Although this process is a type of cloning (nuclear transfer), the resulting egg would still be fertilized by sperm.

Cloning that involves transfer of the genetic material of a somatic (non-gametic) cell to an enucleated oocyte has also been proposed as a treatment for infertility. An offspring that resulted from this procedure would be a genetic copy of the cell source, thus a "cloned" child. As a remedy for infertility, cloning the cells of one member of a couple might be viewed as a last resort, or it could be regarded as preferable to utilizing donated eggs or sperm when one partner has a fertility or genetic problem and the other does not.

The prospect of various applications of cloning adds to the menu of potential reproductive technologies. Issues regarding research and regulation are magnified as we imagine private providers developing and offering these applications, which, in the case of somatic cell nuclear transfer, are truly new technologies with new ethical and social implications.

The Other Alternative: Abandon Assisted Reproductive Technologies

On the assumption that IVF and other assisted reproductive technologies will continue to be offered and new ones devised, on the supposition that these infertility treatments have become too much a part of our social fabric and expectations to be withdrawn, then there is an obligation to provide the regulation and research that would ensure their safety as well as their ethical practice. There is a different alternative, however, and that is to question the initial assumption. All of the high-tech reproductive techniques are purely elective; we do not have to use any of them. They do not combat life-threatening diseases or lessen the risk and pain of chronic diseases. In fact, they do not even treat the condition of infertility in the sense of correcting its physiological causes. Rather, they propose to bypass these conditions and to achieve a pregnancy without remedying the underlying functional deficiencies.

In an essay in *Embryo Experimentation*, the alternatives are starkly enunciated: "Cease using these techniques (even though they could become validated if proper testing were permitted) or do the necessary embryo research to validate procedures before transferring embryos created in that way to women."[46]

If the choice were presented this way to politicians and the public, I believe their reaction would be different from what it is currently. Rather than a moratorium on federal funding of IVF research, we would have a moratorium on clinical use of high-tech infertility treatments, or at least a moratorium on every procedure that goes beyond basic IVF (using an unstimulated hormonal cycle, partner gametes, and one embryo transferred at a time). Although success rates and qualifying candidates for this basic procedure may be low, the unknown risks and harms of other protocols would be avoided until appropriate studies of safety and effectiveness could be conducted.

As someone who is highly skeptical of the burgeoning practice of high-tech treatment for infertility, which involves both scientifically and socially questionable practices, I could support a moratorium on procedures whose risks and outcomes have not been adequately studied. (Here I include practices like surrogate motherhood as well as technologies like IVF.) Minimally, experimental practices should be permitted only within the context of research studies or as part of a clinical trial to test their safety and effectiveness.

Conclusion

American public policy finds itself at an impasse regarding embryo research and reproductive technologies. Federal funding of infertility and embryo research is highly unlikely, and thus the regulation and safeguards that would accompany such funding are equally unlikely. It is also unlikely, however, that the provision of new and as-yet-untested reproductive technologies, including applications of cloning, will be curtailed at the federal level.[47] Because it is both ethically and scientifically unacceptable to offer elective procedures whose safety and efficacy are in question, and because adequate testing is unlikely without federal funding and federal mandates, we have a situation in which society as a whole has simply decided not to take responsibility.

Whose responsibility is it then? The guidelines of professional societies like the American Society for Reproductive Medicine are helpful, but tend to be more a description of current practice than definitive norms. Also, their implementation depends on the professional integrity of individual practitioners because the guidelines have little force beyond voluntary compliance. The National Advisory Board on Ethics in Reproduction (NABER) was founded in 1991 to provide an independent forum for consideration of ethical issues on topics such as egg donation, the use of fetal oocytes, and the commercialization of reproductive technologies. After 7 years of substantial research and publication, the NABER went out of existence in early 1998 due to lack of adequate funding.

One of the NABER's continuing recommendations was formation of a national supervisory body that would develop and implement regulations on reproductive technologies. The NABER suggested a structure similar to the British and Australian models and the proposed Canadian commission.[48] Lori Andrews concludes her strong plea for a government oversight body authorized to license fertility clinics and carry out regulatory functions by asking the fundamental question: "We need to give serious thought to whether our *laissez-faire* market mechanisms are the best determinants of how children should be brought into the world."[49]

10

Consensus, Ethics, and Politics in Cloning and Embryo Research

JONATHAN D. MORENO AND
ALEX JOHN LONDON

Within hours of the announcement that scientists in Scotland had succeeded in cloning an adult sheep by a method that subsequently became known as *somatic cell nuclear transfer* cloning, the President of the United States asked the National Bioethics Advisory Commission (NBAC) to examine the legal and ethical issues associated with the use of this new technology. The advent of cloning is remarkable, therefore, not only because of the possibilities it presents for the cloning of adult humans, but also because of the speed with which a public bioethics body was commissioned to evaluate the social, ethical, and political ramifications of these possibilities.[1]

The alacrity with which the NBAC was charged with examining this new advance is an example of the growing role of bioethics panels in America's civil life. It is also emblematic of the institutional character that public bioethics has taken on in recent years. As we develop these institutions, however, and as their voices come to play an increasingly important part in our moral and political deliberations, we need to look critically at the role that such groups can and should play in our civic life. We need to scrutinize our expectations of the ability of such bodies to grapple with and to settle important and often divisive issues. In particular, the public, and the members of these bodies themselves, should understand both the nature and the limits of the contribution such bodies can make to public debate.

In what follows we address these issues by examining the work of two such public bioethics committees, the NBAC and the Human Embryo Research Panel (HERP). Both of these groups were commissioned to deal with issues raised by reproductive technology, issues that are of enormous importance and about which heated and often divisive debate persists. As such, their work represents the latest bout in the ongoing struggle to understand the role of reproductive research and technology in our communal lives. Nevertheless, even though they dealt with very similar issues, these two groups faced very different challenges both in the course of their individual deliberations and in fulfilling their role as public advisory groups. As a result, the experience of each exemplifies the complexities and pitfalls that characterize the intersection of ethics and public policy making.

To highlight and then to assess the ways in which these groups dealt with the different challenges they faced, we will examine their work within the larger framework of the role of consensus in public bioethics. The goal of achieving consensus is ubiquitous in bioethics and often structures the deliberations of such groups as well as the way they present the results of their deliberations to the public. After offering some brief remarks about the role of consensus in bioethics in general, we will examine the work of the HERP and the NBAC and argue that the current focus on consensus as an end point for such committees is a good one. Furthermore, we will argue that the central function of such advisory committees should be to help in the formulation of stable and fair public policy and that such bodies go wrong when they try to present their findings as moral arguments. In the end, we hope that this investigation will shed important light not only on the role of consensus and the importance of compromise in public bioethics but also on the kinds of expectations that it is reasonable to have for the work of public bioethics.

Consensus as closure and as concealment

Elsewhere one of us (J.D.M.) noted the ubiquity of appeals to consensus in bioethics.[2] Whether in academic settings or in the media, the importance of reaching consensus on a vexing bioethical problem is a common assumption. One cause and consequence of bioethics' consensus orientation is that it is an applied field that spurred (or, perhaps, consolidated) reform in the informal rules that govern physician–patient relations: The defeat of "paternalism" in the social ethics of medicine is often attributed to the triumph of bioethics, whether accurately or not.

Another factor that makes bioethics friendly territory for consensus is that bioethics as a social institution manifests itself in a variety of small group settings, including ethics committees and commissions. Although the conclusions of these groups are always subject to analysis and critique, groups both small and large tend to value moral consensus as a primary indication that deliberation may cease, and ethics panels are no different. Not only ethics panels but also groups formed for countless purposes have good reason to value consensus, whether their primary concern is relevant to moral values or not. Particularly in enabling individuals to work together for highly complex objectives that are widely recognized as value laden, moral consensus operates as a kind of lubricant of social relations.

To be sure, there are alternatives to moral consensus as an end point, including a determination only to identify issues and the evidence and arguments in support of various positions. Ethics panels appointed by government agencies— an important source of the current prestige of bioethics—rarely, however, have the option of operating like a public graduate seminar. Their very *raison d'etre* is, after all, to help resolve some policy problem, not merely to clarify it. Moreover, to the extent that it is possible, resolution implies that panel members must achieve consensus among themselves and create a conceptual framework that can help build a public consensus.

The goal of achieving consensus within an advisory body and then working to extend that consensus to the public at large was explicitly embraced by the leadership of the President's Commission on Ethical Problems in Medicine and Biomedical and Behavioral Research (1980–1984). The President's Commission was the most ambitious instance of a government ethics panel before the NBAC (which began its work in 1996), and both the chairman and executive director described and defended the commission's commitment to finding consensus whenever possible. In at least one case, the report on access to health care, determination to reach consensus is said to have nearly caused a serious breach between the staff and several more conservative commissioners.[3] The most basic criticism of the President's Commission in this regard, however, came from Jay Katz, who pointed out that reports of group consensus tend to paper over interesting and sometimes important disagreements. In a revealing response, Chairman Morris Abram argued that a commission's only weapon in the effort to see its recommendations realized is persuasion, which would presumably be impaired if too much was said about internal disputes on the way to consensus.[4] We will have more to say about the demands of consensus building in a moment.

Ethics panels and the professionalization of bioethics

In retrospect, the President's Commission was given a broad range of issues to consider, from genetic engineering to informed consent to resource allocation. The commission's bioethical expertise was provided mainly by its staff. Subsequent government bioethics panels have, however, been charged with more targeted, if no less ambitious, goals, and the membership itself has included a healthy dose of experience in bioethics. This was true in the mid-1990s of presidential advisory committees on human radiation experiments and Gulf War veterans' illnesses, as well as the NBAC itself, which immediately established focused subcommittees on genetics and human subjects research. About half of the membership of the HERP included individuals who have been recognized as "ethicists" at one time or another in their careers. This development reflects the increasingly specialization and professionalization of bioethics. Accordingly, one can expect that many of the tacit assumptions in the field of bioethics will find their way into the consensus of these panels.

The background consensus of bioethics as a professional field includes many propositions that are not always well articulated. Some, such as the moral right of personal autonomy, are often stated, but in a policy context a commitment to autonomy also implies a commitment to pluralism, especially in a multicultural society like the United States. In turn, pluralism carries with it some implications for decision-making processes, such as diversity of representation. These details are important because pluralism is much more likely to be satisfied in an ethical framework that involves "weighing" or "balancing" various views than in one that emphasizes a relatively uncomplicated moral imperative. Thus, among Western ethical traditions, theories that derive from utilitarian, empiricist, and mercantile sources (*weighing* and *balancing* are metaphors borrowed from the marketplace) are more likely to find their way into the consensus of ethics panels than theories based on deontological, rationalistic, and religious sources. Along these lines, ethics panels freighted with these background assumptions are likely to view ethical standards from faith traditions as useful insights and reference points, but not as decisive owing to their particularistic origins.

We offer these observations about the consensus background of bioethics for two reasons: First, to make the point that in general one can expect to see certain patterns of reasoning issue from bioethics panels as the professionalization of the field continues; and second, to prepare the way for understanding why the HERP was driven to adopt a pluralistic ethical framework even though, as we shall shortly argue, it abandoned this framework when expressing the results of its deliberations.

There should be nothing startling in these observations about the background consensus of bioethics or the way it operates. H. Tristram Engelhardt, Jr., essentially made this point when he observed that bioethics has become a kind of *lingua franca* of modernity, and this has occurred not only within the professional field but also in public discourse about ethical issues.[5] Along with the increasing professionalism of bioethics and the increasing use of technical language in the conduct of bioethical inquiries comes a more or less distinctive set of presuppositions that set the framework for discussion.

To make the latter point as clearly as we can, the "public" bioethics that takes place in such contexts as government ethics panels is not ethics. It is policy making with ethical deliberation as a necessary but not sufficient condition. The conceptual frameworks developed by these panels should not, therefore, be presented as ethical in anything like the way that ethical arguments are presented in academic journals. To do so misstates the case, undermines the consensus-building function of ethics panels, and leaves them open to charges that their ethical framework is unsound. We will elaborate on the way this problem applies to the HERP when we look at the relationship between the way in which the panel arrived at its own internal consensus and the very different way in which it tried to encourage external consensus.

Distinguishing compromise and consensus

The bioethics literature tends not to distinguish between the concepts of consensus and compromise. Yet there are important differences that are easy to overlook because both concepts are processual in nature, a fact that is concealed by the popularity of these terms as nouns, as in "reaching a consensus" or "settling on a compromise." Once the processual nature of consensus is recognized, it can be seen that there are certain preconditions for success, including "formal" conditions like mutual respect among the parties and "substantive" conditions like agreement on certain facts that characterize the problem.

Compromise takes place when disputing parties "split the difference" between irreconcilable points of view,[6] but consensus need not involve that kind of bargaining. Rather, consensus in the full sense may take place, and consensus processes are at their most vibrant, when parties are genuinely uncertain as to the right course of action and through a deliberative process come to some generally acceptable conclusion. The "genuine uncertainty" of which we speak need not be a Rawlsian veil, nor does it demand that the parties come to the table unfettered by any prejudices or self-interest or even prior views. Rather, it requires a seriousness of purpose, authentic doubt about the best outcome, and openness to alternative points of view. Although it is surely possible to expect too much of consensus processes,[7] we believe that this is the kind of posture expected in the "real world" when we assess one another's sincerity in the midst of a problematic situation that seems to require a difficult choice. It is exemplified in the Biblical injunction, "Come, let us reason together."

Internal and external consensus

Ethics panels may engage in two kinds of consensus building, one having to do with their internal dynamics and a second with their external environment. Internally, some ethics panels may arrived at a decision through majority rule rather than through consensus. Technically, Institutional Review Boards can operate on a majoritarian basis, and at least a few hospital ethics committees and even government panels may do so. In the main, however, consensus seems to be the preferred arrangement, for several reasons. As a more ambiguous standard than majority rule, consensus helps preserve the group's internal amity, especially important if the panel is not ad hoc and its members know they will probably have to work together for some time.

Consensus may also be preferred to majority rule owing to the kind of issue at stake. If the issue is seen as a moral one, many people are uncomfortable with the idea that one vote more than half can "decide" an ethical issue. Rather, our society, at least, seems more comfortable with the idea that the morally right course emerges from the joint deliberation of well-meaning people. Institutions will often go to great lengths to maintain at least the appearance of a deliberative model in what are perceived as ethical questions. It is interesting that the only committee of the United States House of Representatives that does not have a majority of members from the party in power, but have rather an equal number of members from each party, is the ethics committee, as though structuring a committee with such a name according to partisan lines would be too obviously unseemly—even for Congress.

Ethics panels and external consensus

Whether a panel operates according to a consensus orientation or not, it needs also to be aware of its relationship to its external environment. Some panels are expected to help build a consensus within the public from which it is drawn, as though its deliberations are surrogates for those that might be conducted if the whole society could fit into a single hall, like a New England town meeting. Perhaps government-appointed ethics panels tend toward consensus because the panel's internal consensus processes are easily conceptualized as the society's consensus processes writ small: How can the society be expected to reach a consensus if the panel can only achieve a majority? Ethics committees or task forces appointed by professional organizations, on the other hand, may not have the same persuasive function and may feel less obliged to operate according to consensus, although they may do so anyway for reasons of collegiality.

We will not dwell here on what has been called the "authority problem," namely, how the conclusions of consensus-oriented ethics panels come to deserve a stature to which society defers. This tough issue in moral epistemology turns on whether the moral authority of consensus resides outside the consensus activity or whether it emerges from the nature of consensus processes themselves.[8] However one treats the authority problem, in the case of government-appointed "expert" panels on ethical issues moral authority in itself is probably not going to be enough to bring a commission's proposals to realization. Depending on the issues, a heavy dose of political sophistication is required of those who seek to shape government policy by building a moral consensus external to the panel.

One cannot generalize about the relative importance of internal versus external consensus building in ethics panels. Circumstances determine the task at hand. For example, a local hospital ethics committee that happens to include many of

For example, a local hospital ethics committee that happens to include many of the most powerful members of the staff and administration may worry little about shaping opinion in the rest of the institution, so seriously are its recommendations taken. The same may be true of a national ethics commission composed of influential figures working mainly on issues that are not terribly divisive and at the behest of an agency eager to receive and to begin to implement its proposals. Such circumstances offer the group the luxury of focusing on internal processes rather than worrying about persuading officials or the public at large.

The circumstances of many other ethics panels, however, offer no such luxury. Congressional and presidential advisory bodies (and many more local ones) are likely to be characterized not only by diversity of internal opinion (at least at the beginning) but also by the challenge of consolidating public opinion about matters that are often arcane and complex. Relevant to this phenomenon is a special form of consensus building that can be called "consensus extending." In such processes, the deliberative body identifies views or values that are known to be already widely held and attempts to infer from them some other views that should also be acceptable to the public. One advantage of this strategy is that it avoids confronting the potentially divisive main issue head on and instead attempts to find clues that might yield a justifiable resolution likely to find public acceptance. As we turn to the HERP report, we will see that it adopts this strategy by noting the public's acceptance of three propositions: the importance of research, the serious moral consideration due preimplantation human embryos, and the need for federal review of research with embryos. As we will also see, however, by failing to appreciate the nature of its own contributions, the HERP was unable to fully extend its own internal consensus.

Compromise, consensus, and ethics in the human embryo research panel

Despite some disagreement, the HERP committee members generally concurred that acceptable research included methods for improving the possibility of pregnancy, fertilization, egg activation, egg maturation, egg freezing, preimplantation genetic diagnosis, and the development of embryonic stem cells. Cloning egg cells without transferring them to the uterus was deemed to require further review, and cloning and experimenting with egg cells and then transferring them was deemed unacceptable research.[9]

To its credit, the HERP made clear where there was only a narrow majority, especially in its discussion of which categories of preimplantation embryo research are "acceptable" for funding by the federal government, which require further review, and which are unacceptable (pp. 75–83). Three individual statements were also appended that express reservations some members had about specific recommendations and provide further insight into the HERP's deliberative process. Yet the main body of the report was evidently phrased carefully sought to preserve consensus by enabling members to formulate individual statements that were appended to the text, thus providing members with enough flexibility that they did not feel they had to dissent from the report as a whole. It is also important that the statements were not called "dissents," as they well might have been, which would have somewhat impaired what was in the main an appearance of solidarity. In this respect, the HERP achieved both consensus and openness.

We believe that, once the HERP members reached their internal consensus on the moral justifiability of human embryo research, they adopted the right conceptual framework to advance its view. That framework stressed a pluralistic justification for human embryo research within carefully drawn limits and attempted to respect the view that all fertilized human eggs have some moral status. In determining that the potential benefits of embryo research to women, children, and men outweighed the preimplantation embryo's moral standing, the HERP settled on what might be called a "consensus compromise," an agreement on one way of attempting to respect multiple principles. The HERP also navigated the problem of overselling its own consensus by acknowledging its unease about some issues, such as that on the deliberate creation of "spare" embryos for research. For these accomplishments and more, the HERP is to be commended.

Unfortunately, because the role of such bodies in building moral consensus is not well understood, the HERP faltered at one sensitive point: It seems to have felt obliged to present an ethical argument in support of the view that some embryo research may take place rather than a policy argument with ethical implications. In actuality, the panel did not present an ethical argument, although it said it did. Like others, we are critical of the way in which the panel's proffered conceptual framework was put forth as the result of an ethical argument, but we approve of the framework as the basis of a policy argument. The latter sort of argument has the burden of building consensus in the actual sociopolitical environment external to the panel, a burden that an ethical argument may not have.

In especially controversial matters, consensus in the full sense may be impossible because parties may come to the table with prior views that are fixed. The HERP was fated to be unable to formulate a consensus in the full sense (at least not one that would be acceptable outside the HERP), because some members of our society hold a fixed position on what counts as the beginning of personhood. Although the HERP might have reached a full internal consensus on this point, the unwillingness of large portions of the population of the United States to change their position on such matters meant that the panel could not achieve an external consensus on behalf of society as a whole.

Furthermore, because the HERP's recommendations do not accept that human life with full moral standing begins with the union of sperm and egg, compromise was inevitable. Because many Americans hold the view that full moral standing begins with conception, the best the HERP could have done is to achieve a ing begins with conception, the best the HERP could have done is to achieve a consensus compromise. For this reason, despite the depth of experience of its members, the HERP may have misjudged the political environment when it recommended that the creation of research embryos should be permitted. Not only did this judgment detract from the HERP's internal consensus, it presented an easy target for critics of the very idea of human embryo research. Instead, the HERP could have merely indicated that it did not find the objections to this practice to be conclusive. Not wanting to appear to engage the abortion issue at all, the HERP attempted instead to argue that no single ethical criterion for resolving the problem of the embryo's moral status is up to the job. As we shall show, however, their argument was not an ethical one, and thus the central issue—coming up with a consensus when there could not be full consensus—was somewhat obscured.

Despite our general approval of the tone and execution of the HERP's report, it includes an unfortunate confusion that illustrates the importance of a better understanding of the role of ethics panels and the nature of the consensus process in which they engage. What is especially unfortunate about this confusion is that it is utterly unnecessary, for it occurs only in the chapter that deals with "ethical considerations," not in other chapters.

The panel's chapter on "Ethical Considerations in Preimplantation Embryo Research" is presented as an ethical analysis grounded in values that underlie consensus ethics, such as an appreciation of cultural pluralism and moral diversity. A careful reading, however, shows that it is not an ethical analysis; rather, it is a policy analysis. That is, the chapter is not "an assessment of [the preembryo's] moral status" (p. 40), as it purports to be, but an assessment of how a pluralistic society can best encompass various views about the pre-embryo's moral status. Thus, although the chapter is in fact a consensus-oriented analysis, it presents itself as a standard ethical analysis, thereby masking the important policy work it attempts to do.

To see this, one need only consider the way the chapter contrasts what are called *single criterion views* of the moral status of the human embryo with what are called *pluralistic views* of its moral status. In any subject matter, single criteria are almost sure to be too limited to do the conceptual work required of them (what is the single criterion for being a work of art or being a rock?) or more complex than the word "single" suggests (the third "single criterion" for personhood mentioned is that of "well-developed cognitive abilities" [p. 37]). The single criterion approach seems to have been created mainly to do the rhetorical job required of it in the HERP report's narrative.

If the reader did not already have a sneaking suspicion that the single criterion approach is a loser, he or she could simply turn the page and learn that the pluralistic approach "emphasizes a variety of distinct, intersecting, and mutually supporting considerations." Happily, a pluralistic approach can embrace a num-

ment, sentience, brain activity, and degree of cognitive development."
Unfortunately, as the text acknowledges, none of these is by itself a sufficient
condition for personhood, but together "at some point" they give an entity full
moral status and entitlement to "protectability" (p. 38).

The report then considers "implications for public policy," noting that
Americans hold "widely different views" on the moral status of prenatal life and
that the goal of public policy is "a reasonable accommodation of diverse interests," taking into account "the diverse moral sensibilities that exist in the community." Pluralistic views are said to do this better than single criterion views because the former "is less subject to the specific criticisms leveled at each of the
single criterion views" and "corresponds with the steady increase in moral respect many people give to prenatal life in its various stages from conception to
birth" (p. 40).

The first supposed advantage of pluralistic views is again a rhetorical one that
might be called "safety in numbers": The more criteria are included in a framework, the more likely the framework will survive criticism. The second alleged
advantage is the correspondence of a pluralistic view with what "many" think
about the issue. Neither advantage mentioned is part of an ethical analysis. Both
are strategic, in terms of likelihood of public embrace of a certain approach, and
meta-ethical, in the sense that these advantages range over and characterize different ways of attempting to gain a widely acceptable theory.

We have said that the HERP report's pluralistic framework is not a moral argument, but rather an effort to build a consensus compromise through a policy
argument with ethical implications. In other words, one might say that the HERP
was attempting to formulate a story about the human preimplantation embryo
based on themes with which most Americans could feel comfortable, including
that preimplantation embryos have some moral status. Although a few will not
be happy about the way the story comes out, their reservations, however grave,
are not supposed to undermine the general satisfaction with the story. That, at
least, is the hope.

Thus, the chapter on "Principles and Guidelines for Preimplantation Embryo
Research" states in its introduction:

Throughout its deliberations, the Panel considered the wide range of views held by
American citizens on the moral status of preimplantation embryos. In recommending public policy, the Panel was not called upon to decide which of these views is correct. Rather,
its task was to propose guidelines for preimplantation human embryo research that would
be acceptable public policy based on reasoning that takes account of generally held public views regarding the beginning and development of human life. (p. 65)

This statement reflects an appreciation of the need to extend the public moral
consensus to embryo research by calling on well-established views in other areas
so as to formulate a consensus compromise on embryo research. Because the report's "ethics" chapter confuses the nature and purpose of its pluralistic frame-

port's "ethics" chapter confuses the nature and purpose of its pluralistic framework, however, it is open to the charge that it fails as a moral argument, as indeed it does.

In their criticism of the panel's report, George Annas, Arthur Caplan, and Sherman Elias point out that, for the framework to explain how moral standing is conferred on embryos, it must explain why the particular properties included in the framework confer moral worth. The report does not do that, and so it fails as a moral argument. Annas, Caplan, and Elias argue that "inability to define the moral status of the embryo convincingly is the crucial failure" of the report and is also why so many Americans have reservations about embryo research.[10]

The panel's framework would have been less open to criticism, in our view, if it had announced its aim as frankly consensus oriented rather than as an effort to assess moral arguments. All of the elements of the former sort of presentation are in the report, such as reference to the nation's cultural pluralism and to its diversity of moral and religious beliefs, and they are summarized well elsewhere in the text.

The confusion between formulating ethical arguments and developing an intellectual basis for consensus building appears even in the executive summary, which states: "the Panel concludes that sufficient arguments exist to support the permissibility of certain areas of research involving the preimplantation human embryo within a framework of stringent guidelines." (p. x) On the approach we recommend, it would state, "the Panel concludes that, taken as a whole, our society's moral values support the permissibility of certain areas of research involving the preimplantation human embryo within a framework of stringent guidelines." Again, the emphasis is on the panel's analysis of the values of the society of which it is a part, not on its judgment from on high.

The HERP's charge permitted the approach we suggest. According to the report's executive summary, "its task was to propose guidelines for preimplantation human embryo research that would be acceptable public policy based on reasoning that takes account of generally held public views regarding the beginning and development of human life" (p. ix). A consensus-building strategy would emphasize those "generally held public views" more than a moral analysis based on those views, for the latter is almost sure to be subject to criticism on philosophical grounds. An account that hews closely to "generally held public views" accentuates description rather than prescription.

Some might see our position on this matter as political in the prejorative sense of cynical manipulation of the policy process and that we also want to take the ethics out of bioethics. These criticisms would misunderstand our view, which is not that ethics is dispensable but that public bioethics is, like it or not, a public policy creature. The goal of deliberating about public policy is to make public policy. In this instance, because a consensus in the full sense was not in the cards, it might have been better to see the job as one of formulating a consensus com-

Consensus building about a compromise that involves a moral view deeply held by some members of our society is bound to be a messy business. The alternative is to stick close to the seminar room and to refrain from engaging in public bioethics concerning controversial issues like those pertaining to human reproduction. Some may prefer this locale, but, for better or for worse, bioethics is in fact a player in the policy arena, and it is not clear that it can pick and choose its issues. Calling a framework an ethical argument when it is not, however, is no solution.

Compromise, consensus, and ethics in the National Bioethics Advisory Commission

Unlike the President's Commission, say, the NBAC was charged with the narrow task of evaluating a single new and relatively untested technology. In its report, the NBAC concluded that the cloning of human beings by means of somatic cell nuclear transfer was morally unacceptable at this time because of the unacceptably high risks posed to the resulting fetus and child. As a result of this consensus, it recommended a continuation of the existing moratorium on the use of federal funds for human cloning and called for a moratorium on all somatic cell nuclear transfer cloning with the intent of creating a child. It also called for the inclusion of a "sunset" clause so that at the end of a 5-year period these issues could be re-evaluated by a suitable oversight body and the moratorium either rescinded, augmented, or reinstated.[11]

Although the questions surrounding the cloning of human beings may be no less controversial than those surrounding embryo research, the NBAC was able to reach a clear consensus without having to engage in any form of compromise. This fact, however, is not the result of our having made substantial progress on these issues since the HERP convened in 1994. Nor is it the product of widespread agreement on the illicitness of cloning human beings. Rather, it is the result of the relative lack of information about the safety of somatic cell nuclear transfer. The judgment that somatic cell nucleus transfer cloning is morally unacceptable was built on the "virtually universal concern regarding the current safety of attempting to use this technique in human beings."[12] As we will see later, the NBAC did not seriously engage with the more substantive questions concerning the acceptability of cloning humans as such. Had it done so, it is highly likely that it would have found itself in much the same situation as the HERP. As a result, the NBAC report may not suffer from the same shortcomings as that of the HERP, but, as we will see, the NBAC report raises important issues concerning the role of such panels in its own right.

As we noted earlier, there was no need for compromise within the NBAC because it readily achieved an internal consensus on the problem of safety. For this reason, some have hailed the NBAC report as a "significant achievement" not only because it was able to reach a consensus on a controversial issue within the reason, some have hailed the NBAC report as a "significant achievement" not only because it was able to reach a consensus on a controversial issue within the allotted 90-day period but also because the report makes a concerted effort to lay out the relevant moral topology and to provide a kind of prolegomenon to the national conversation about the licitness of cloning human beings that it hopes will follow in its wake.[13]

The NBAC should be commended for taking seriously its role as a consensus-oriented, public policy–centered body. For instance, it justifies the considerable attention paid to the views of various faith traditions concerning the licitness of cloning humans by noting that an acceptable public policy will have to be not only morally justifiable but also politically feasible. Any public policy that runs counter to the deeply held beliefs of these religious traditions will likely be the subject of widespread opposition, thereby possibly running afoul of the feasibility requirement.[14] Similarly, in its section on "Legal and Policy Considerations" it admits that

Members of the Commission could not come to a common evaluation of each of these [moral and theological] objections, as they are partly speculative, partly theological, and partly based on particular values or world views that are commonly, but nonetheless not universally, shared by all Americans. On the other hand, the collective force of these objections makes a strong prima facie case for a political judgment that creating a child in this manner would violate the deeply held views of many Americans.[15]

Although moral and theological questions are important, the NBAC is forthright in its view that such considerations must be integrated within a political framework that includes the disparate views of a pluralistic, democratic community. These arguments may not establish the conclusion that cloning humans is unacceptable, but their prevalence within the larger community represents an important factor that must be taken into account by any feasible political judgment.

As laudable as these accomplishments are, however, a much less sanguine view of the NBAC report sees them as being purchased at the price of a larger social responsibility. Not only did the NBAC not attempt to forge a consensus around ethical and social issues other than safety, but, as one member has put it, "Consensus on the safety argument meant, however, that NBAC did not have to try to resolve the larger debate about the probable impact of acts and especially widespread practices of human cloning on social values that are not reducible to harms or wrongs to individuals."[16] From the narrow perspective of its immediate charge, this is true; once the safety issue was settled, the NBAC could make a recommendation without becoming mired on volatile social, ethical, and theological issues.

Nevertheless, where the HERP was forced to engage in what we have called the consensus-extending process, the NBAC demurs, and its unwillingness to grapple with more substantive questions concerning cloning as such has led to a some underlying issues at the heart of the debate about cloning. The NBAC's report puts itself forward as beginning a national debate that needs to ensue if we are to come to a broader consensus about the appropriate uses of this new technology. What kind of contribution to this national debate, however, does the NBAC's report really make?

When it comes to issues other than safety, the NBAC's report reads more like a fact-finding study than a document with normative import aimed at shaping public debate or public policy. In some cases, the facts that were uncovered are genuinely important. For instance, it is significant that there already seems to be a consensus in various faith traditions that a child who resulted from the cloning process would not be diminished in its humanity and would be entitled to "the same moral protections that already apply to other persons created in the image of God."[17] This is a fact about the beliefs of major faith traditions in this country that has significant normative import. Because it did not have to engage in a process of consensus compromise or consensus extension, however, this fact is left largely unexplored. Similarly, when it comes to issues of greater disagreement, the report is often content simply to note the existence of controversy, the nature of the relevant disputes, and to move on.

Thus, although the report notes that there are a number of complicated and conflicting views on many difficult issues, it does very little in terms of suggesting how public policy should be shaped by these debates or even to suggest strategies for confronting these issues so as to make the creation of a workable public policy more feasible. This is unsatisfying for those who are well versed in the nuances of these debates as well as for those who are not, but who are looking to the report for normative guidance. As the question of safety recedes into the background, the NBAC's report has relatively little to contribute to the shape of the national debate. This is not to say that the NBAC should have tried to provide substantive answers to the thorny moral and political questions lurking just beyond the safety issue. It is simply to say that the report could have gone some way toward shaping the context in which this debate should occur.

For instance, because it does not attempt to set out the framework of a consensus-extending process, the NBAC report is open to the charge that it deals with somatic cell nuclear transfer cloning outside of the broader context in which it arose and within which it would be utilized.[18] This is, after all, one new reproductive technology among many, and dealing with it as an isolated innovation obscures the fact that the field of reproductive technology is itself in need of serious regulation and review. We have learned to adapt readily to the scientific advances we have achieved in this century, and some have already begun to wonder how long it will take before the outrage over the possibility of cloning humans will seem "as misguided as medieval bans on dissecting cadavers in medical schools."[19] If human cloning is just an incremental step beyond what is already being done with the array of fertility drugs, in vitro fertilization, artificial

ical schools."[19] If human cloning is just an incremental step beyond what is already being done with the array of fertility drugs, in vitro fertilization, artificial insemination, and our extant practices of genetic manipulation, then it will become increasingly difficult to see why cloning should be singled out for special regulation once we become more adept at, and inured to, the cloning of sheep, cows, and monkeys. In fact, one worry that many people had about the use of cloning, the creation of a delayed twin, has already been partially realized through the use of existing reproductive technology. Using one of her own frozen embryos, a woman gave birth in February 1998 to a baby boy born 7 years after its non-identical twin brother.

Noting the analytical similarity between cloning and our existing fertility enhancement practices, Laurence Tribe cautions against using the law to condemn or outlaw certain "patterns of human reproduction." He argues that "to ban cloning as the technological apotheosis of what some see as culturally distressing trends may, in the end, lend credence to strikingly similar objections to surrogate motherhood or gay marriage and gay adoption."[20] Tribe is worried about the effects that a ban on cloning will have for the children who may result from illicit use of the technology. Whether these are legitimate reasons to regulate rather than ban cloning remains to be seen. We submit, however, that these are legitimate worries about the possible effects of undertaking a piecemeal regulation of individual reproductive technologies. The point is not that cloning's similarity to our existing reproductive technologies should allow it to be utilized as freely as they are. It is rather that our concerns about cloning should be expressed in the context of a thoughtful deliberation about our use of reproductive technologies in general and that what should be avoided is not the banning or regulating of patterns of human reproduction per se, but the ad hoc way of making public policy that will result from considering individual reproductive technologies in isolation from one another.

Had the NBAC attempted to provide a normative framework in which the debate about cloning should be conducted, it could have done so by placing this new technology within the proper social context and thereby served as a catalyst for a long overdue examination of the use and regulation of reproductive technologies as a whole. This should not be taken as the rather unrealistic objection that a commission with 90 days to make its recommendations should have tried to tackle these broader problems as well as the question of cloning human beings. It is, rather, the more realistic charge that had the NBAC included a chapter in which it tried to forge the beginnings of this national conversation it could have set out the basis of a normative framework in which this conversation should occur and at least gestured at the way that a feasible consensus or consensus compromise might be reached. Although this may have been the more politically daring path, done well, it may have also been the more socially beneficial.

Having said this, however, it is not clear whether these dissatisfactions should the lesson of the HERP is that public bioethics bodies should recognize the political nature of their task and recognize as one goal that of forging a workable public policy, then the lesson of the NBAC report is that, if we are going to look to such bodies for guidance, it will be necessary to give them the time that it takes to engage in the messy business of building a workable consensus.

11

Morality, Religion, and Public Bioethics:
Shifting the Paradigm for the Public Discussion
of Embryo Research and Human Cloning

BRIAN STILTNER

Public ethics bodies play a major role in the development of public policies that govern scientific research and health care.[1] Their tasks include weighing the ethical ramifications of forms of research, educating the public about the research and its likely benefits, and recommending directions for institutional practices and legal policies. Much debate about public ethics bodies has concerned the mode and level of their ethical reasoning. Should public ethics bodies develop substantive moral arguments on issues that are subject to widely divergent moral and religious interpretations, such as the status of the human embryo? To develop such arguments would, of course, require ethics panels to consider the ethical and philosophical arguments about the status of the embryo as well as arguments about the dignity of the human person, the symbolic and social value of procreation, and so on. Is this something we should expect ethics panels to do?

The question can be framed thus: Should public bioethics committees develop substantial moral arguments or make only procedural arguments about the competing interests involved? Ethics bodies wrestling with these controversial questions face a quandary: To what extent and in what way should they attend to the pluralism of moral and religious views in society? If an ethics body is sensitive to such views, even the most common ones expressed in the society, and seeks to rely on them for insight, it will have a difficult time drawing these multiple threads into a unified conclusion that can speak to all citizens. Yet if the ethics body limits its engagement with moral and religious views in the hopes of delivering clear recommendations acceptable to a broad public, it runs the risk of antagonizing various interest groups and perhaps a large segment of the public who expect to see the report firmly grounded in moral or religious principles or both.

To explore this question, this chapter considers how moral and religious arguments were employed in the reports of two bioethics committees: the 1994 report of the Human Embryo Research Panel (HERP) and the 1997 report on human cloning of the National Bioethics Advisory Commission (NBAC). Through a reading of the ethical sections of the HERP report, I will explore the tensions between the substantive and procedural modes of ethical argument. Although the HERP commendably developed an ethical framework to guide its policy recommendations, its framework is pulled between the competing demands of the two forms of argumentation. The panel hoped to avoid the policy-making stalemate it thought would occur if it put forth a substantive argument concerning the moral status of the human embryo. Its thought was that such an argument would then be contested by citizens opposed to embryo research for substantive reasons, and there would be no way to resolve these differences in a political forum. In my view, not only does this strategy not work, but the report displays the panel's confusion about the kind of argument it was making. Indeed, the panel makes substantive arguments about the embryo, but wants to keep these arguments immune from the contest of substantive debate.

After discussing the HERP report I will consider the NBAC's exploration of religious arguments about cloning. The commission exhibits far less skittishness than the panel about engaging substantive arguments; indeed, it explores religious traditions as sources of insight for the policy debate. Yet the same problem is evident in the NBAC report: The commission does not make clear what role these particular moral arguments should play in policy formation, nor does it persuasively connect these arguments to its own recommendations, which take a largely procedural tack. Both reports are hampered by an outlook that seeks to constrain public bioethics either to procedural arguments alone or to a certain kind of substantive argument that tries not to rely on any particular moral or religious worldviews.

I will argue that it is misguided to drive a wedge between substantive and procedural modes of argument, since they have a natural and necessary connection to each other and tend to work best in conjunction. As an alternative to the two committees' approaches to public policy, I outline a different model—a common good approach to policy formation in which procedural and substantive argument each have a place. I suggest that public ethics bodies can use religious arguments and perspectives as a legitimate resource for policy making in four ways: by reflecting back the arguments and values that citizens use in making up their minds on issues, by showing how religious considerations would support or undermine various policy options, by appreciating that religious groups play an important political role both when they challenge a reigning social consensus and when they support it, and by envisioning concrete roles for religious organizations in the public debate.

In the common good model, particular religious and moral traditions are seen as potential contributors to public debate instead of divisive voices to be excluded. To develop such a model is by no means simple. In general, this model would pluralize and broaden policy discussions extensively; it views bioethics committees less as definitive decision-making bodies and more as the generators and synthesizers of a wider public debate. This process of policy formation will be slower and more chaotic than other options; yet in the long term it is likely to be both more effective and more beneficial to the public good.

The double-bind of the Human Embryo Research Panel

The HERP was charged with sorting through the scientific, therapeutic, and ethical questions associated with federal funding of research in preimplantation human embryos. Harold Varmus, the director of the National Institutes of Health (NIH), asked the panel to assess the types of research that should and should not be acceptable for federal funding and to propose any warranted guidelines for research beyond those already in place.[2] The HERP's charge was thus fairly focused both as to the scientific subject matter (research on the preimplantation human embryo) and as to the scope of guidance sought (in what forms and under what conditions such research could be funded).

The HERP report makes sure to note the limited scope of the charge; in particular, research with in utero fetuses and fetal tissue transplantation were outside the panel's scope, for these matters are already forbidden federal funding.[3] At the same time, "Panel members were given wide latitude in identifying the specific issues and questions that needed attention and the approach they would take in analyzing and addressing them."[4] Therefore, while commentators should resist criticizing the HERP for not addressing issues outside its purview, they may justifiably criticize or praise the ethical, political, and scientific framework by which the panel analyzes the issues, for these were matters of the panel's choosing.

My interest here is with the ethical framework that underlies and justifies the HERP's recommendations and how that framework is thought to relate to the broad range of moral views in the United States. The panel identifies three major ethical considerations under which it finds certain forms of preimplantation embryo research acceptable.[5] First, the prospect of significant scientific and therapeutic benefits provides a strong reason to pursue and fund promising areas of research. Second, the human embryo "warrants serious moral consideration as a developing form of human life," but, as its moral status is not on par with an infant or adult, this consideration should guide and limit embryo research rather than ban it altogether. Third, because embryo research will occur with or without federal funding, it is better that the government involve itself by providing funding, to which it may then attach conditions and restrictions.

What are the theoretical justifications for these ethical considerations? The fundamental goods the HERP seeks to promote are (1) human health, to be achieved especially through the correction of diseases and the removal of impediments to physiological functioning; and (2) personal autonomy, to be facilitated by ensuring informed consent in research, protecting patients from unwarranted health risks, and promoting procreative liberty. Hence, we notice a primary stress on individual rights and well being. These goals are advanced in a public policy framework that is largely consequentialist: It involves weighing benefits against risks and then determining the policy that will produce the best overall balance of results. The framework is not thoroughly consequentialist, for sharp boundaries are set by individual rights (the rights of bodily safety and procreative liberty are strong in this framework), while softer limits are set by public sensitivities over such matters as the moral status of fetuses, the nature of families, and the integrity of procreation. Communal needs have only a weak role in this framework; they appear most notably through the concern for public sensitivities. The public's health stands in the background of the whole analysis, for the advances made through research can potentially benefit any member of society. Yet all of these claims about communal goods are weakly defended, if at all. No attention is given to such issues as the just distribution of health care resources, what the nation's research priorities should be, how embryo research might improve the health and well-being of children and families as a whole (rather than as individuals), and how the public can become further involved in these deliberations.[6]

Having examined the general ethical framework of the HERP report, let us look at how it handles particular moral viewpoints. Several important ethical issues are implicated in such research, including the protection of human subjects, the right of reproductive liberty and its scope, the aspirations and well-being of infertile couples, the needs of persons with genetic illnesses, justice in the distribution of medical resources, and many others. Yet by far the most sensitive and contentious issue the HERP had to face was the moral status of the human embryo. The American public exhibits a wide range of ethical opinion on this issue. In light of the strong feelings and organized political support for the pro-life cause, the panel had good reason to fear that its recommendations would be drawn into the political fray over abortion. The panelists tried to avoid this result by the way they went about their task. They maintained a narrow focus on the preimplantation embryo, deferring to existing protocols and laws regarding the postimplantation embryo. Also, they invited and listened to pro-life representatives in their public hearings, perhaps to convey their appreciation that there are strong pro-life concerns about this research.

As can be expected, the panel's desire to sidestep the abortion issue influences its ethical argument. Let us briefly look at the HERP's identification of a principle of moral concern for the human embryo that is worthy of increasing respect over the course of its development. The panel finds problematic many substantive determinations of the embryo's status, namely, those that determine moral personhood according to a single criterion. Single criterion approaches propose one characteristic or power of a human being, possession of which is sufficient for moral personhood and moral protectability.[7] The panel gives the most attention to the criterion of possessing a unique diploid genotype, which a human embryo has once fertilization is complete; this view is more popularly expressed as the conviction that personhood begins at conception. Many other qualities can serve as a single criterion, such as the presence of brain activity, the ability to feel pain, or the possession of well-developed cognitive abilities. The panel briefly describes the conceptual problems that each of these proposed criteria face if established as the sole sufficient criterion for moral personhood.

The panel prefers a second broad approach to establishing moral personhood, a pluralistic one. This approach "emphasizes a variety of distinct, intersecting, and mutually supporting considerations. According to this view, the commencement of protectability is not an all-or-nothing matter but results from a being's increasing possession of qualities that make respecting it (and hence limiting others' liberty in relation to it) more compelling."[8] The HERP uses this framework to affirm all of the previously mentioned qualities and others, too, as relevant to appraising the increasing moral status of the fetus over the course of its development. Moral respect begins minimally with fertilization and increases gradually "until, at some point, full and equal protectability is required." The HERP does not say where that final point is, because it does not need to: For its purposes, the preimplantation embryo clearly does not meet enough criteria to warrant protection against research. Nonetheless, the panel feels that for public policy purposes, some clear line is needed as a time limit after which preimplantation embryo research may not continue. The panel established the time of the appearance of the primitive streak at 14 days as that limit. This characteristic is not a firm marker of moral personhood, but it does mark a new developmental stage, after which neural material (a physical condition for sentience) begins to develop. Based on this ethical factor and other considerations, the HERP settled on the 14 day time limit "as a compromise among competing viewpoints."[9]

Now compare these reflections on the embryo's status with the HERP's stated desire to remain neutral with respect to various views about that status:

Americans hold widely different views on the question of the moral value of prenatal life at its various stages. These views are often based on deeply held religious and ethical beliefs. It is not the role of those who help form public policy to decide which of these views is correct. Instead, public policy represents an effort to arrive at a reasonable accommodation of diverse interests. To the extent possible, it takes into account the diverse moral sensibilities that exist in the community. Even constitutional reasoning acknowledges the importance of diverse but deeply held views. Public policy employs reasoning that is understandable in terms that are independent of a particular religious, theological, or philosophical perspective, and it requires a weighing of arguments in the light of the best available information and scientific knowledge.[10]

According to this paragraph, the panel wishes to establish bioethical policy with an appreciation of moral diversity, but on the basis of publicly accessible reasons. Is this statement of principle compatible with the argument for moral respect? Can the panel assume a stance of respect for the embryo while remaining neutral about its moral status?

We must first note that the paragraph above is not an aberration. Both in the cover letter to the final report and in its Executive Summary, the HERP claims that it was not called on to adjudicate among competing understandings of the embryo's status and that it did not try to do so.[11] The panel is at pains to make this claim for neutrality. Yet it is undeniable that the HERP's recommendations are guided in large part by its ethical analysis, an analysis that includes an examination and interpretation of competing views of the embryo's status. The panel's ethical judgment, in essence, is that the preimplantation embryo deserves some respect, for it has the potential to acquire the characteristics that will eventually grant it moral personhood; yet it is impossible to specify how much respect, except to say that it is more than no respect at all and something less than the full moral respect due to a (born) person. Beyond this general determination, the HERP believes that it has no special knowledge or authority such that it could ask all Americans to accept its view of the matter. So, indeed, the HERP is *not* refusing to take a stand on the moral status of prenatal life; it is *not* neutral about this matter.

This reading fits with the panel's actual ethical analysis, for the panel makes philosophical arguments about why the single criterion view is inadequate, why the embryo is certainly not a person just after fertilization, and why the appearance of the primitive streak marks a time of increased value of embryonic life. Then what are we to make of the panel's statement, "it is not the role of those who help form public policy to decide which of these views is correct," and its other claims to neutrality? To alleviate the inconsistency, the HERP would have to modify one of its two trains of argument. Either it is making a philosophically grounded, ethical argument about the status of the embryo, judging as it does that some moral arguments are better than others; or it is only engaged in the task of balancing competing interests fairly, having no need to develop an argument that the embryo deserves a measure of moral respect.

Part of the inconsistency can be attributed, no doubt, to the fact that the report was developed by a committee of persons with different expertise and ideas—a common enough occurrence and one on which we need not dwell. Yet I also sense a fundamental lack of clarity on the part of the panel about the very nature of the argument it wants to make. What we find in the report is a mixture of substantive and procedural argument. By "argument" I mean a mode of reasoning that articulates and justifies an opinion on a moral issue and a related mode of discourse that explains such reasoning to others so as to demonstrate that the opinion is justified and could command the others' assent. Let me explain how such arguments operate.

A substantive argument reasons about values and principles and then applies them to the issue at hand, seeking a substantial resolution of the ethical matter. Substantive arguments may work from any number of particular religious and philosophical traditions. For instance, substantive responses to the question of embryo research could be developed from Roman Catholic natural law theory and Catholic teaching regarding the protection of unborn life, from Jewish teachings on medicine and the status of the fetus, from a Biblically based Christian perspective, and from any other religious perspective. Likewise, substantive answers could be derived from the frameworks of liberalism, communitarianism, libertarianism, Marxism, feminism, and many other philosophical schools and traditions. What makes any given approach substantive is the conceptual framework from which it is advanced: if that framework involves comprehensive accounts of human beings and what is of value to them, including nonpolitical goods and values, then that framework is substantive.

An alternative is to eschew the moral questions that are essentially based on particular worldviews and to take a procedural approach to the policy questions. A procedural mode of argument weighs the expected benefits and potential harms for all parties involved and tries to come up with a solution that is just. A strong form of procedural argument holds that questions of justice (how to maximize benefits to the public while being fair to all affected parties) and questions of procedure (whether the decision-making process is democratic and fair) are the only considerations for public ethics bodies.

Where does the HERP report fit? It is clear that the panel marshals ethical considerations in favor of its recommendation to fund some embryo research. Is the form of its ethical argument substantive or procedural? R. Alta Charo, a panel member who unsuccessfully argued in favor of its taking a procedural approach, later termed the panel's method "deductivism," the process of reasoning from an ethical theory—or, better, from philosophical principles that are not beholden to any particular philosophical method—to specific applications. She finds this method flawed:

The usual deductivism of public bioethics is doomed in the absence of an agreed methodology for resolving conflicts among competing ethical theories. Indeed, the deductivist form of public bioethics becomes most useless precisely when it is most needed, i.e., when fundamental principles grounded in faith-based moral systems (e.g. the sacredness of human life) conflict with appeals to empiricism and consensus-based values.[12]

In short, the panel makes an ethical argument that it hopes will not mire it in adjudicating among diverse ethical values—a project Charo thinks is sure to fail.

Charo proposes an alternative method that seeks a purely procedural approach. In what she calls a "political ethics analysis," a public ethics body such as the panel should deem the question of the fetus's status irresolvable in a pluralistic public forum. Rather, it should weigh the interests of "already born members of the population" and ask "whether ethical principles of justice require that one or another of their interests be given preference."[13] A political ethics analysis considers the harms and benefits that are likely to attend different policy options. The weighing will consider medical benefits and harms as well as the emotional and political ramifications on all interested parties. For instance, a committee should be concerned with the pain that will be felt both by infertile couples if fertility research is stymied and by pro-life–oriented citizens if embryo research is approved. In such an analysis, the particular moral viewpoints *do* matter—not to establish a substantive position (the status of the fetus), but because they affect the interests of those who hold them.

The balancing should also consider to what extent the interested parties have access to the means to fight for their viewpoint in the public forum. Political ethics is concerned with the vitality of the political process and fairness to all interested parties; hence, Charo maintains that this approach would give greater deference to the views of those who lack the political strength to defend their interests. In this way, political ethics is quite unlike political pragmatism.[14] With Charo's argument in mind, one can easily see her influence in those passages of the HERP report that abjure taking any stand on the moral status of the embryo. Because the panel did not embrace fully the political ethics approach, however, it exacerbated the sense of indetermination between the two approaches.

Some commentators, while agreeing with Charo that the HERP tried to make a substantive argument and did not succeed, render very different advice to the panel. George Annas, Arthur Caplan, and Sherman Elias believe that the HERP got caught between its need to address the status of the embryo and its desire to avoid becoming a judge of substantive moral viewpoints. In their view, the way out of the bind would have been for the panel to offer a fully developed, substantive moral argument. They write:

The reason the panel's recommendations have been more or less ignored has little to do with its generally reasonable conclusions. Rather, in our view, it is because the panel did not make a persuasive moral case for the conclusions. Unless a strong moral framework is presented that recognizes and addresses the concern of those troubled by the use of human embryos for research, such research is unlikely to gain the political acceptance needed for it to receive federal funding.[15]

For these authors, the panel persuasively made the basic claim that the embryo does not have rights at the moment of conception or during its early development. Yet they take issue with the HERP's use of the pluralistic approach, for they find that the panel did not give sufficient argument to make this framework convincing:

[T]hat framework requires a detailed analysis that explains why the particular properties cited confer moral worth, or to what degree each property cited is necessary and sufficient. Without such an underlying rationale, the framework looks like an attempt to rationalize a desired conclusion—namely, that some research on embryos ought to be permitted—rather than to derive a conclusion from an ethical analysis.

. . . Without knowing why certain properties count, we cannot draw clear boundaries between acceptable and unacceptable types of research. From a pluralistic perspective, we cannot tell whether it is right to prohibit research after the primitive streak appears at 14 days' development. Why should research on older embryos not be allowed, if it would benefit other embryos, fetuses, children, or adults?[16]

Annas, Caplan, and Elias put forth this argument precisely because they want to see valuable research in this area go forward: They believe that the political terrain of abortion is so sensitive that an argument for embryo research has to be carefully disentangled from the abortion debate. That cannot happen unless a "strong" and "persuasive" moral argument is made; moreover, this argument should be one that takes account of citizens' moral qualms and convictions.

Until it is demonstrated that embryos are owed moral consideration, concern about the ethics of research on embryos can be dismissed as "nothing more than fights over symbols." However, such curt dismissals completely fail to respond to the deep moral reservations about such research held by many Americans, including the President. By adopting a bald political compromise on a moral issue, the panel guaranteed that its report would have no effect.[17]

At the end of this quotation, Annas, Caplan, and Elias cite the article in which R. Alta Charo advances her criticism of the HERP report, although it is not clear to what extent they are affirming Charo's analysis. Certainly Charo would not agree that the panel should have made a fuller substantive case for the embryo's status; on this matter she advocates an approach closer to political compromise. Except for their suggestions that the panel needed to display greater sensitivity to those citizens who are troubled by embryo experimentation, these two interpretations of the HERP report stand opposed. Listening to such criticisms, the panelists might well feel, as the old saw puts it, that they were damned if they did and damned if they didn't. Charo criticizes the panel for trying to make a substantive moral argument *at all*; Annas, Caplan, and Elias fault it for not making *enough* of a substantive argument; and various politicians, interest groups, and citizens complain that it made the *wrong* substantive argument. Clearly, the HERP was subject to many expectations and could not have hoped to please everyone, yet the double-bind I have identified—that the HERP wanted to eschew substantive argument but ultimately could not—was of its own making. So what could the panel have done differently?

I suggest that we do not have to choose between the substantive and procedural approaches. Indeed, I doubt that we can. For procedural arguments about justice necessarily depend on a deeper level of substantive reasoning about the persons and the community involved. Debates about justice may *focus* on fairness, but they are never *simply about* fairness. We cannot truly know what it means to be just unless we have some idea about who counts as a member of the community that is trying to set up fair procedures and unless we have some vision of why it matters to be just in the first place. To have some idea about these matters, one has to reason within a substantive ethical framework, or at least be prepared to appeal to one. Certainly not every discussion and debate about justice in our society has to delve into these fundamental questions, but we ought to be aware that procedural arguments ride on the shoulders, as it were, of substantive arguments and agreements.

In arguing about justice and public policies with our fellow citizens, we will often find it unnecessary to appeal to our substantive frameworks. Yet it happens that impasses are reached when all sides know that the source of disagreement lies at the substantive level. At these times, the debate is not advanced by the parties continuing to push their claims about procedural rights. I agree with Annas, Caplan, and Elias that what is needed at these times is not less substantive argument, but more. In the third section, I will develop an approach to public policy that brings together the two approaches in a coherent and mutually strengthening fashion. Before proceeding to that, I will explore in the next section how the NBAC intimates a more promising approach in its report on human cloning by exploring, in much greater depth than does the HERP, substantive ethical and religious perspectives on the technology in question.

The more promising approach of the
National Bioethics Advisory Commission

The NBAC's work was similar in many ways to that of the HERP.[18] Both panels held a series of public meetings during which they discussed the general approach they would take to the issue, heard from members of the public and various experts to inform their deliberations, and, through a process of delegated writing, group editing, and voting, produced reports of approximately 100 pages. Similarly to the HERP, the NBAC tried to focus its questions and method of proceeding so that the issue could be effectively addressed. The NBAC chose to focus on the specific question of the propriety of cloning a human being through somatic cell nuclear transfer with the goal of creating a child. Like the HERP, its report contained chapters surveying the scientific, ethical, and policy issues.

There are instructive differences between the two bodies as well. Unlike the HERP, the NBAC also devoted a chapter to religious perspectives on the issue. The NBAC tended to survey a wider variety of pro and con perspectives on the use of cloning and did not push to come to a definitive resolution of most of the major questions. In large part because the issue of cloning was so new (or at least seemed to be), the NBAC did not feel able or required to make strong policy recommendations. In a way, the commissioners were trying to say: Both the public and experts have not had enough time to think the issue through; therefore, to speak of a public consensus on most of these matters would be premature. At the same time, however, they recognized an operative public consensus on a few fundamental issues: (1) The issue is new and needs to be discussed and investigated further and (2) our lack of knowledge about the safety of cloning indicates that the technology should not be used to create human embryos, especially with the aim of bringing them to term.

In this section, I will argue two points: that the NBAC's engagement with substantive moral frameworks, particularly religious frameworks, makes a fresh and useful contribution to the public debate about cloning, but that the NBAC puts itself in a bind similar to the HERP's by failing to provide a thorough rationale for its ethical recommendations. I will develop these claims by exploring the NBAC's treatment of religious arguments about cloning.

A distinctive feature of the NBAC report, in contrast to reports by the HERP and other public ethics bodies, is that the commissioners devote a chapter to religious perspectives. This chapter, the third in the report and roughly as long as the chapter on ethical considerations that follows it, surveys cautionary and affirmative arguments about human cloning in Western religious traditions. Christianity (both Catholic and Protestant), Judaism, and Islam are the focus of attention, although the commission also looked at Eastern religious views during its research. The NBAC opens this discussion by noting three reasons for investigating religious views at all.[19] First, it is important to look at religious views because these inform many citizens' opinions, and they can be a source of enrichment in the broad public debate. Second, the commission wanted to see if religious reasons overlap with secular reasons and might thereby contribute to a rough social consensus on certain matters. Third, the NBAC realizes that the strength of religious views in opposition to a policy may make that policy unenforceable; hence, there is a practical need for policy makers to know which policies citizens are willing and unwilling to support, and why.

The report goes on to explore at some length broad theological themes in Western religions, such as human beings as creatures of God, responsible dominion over creation, human dignity, and the meaning of procreation. The report presents the range of interpretations given to these themes and applies them to cloning. A complex picture develops. On the one hand, several fundamental beliefs in Judaism, Christianity, and Islam caution against cloning and condemn a variety of motives that would lead to its use. On the other hand, some interpretations within all three religions suggest the possible propriety of the technology for certain reasons and within certain limits. The NBAC summarizes the positive and negative assessments:

Specifically with regard to cloning humans to create children, some religious thinkers believe that this technology could have some legitimate uses and thus could be justified under some circumstances if perfected; however, they may argue for regulation because of the danger of abuses or even for a ban, perhaps temporary, in light of concerns about safety. Other religious thinkers deny that this technology has any legitimate uses, contending that it always violates fundamental moral norms, such as human dignity. Such thinkers often argue for a legislative ban on all cloning of humans to create children. Finally, religious communities and thinkers draw on ancient and diverse traditions of moral reflection to address the cloning of humans, a subject they have debated off and on over the last thirty years. For some, fundamental religious beliefs and norms provide a clear negative answer: It is now and will continue to be wrong to clone a human. Others, however, hold that more reflection is needed, given new scientific and technological developments, to determine exactly how to interpret and evaluate the prospect of human cloning in light of fundamental religious convictions and norms.[20]

The NBAC does not try to show whether some religious arguments are better than others, saying that such assessment would be beyond its competency and purview, but tries rather to understand better (and to help Americans understand better) the diversity of religious views. The commission comes to the conclusion that "the wide variety of religious traditions and beliefs epitomizes the pluralism of American culture. Moreover, religious perspectives on cloning humans differ in fundamental premises, modes of reasoning, and conclusions. As a result, there is no single 'religious' view on cloning humans, any more than for most moral issues in biomedicine."[21]

It is certainly true that there is no single religious view on cloning humans, only various religious views. The NBAC suggests that its proper role is to survey these views, but not to employ them substantially in its own evaluation. The reason, apparently (for the NBAC never says as much), is that such use would put the commission into the difficult and controversial position of judging which religious interpretations of human cloning are best. How can it do that in light of the wide diversity of views within American society and within religious traditions themselves? How can it do that and still respect the right of citizens to hold any religious or irreligious views they wish?

My first approach to this question is to note that the investigation of religious arguments plays a more significant role in the commission's analysis than it admits or perhaps even realizes. Consider its five key recommendations, which are presented in the Executive Summary of the report. The religious views surveyed, especially on the matter of human dignity,[22] certainly contribute to the consensus on caution and the mandate to ensure the safety of children and all human subjects before any research may proceed (recommendation I). The temporary ban on funding recommended by the NBAC (recommendations I and II) fits with religious calls for banning or significant restriction on the use of cloning.[23] Most religious views are supportive of genetic research for the purposes of therapy and basic scientific knowledge,[24] so these views would likely support the narrow purview of such a ban (recommendation III). The NBAC explicitly cites the pluralism of religious and ethical views in its call for a national dialogue (recommendation IV). It is not clear from the chapter on religion whether participation in public dialogue is important to religious groups themselves, yet we may surmise that being able to participate in the public debate matters to those religious groups, scholars, and citizens who make public statements on issues. Finally, the need for more public education about cloning (recommendation V) is mentioned as an activity that religious thinkers support.[25]

The way the NBAC employs religious perspectives corresponds to the rationales for investigating them in the first place. For one thing, religious views can and do enrich the ethical and political discussions about cloning. Religions such as Judaism, Christianity, and Islam bring long-standing theological and legal traditions to bear on biomedical problems. Religious views can supply important overarching visions to the debate: Some generic ones that emerge in the three religions are the sanctity of human life, the value of nature, human responsibility to care for nature, and warnings against human hubris and shortsightedness. To be sure, these visions are not definitive foundations on which to draw up scientific policy, and policy makers must be careful in how they rely on religious arguments in their decisions. Yet these visions can be very valuable just because they present an alternative way of looking at things: They may press into the debate a consideration of values—such as the well-being of vulnerable persons or the quality of society's common good—that have not been given their due in the discussion up to now.

Religious views can also be valuable in their contribution to a broader public consensus, which is the NBAC's second rationale for exploring religion. Here we see that the religious traditions studied, whether they find human cloning unacceptable or potentially acceptable, all raise a basic concern about the safety of human subjects. The NBAC found that this was an ethical consideration that establishes common ground between religious and secular perspectives, as well as between multiple religious perspectives themselves.

The NBAC's third rationale for listening to religious views was that policy makers might better understand the political feasibility of proposed policies. The public dismay that would be caused by government support for a technology such as human cloning is a "social cost" that must be placed in the cost/benefit equation considered by policy makers. The connection to religion is that religious communities might be the locus of strong opposition to particular biomedical policies, as some have proved to be in the past. With this angle in mind, the NBAC concludes that the tenor of religious opinion in the United States moves against human cloning, although this opposition is not monolithic. As far as reception by religious groups is concerned, the NBAC's recommendation for a temporary ban with a sunset provision could be seen as trying to satisfy both clusters of religious opinion—those against and those cautiously for cloning.

The benefits of attending to religion are encompassed, the NBAC believes, in these three rationales. Are these benefits enough, however, to justify the risk and difficulties that the use of religious arguments entails? The risks I have in mind are those well-worn claims about the problems of achieving consensus in a pluralist society. The fear is that religion is too personal and involves too many non-rational elements to serve as a factor in public deliberation. To avoid the complications and passions that might be aroused by religious rhetoric, many would say that we are best served by keeping public bioethics firmly on publicly accessible, and thus secular, grounds.

We have evidence of this attitude in the HERP report. The NBAC's reluctance to draw explicit connections between its detailed, informative survey of religious views and its recommendations to the President may indicate a similar worry about employing substantive arguments in the public forum, especially arguments that originate in religious frameworks. Yet, of course, religion is not and need not be anathema in politics broadly conceived, in the "public square," if it plays an appropriate role. I think some benefits both procedural and substantive can be seen by the NBAC's attention to religion, although the commission itself only acknowledges the former. The primary procedural benefit is that citizens who rely on religious belief and principles in forming their political and moral opinions will see that there are ways they can connect their reasoning and ideas to the public debate engendered by the report. There is a pragmatic side to this: Religious citizens might feel that their concerns were "heard," were taken at least more seriously than they normally are by public ethics bodies considering sensitive matters. Such reception would be particularly important in mollifying religious opponents of abortion, although I would not say that this should be the reason for attending to religious views.

Going further, we could argue that including religious voices is a boon to democratic deliberation: It models how religious arguments can be thoughtfully and thoroughly explored. Appreciative understanding of another's opinion is requisite for a genuine dialogue to occur. Such understanding has proved hard to attain in the sensitive areas in which religion and politics have mixed in recent years. The NBAC report shows its readers that it is possible to talk about religion as part of policy-oriented debates and to do so civilly.

Claiming these procedural benefits is not controversial, but identifying substantive benefits might be. To claim that there is a substantive benefit entails, at the least, that including religious perspectives improves the quality of argument in the report. A stronger claim is that religious opinions bring to the table some ethical and political arguments and values that would not otherwise receive sufficient consideration. To many readers, it may sound far-fetched to make such claims for the NBAC report. After all, how differently would the report read if the chapter on religious perspectives was not there at all? I believe the answer is "not much differently."

The NBAC would not have offered substantially different arguments and recommendations had it not considered religious views as thoroughly as it did. This is not to say that the consideration of religious views had no impact on its deliberations, but to suggest that the consideration of religion confirmed rather than significantly challenged the commission's ethical and policy analyses. Some substantive moral values encountered in the religious chapter, especially human dignity, seem to have shaped the commission's recommendations for caution and a temporary ban by confirming and supporting an analysis it made on secular grounds. This confirmation is not unimportant, yet the NBAC is so restrained in employing its investigation of religion that the chapter's impact on the report is negligible. The NBAC barely begins to draw on the rich insights that could be derived from a theological concept of human dignity in distinction to a philosophical concept. The NBAC lays out the religious perspectives in the manner of "on the one hand . . . on the other hand," making hardly any attempt to show how citizens might actually work with these diverse religious opinions and think their way through them. The chapters on ethics and public policy lay out similar sets of pro and con arguments, but in these instances the NBAC uses the differences to present some of its own considered interpretations and conclusions. Thus, the report is unbalanced. Religious perspectives are given a central place, but their implications are not worked out in any detail. Courtney Campbell, who prepared for the NBAC a commissioned paper on religious views of cloning, holds up a similar criticism of the commission's attention to religion: "My own sense," Campbell writes, "is that, in the NBAC hearings, the contributions of religious perspectives were deemed politically important and ethically insignificant."[26]

The NBAC began to demonstrate a constructive way of involving religion in public policy discussions. Its report goes a few steps down a more promising path, but does not carry its use of religious perspectives to an effective conclusion. What I am asking of public ethics bodies—and it is a tall order, I admit— is that they be open to discussing religious perspectives on the issues at hand and strive to make religious insights operative throughout their analyses and recommendations. How they can do so within the domain of a pluralist, democratic polity will be the focus of my final section, in which I will sketch a common good model for forming public policy. Continuing to focus on the areas of embryo research and human cloning, I will say more about the use by public ethics bodies of procedural and substantive moral arguments and of religious discourse as a form of substantive argument. What follows might be taken as general suggestions for how to develop the work started in the NBAC report.

A common good approach to policy formation

Recall that my purpose has been to find the best model of public discourse, one that befits a democratic, pluralist culture and can help the discussants move closer to the political common good in ways appropriate to the topic they are debating and deciding. The common good means a beneficial way of life for a society and its members; more specifically, it refers to the social conditions that improve citizens' well-being and help them live together peaceably. I am convinced that the common good remains a viable goal for a liberal democracy and an accurate way to describe what any instance of politics should ultimately be about.

Fundamentally, citizens of a political society seek to have a good life together. When we specify that the society is a liberal society, we are saying that certain limitations have been placed on the public's pursuit of the common good out of respect for the goods of personal autonomy and the diversity of human thought. When we specify that the society is democratic, we mean that there are certain political structures and methods through which the common good should be pursued. Both of these qualifications can be incorporated into the classical theory of the common good to keep it relevant and workable in modern societies.[27]

Understandably, the fact that citizens in a liberal democracy hold a variety of religious and moral viewpoints presents a challenge to identifying and pursuing a common good, at least in the substantive sense that the common good picks out shared ideals of the good human life, shared virtues and values. Charo is responding to this challenge when she proposes that public bioethics should focus on procedures that will achieve fair, just, and democratic decisions. I think she has one piece of the solution. Fair procedures and the resulting decisions are certainly part of society's commonweal, although in this case they are the procedural elements of the common good. Some would propose that the common good for a pluralist, democratic society is to be understood only as a procedural common good. As I have suggested in discussing both the HERP and the NBAC reports, I do not believe we have to choose between procedural and substantive discussions of policy issues or, by extension, between a procedural and a substantive common good. Rather, I hope to show that the two forms of argument need to work together because of their intrinsic connections and, moreover, that the right use of substantive argument can strengthen the practice of public bioethics.

What needs to be acknowledged from the outset is that we cannot avoid substantive argument in the political arena. The presumption that we can leads to facile claims, as when Steed Willadsen, a cloning researcher who works at St. Barnabas Hospital in East Orange, NJ, says, "The fact is that, in America, cloning may be bad but telling people how they should reproduce is worse. . . . America is not ruled by ethics. It is ruled by law."[28] His claim is simply incoherent, for an ethical framework undergirds our law, and implicit in our political policies are ethical assumptions. If our society is to think through the cloning issue adequately, we must engage the ethical foundations of our law, the ethical assumptions of current policies regarding medicine and research, and the ethical implications of any proposed policies. We should not rule out any views just because they may be characterized as religious, ethical, or particular to the thinking and traditions

194 PUBLIC POLICY ISSUES

of a particular subcommunity within society. The mistake is to think that there is some purely neutral ground on which scientific policy can be created.

A related aspect of our political culture is that citizens do use substantive moral and religious beliefs to come to their political decisions. Therefore, it is appropriate for public ethics bodies to make correlations between the arguments they employ and those that are represented in the society at large. I do not mean that ethics bodies have to use only arguments that can be found in the wider culture or that they have to fit their reasoning to someone else's; I simply mean that they will do the public a service by locating their arguments within the context of the ethical, religious, and technical arguments that are commonly found in the public forum. The NBAC did something to this effect by surveying religious and ethical perspectives, but it should have taken the additional step of showing where it found those perspectives compelling in its own reasoning. (This use of religious perspectives goes beyond the position attributed to commissioner Thomas Murray in a news story, that the NBAC's task was not to decide the validity of ethical arguments, but simply to reflect the public's concerns in its report.[29]) By listening to diverse ethical arguments, giving them expression in their reports, and engaging them as worthy of response, public ethics bodies might contribute to a less antagonistic relationship between themselves and oppositional members of the public. These actions might help some citizens and groups feel less alienated and show them that their participation is welcome. Here the procedural dynamic comes into play: A fair, open, and just process requires giving ample room to diverse and dissenting voices.

I hold as central to a common good approach the claim that substantive moral and religious viewpoints can be used as a resource in public bioethics. This use can be justified in several ways. First, we can identify the positive contributions that religious citizens and groups do in fact play in public life. Second, we can note that substantive viewpoints do not pose the same difficulties at every level of politics: Judges and elected officials, acting in their official duties, need to exercise care to base their decisions on reasons that citizens could find reasonable. At lower levels of political authority, though, the room for multiple rationales and discourses increases, opening the door for both citizens and politicians to rely on religious beliefs and arguments in making their cases in the public square. This reliance is legitimate within a liberal democracy.[30] The third and most robust argument for religion's role in politics would involve drawing out the ethical and religious aspects of American political culture and of liberal democracy itself. Such a discussion would, however, take us too far afield.

Central to an argument that seeks a principled role for religion in a liberal democratic society is the one I have been making: Substantive and procedural arguments have a necessary connection in that procedural arguments rely on a more fundamental substrate of substantive arguments and agreements in a community. Agreements—and even most disagreements—about justice depend on tacit and deep-seated cultural agreements on matters of the good such as duties, values, and virtues. Michael Walzer illuminates this relationship when contrasting moral maximalism, the "thick" morality of groups, with moral minimalism, the "thin" appeal to universal concepts such as justice, fairness, and truth telling. Walzer writes: "It is popular these days to think of the minimum in procedural terms—a thin morality of discourse that governs every particular creation of a substantive and thick morality. . . . Minimal morality consists in the rules of engagement that bind all the speakers; maximalism is the never-finished outcome of their arguments."[31]

This proposition is flawed, however, for two reasons. First, the procedural rules that make the pursuit of the common good possible in a democracy are already quite thick—they are not something timeless, given in our nature and shared by all cultures, but they are actually "a way of life," a product of our particular political history.[32] Second, the proposition gets the order backwards: It suggests that the procedures logically and chronologically precede the development of a substantive morality, when in fact a society requires a substantive morality as the context in which any rules of engagement can be developed. Walzer's general picture of how thick (substantive) and thin (procedural) moralities are related is this: Cultures and their members at any given point find themselves in possession of a substantive morality; from this thick morality they can distill out a thinner, procedural morality as circumstances require. Thin morality is needed for a variety of reasons: Among other things, it facilitates conversation in pluralistic and cross-cultural contexts. The point I take from Walzer's argument is that procedural morality is a tool we can use effectively in a democracy, but we deceive ourselves if we think that it is all we have. We need to remind ourselves of the richer moral traditions and commitments to which we have access. As Annette Baier puts it, speaking of the component of thin morality known as rights: "Rights are only the tip of the moral iceberg, supported by the responsibilities that we cooperatively discharge and by the individual responsibilities that we recognize, including responsibilities to cooperate, in order to maintain such common goods as civilized speech and civilized ways of settling disputes. For it takes more than rights to settle disputes about rights."[33]

If this picture of procedural morality riding on the shoulders of substantive agreements is accurate, then policy making must pay more attention to citizens' religious and moral beliefs and the ways these support or challenge a liberal society's working consensus on a procedural morality. When debates about justice and rights come to an impasse, the only way through may be to broaden the scope of the public conversation rather than narrow it. In sum, public bioethics committees should hold substantive and procedural arguments together by surveying the many religious and ethical perspectives that inform public debate (as the NBAC did), taking firm stands on the ethical arguments (as the HERP did), and defending those positions in the court of competing arguments (which neither committee did in any depth). Since these committees speak for the public, they should show significant engagement with the multiple perspectives found in the society at large. Such use is procedurally fair when it is wide and representative; it is substantive when those perspectives influence the deliberations and conclusions of the committee.

My final task is to explain in more detail the most controversial part of this argument: a public ethics body's use of *religious* perspectives and arguments to shape its deliberations and conclusions. Certainly there are inappropriate ways of doing this; let me identify four appropriate ways to use religious views. First, these bodies should attend to the importance of religion in the deliberations of citizens. That is, they should help the public and policy makers recognize that religious traditions constitute a resource that informs ethical and political values in our public culture while delivering complex and various verdicts on any given issue. As we have seen, the NBAC does this more so than the HERP. Second, public ethics bodies should show clearly how the religious considerations they survey work to support or undermine certain policy options. Again, the NBAC lays these out better than the HERP, but the NBAC does not make these considerations operative in its recommendations. Third, public ethics bodies should discuss religion with sensitivity to the ways that religious views might modify and challenge a secular consensus rather than merely overlap with it. Neither committee does this. Finally, public ethics bodies should envision a concrete role for religious organizations in the public dialogue. The NBAC suggests such a connection, but goes no further than to say that a national dialogue should occur.

We have encountered the first two ways of using religious arguments earlier in this chapter, but the third and fourth are new claims that require defense. I think the commissioners' intuitions are right that religion should be a part of the national dialogue on cloning and that religious views can play a valuable role in public bioethics. It is fair to surmise that the NBAC is wary of cashing out the religious perspectives to any significant degree because of the risks of bringing religion into political deliberation. Can religious views really have a place in the discourse of governmental institutions? Well, of course; they do in the NBAC report itself. More to the point: Can religious arguments appropriately be used as reasons for policy decisions? The four ways of employing religion I have just described violate neither constitutional principles regarding the separation of church and state nor the spirit of a liberal democratic society, properly understood.[34]

Note that these methods do not in fact seek to base a policy decision on religious reasons; they do seek to introduce the religious arguments that citizens themselves employ into the discussion and deliberation that lead to policy decisions. I hold, then, that there is a crucial difference between employing religious arguments as *resources* in policy making and using them as the *foundations* for policy making. In using religious views as resources, public ethics bodies will be looking for ways that religious traditions can contribute to a public consensus in conjunction with secular approaches. They will also be looking for ways that religious traditions can enrich the ethical, scientific, and policy discussions.

The NBAC sought to do both,[35] although it was vague on what it found enriching for its own analysis in those religious interpretations. The commissioners might have made more explicit how some general trends in the religious traditions studied cohere with and support the recommendations they make. They might also have noted that the way they seek an overlapping consensus tends to put secular considerations in the driver's seat and that this approach has its limitations. Religiously motivated citizens have sometimes performed a valuable public service by challenging the reigning public consensus rather than simply supporting it to the extent that their views overlap with it.

One might respond that this request to make religious arguments operative is asking too much of the NBAC or any other public ethics body because they have a difficult enough time bringing together the diversity of ethical arguments into a coherent policy recommendation. Yet, by the same token, the commission asked a lot of the religious scholars who testified before it when it pressed them to translate their arguments into publicly accessible terms.[36] Courtney Campbell writes that those who testified faced the "translation" problem that generally confronts religious scholars' attempts to participate in a public policy forum. Their dilemma is whether to remain distinctive to their traditions and risk irrelevance or to attempt the translation and risk diluting the content of their tradition's wisdom. Campbell finds it unfortunate that the commissioners "continually invited the religious thinkers to delineate the significance of their claims about cloning for a public that did not necessarily share the belief system and narratives of a given faith tradition," because this invitation makes two mistakes—it presumes that there is a "public" with a settled consensus on values, and it "imposes a higher burden of relevance" on religious thinkers than on others.[37]

The religious scholars appearing before the NBAC did as well as they could to meet the challenge, but we should stop to consider what gets lost if everything a religious leader or citizen says in the public square has to be translated. My way of understanding the matter is as follows.[38] Religious groups and citizens contribute to society's common good in several ways. One is by offering intellectual resources to public debates. In this role, religious thinkers will want to make the most effort to translate, for they have to make their views at least intelligible (not necessarily reasonable) if they hope to influence political deliberation. Even so, there may be reasons they cannot or do not want to translate: Although a concept like human dignity conveys its meaning effectively in both religious and secular contexts, the concepts of proper stewardship and humility before the Creator will lose some of their meaning and power if translated to a nonreligious context. I would not want to see a religious speaker's conceptual vocabulary reduced by the need continuously to translate for the sake of relevance.

Two other ways religious groups and citizens promote the common good are by creating conditions for social harmony through service and by promoting goods for persons and society that are neglected or marginalized in the political status quo. This last contribution is an aspect of religion's prophetic task. Here, again, religious groups may find that it advances their mission when they translate their language into publicly accessible terms, but they may also find that such translation attenuates the distinctive vision of the common good they want to present. In their prophetic role this is especially true. At the same time, my argument does not entail that prophetic discourse has only a critical and never a constructive task. Indeed, a religious group's efforts to foster public dialogue and draw out common values in the culture may be a prophetic act. As Campbell puts it:

Part of the prophetic task of the religious tradition is to enable the *discovery* of values that seem shared across the pluralism of a society's diverse moral traditions, and to participate in the *retrieval, selection,* and *interpretation* of such values as a basis for moral discourse among citizens. This was the force, I believe, of the recurrent religious appeal in the NBAC hearings to the "common good" in considering the ethics of cloning. . . . [39]

The implication for public ethics bodies is not that they should adopt the prophetic discourse of one or more religions but that they should acknowledge that religions contribute in more ways than by translating their ideas into secular discourse.

Public ethics bodies might serve the common good most effectively by promoting national dialogue, their contributions to which can include initiating public dialogue, synthesizing and expressing an operative public consensus, trying to create a public consensus, or feeding information and recommendations into a political body. Often an ethics body may have or take on several of these tasks, a situation that makes its job more complicated by giving rise to competing expectations on the public's part. Of course, it is much easier to synthesize a public consensus rather than to create one.[40] One cannot expect the NBAC to have done either in the 90 days allotted to it on an issue as new to the public as human cloning; one can only expect the NBAC to have initiated the public conversation that might lead toward eventual consensus.

To get to the point where a consensus could be synthesized, public ethics bodies should think about how a national dialogue can take place and how their own work connects to it. It is regrettable that the NBAC did not have the time to say more about how its vision of a national dialogue could proceed.[41] Clearly, this is a place where religious traditions can and should come into play. The NBAC made a significant contribution by inviting religious scholars to testify, commissioning background studies on religious perspectives, and including a substantial chapter on religious views in its report. Like the NBAC, I affirm the valuable role religious organizations can play in promoting public education and national dialogue. As I have argued, at times their contribution will be to complement a public consensus and motivate their adherents to support it; at other times their contribution could be to challenge the current consensus or the reigning ideologies.

Religious institutions are already involved in the process of civic education on timely ethical issues: This occurs when ministers make applications to those issues from the pulpit; when the issues are discussed in adult religious education classes, the popular religious press, and other forums; when church bodies publish statements; and when para-church organizations mobilize their members to raise public awareness or create social change. In the case of cloning, a number of religious bodies issued public statements in the wake of the announcement about the cloned sheep, and we may imagine that various types of discussion have been occurring in churches around the nation.[42] Thus far, para-church organizations have not made human cloning a major focus of their efforts, except that religious (and nonreligious) pro-life organizations have been tracking the work of the NBAC and other government bodies.[43] Because the American public is just beginning to reflect seriously on cloning and related advances in biotechnology, the greatest need for religious groups is to promote reflection and to educate their members and the public about the underlying moral values and choices.

Public ethics bodies should consider formally involving religious institutions in the work of public education: Churches, seminaries, religious scholars, and the religious media could be very effective collaborators in this project. Public ethics bodies should call on churches as forums for educating citizens on scientific advancements and their ethical ramifications; they should think explicitly about churches as one type of public forum whenever they develop materials that get distributed to community organizations. Ethics bodies might work with religious institutions to improve the "ethical literacy" of the public.[44] As for the specific methods, a starting point could be for the President to ask the National Institutes of Health to create an initiative that engages religious and other community leaders in a collaborative effort at public conversation and public education on bioethical issues. President Clinton's Initiative on Race might serve as a model or a starting point for thinking about the benefits and drawbacks of a bioethics initiative.[45]

Finally, we should not overlook the fact that use of religious argument might influence policy making in some constructive ways. The NBAC's consideration of religious views filtered into deliberations in the United States Congress, particularly when Senator Bill Frist organized a hearing before the Committee on Labor and Human Resources, Subcommittee on Public Health and Safety, entitled "Ethics and Theology: A Continuation of the National Discussion on Human

Cloning."[46] This is one example of how government bodies can employ religious perspectives and arguments as resources in their deliberations. For all the reasons discussed in this chapter, it is appropriate that religious perspectives should have a voice in the political forum as well as the broader public forum.

We cannot expect the process of a national dialogue to be easy. Before we get to consensus, we have to expect confrontation, a confrontation fueled in part by religious groups acting in their prophetic role. Given how often citizens with strong religious convictions are dismissed as unreasonable and an obstacle to policy making, I hope this chapter has succeeded in showing how religious groups can play a constructive role in public policy. It would be misguided, however, to look to religion only when it can play that supportive role; one of my arguments has been that religious groups contribute to the common good even when they call technological progress into question. Public ethics bodies will best contribute to public education and genuine public deliberation if they do not try to keep the controversial arguments to the side by appealing to procedural strictures.

The common good approach to public conversation that I have laid out proposes that substantive arguments, even religious ones, have an important role in public conversation and political deliberation. This model has a better chance than its procedural or deductivist competitors of meeting the challenges that face public ethics bodies and the public as they try to weave a way toward consensus.

ACKNOWLEDGMENTS

My appreciation goes to Dr. Mary Groesch at the Public Health Service of the National Institutes of Health and to Ms. Debbie Stewart at the National Bioethics Advisory Commission for sending me transcripts of testimony before the HERP and the NBAC; and to Sarah McSweeney and Wendy Ward for bringing articles about human embryo research to my attention. I greatly benefited from the suggestions made by Paul Lauritzen, David Clough, and Thomas Scheidemantel on drafts of this chapter.

12

The Law Meets Reproductive Technology: The Prospect of Human Cloning

HEIDI FORSTER AND EMILY RAMSEY

The prospect of acquiring the ability to clone human beings raises a variety of ethical, metaphysical, and legal questions.

This chapter addresses the current legal issues associated with the prospect of human cloning. Samples of proposed legislation at both the federal and state levels are provided and international initiatives are briefly mentioned. United States Constitutional issues related to cloning legislation are then described, and procreative liberty is discussed. Finally, some issues and concerns raised in earlier discussion are addressed, including perceived harms and benefits of human cloning through the use of the somatic cell nuclear transfer technique.

Legal activity at the federal, state, and international levels

Much controversy has surrounded the questions whether to regulate human cloning and what the appropriate legislative format might be. For example, Senator Tom Harkin of Iowa believes that human cloning is "right and proper."[2] Senator Bill Frist of Tennessee, Chairman of the Committee of Public Health and Safety, believes that lawmakers should work toward drafting a bill to regulate human cloning that does not jeopardize possible life-saving research.[3] Harold

An earlier version of this chapter was published in the Valparaiso University Law Review in 1998.[1]

Varmus, Director of the National Institutes of Health, cautioned a congressional subcommittee against premature cloning legislation.[4] Varmus is concerned about anti-cloning laws being too restrictive and thus preventing potentially beneficial research. The controversy has resulted in different initiatives to regulate human cloning technology in the United States at both the federal and state levels and in the international setting.

The Federal Level

After the announcement of the cloned sheep, in the United States there was a frenzy of activity to regulate human cloning at the federal level. In February 1997, President Clinton asked the National Bioethics Advisory Commission (NBAC) to review the legal and ethical issues associated with human cloning. The President asked the NBAC to discuss human cloning issues for 90 days and to draft a final report and recommendations on possible federal action to prevent the abuse of cloning techniques as applied to humans. On February 27, 1997, a bill was proposed in the United States Senate addressing the cloning of human beings.[5] On March 4, 1997, President Clinton issued a moratorium directing that no federal funds be allocated for the cloning of human beings.[6] President Clinton also asked privately funded scientists to halt human cloning research. On March 5, 1997, the United States House of Representatives proposed legislation addressing the issue of human cloning.[7]

Among other issues, the NBAC reviewed the current status of legislation related to human cloning and the possible constitutional arguments if laws were passed to restrict the creation of children through somatic cell nuclear transfer cloning. After an inquiry into and discussion of the matter, the NBAC determined that "any attempt to clone human beings via somatic cell nuclear transfer techniques is uncertain in its prospects, is unacceptably dangerous to the fetus and, therefore, morally unacceptable."[8] Currently, President Clinton's moratorium restricts human cloning only in situations involving federal funds. Thus, no regulations control the use of private funds regarding human cloning. The NBAC recommended that President Clinton continue the current moratorium on human cloning and ask for voluntary compliance from the private sector while federal legislation banning human cloning was further explored and discussed.

Following the recommendations of the NBAC, President Clinton introduced the Cloning Prohibition Act of 1997. President Clinton transmitted this legislative proposal to Congress in order to implement the NBAC's guidelines.[9] The President's proposal would prohibit any attempt to create a human being using somatic cell nuclear transfer technology, but would allow further review of both the ethical and scientific issues surrounding the use of somatic cell nuclear transfer in humans. In reference to the proposed legislation, President Clinton stated, "What the legislation will do is to reaffirm our most cherished beliefs about the miracle of human life and the God-given individuality each person possesses [and it] will ensure that we do not fall prey to the temptation to replicate ourselves at the expense of those beliefs."[10]

Although he would prohibit research on human cloning, President Clinton would carve out an exception for certain types of cloning research. The NBAC had acknowledged the potential medical benefits from cloning research, such as growing new tissue and using genes to prevent or improve the treatment of diseases. Based on the NBAC's findings that cloning technology may be beneficial for producing replacement skin, cartilage, or bone tissues for burn and accident victims and nerve tissue for spinal cord injuries, the President's proposed Cloning Prohibition Act of 1997 would not forbid such research activities. President Clinton's proposal would permit the following research activities within biomedical and agricultural areas: *(1)* the use of somatic cell nuclear transfer or other cloning technologies to clone molecules, DNA, cells, and tissues; and *(2)* the use of somatic cell nuclear transfer techniques to create animals. President Clinton's legislative proposal would also require the NBAC to perform further study and produce another report on human cloning in four and a half years.[11] At that time, the President in office would reconsider how to address the issues of human cloning.

The President's proposed legislation is a typical example of the many attempts to legislate against human cloning. The NBAC suggested that human cloning may be regulated through either federal legislation or other means, such as voluntary participation in a moratorium or a prohibition on the use of federal money to fund human cloning research.[12] In Congress, nine federal bills were proposed in 1998 to regulate human cloning, and two federal bills were proposed in 1999 to regulate human cloning. None of the 1998 bills passed, and the two 1999 bills ended 1999 in subcommittees in the House of Representatives. No new bills have been introduced in 2000. The proposed bills vary in their definitions, prohibitions, and methods of controlling the uses of cloning technology. A few of the different regulatory strategies and sample language are provided.

Like Clinton's moratorium, the first method United States Senators employed was to restrict federal funding for research regarding human cloning.[13] As most research in this country is funded with government monies, this type of restriction would be fairly effective. The technology to create a person through cloning could, however, advance in the private sector. The proposed bill using this tactic to discourage human cloning research defined the term *cloning* as "the replication of a human individual by the taking of a cell with genetic material and the cultivation of the cell through the egg, embryo, fetal, and newborn stages into a new human individual."[14] No federal statutes have been passed that would specifically ban the use of federal funds for human cloning; however, within a few congressional appropriations bills, there are prohibitions against the creation of embryos through the use of cloning technology.

The next approach in the Senate involved making the use of cloning technology to create a human being unlawful. An example of this type of bill proposed making it unlawful for any person to clone a human being or to conduct research for the purpose of cloning a human being or otherwise creating a human embryo.[15] This bill also prohibited federal funds from being obligated or expended to knowingly conduct any research project to clone a human being or otherwise create a human embryo. Furthermore, it set forth a civil monetary penalty. Any individual in violation of the legislation would be fined not more than $5000 and would be prohibited from receiving any federal funding for research for a period of 5 years after such violation. This particular bill also incorporated a statement of the federal government's role in promoting its ethical stance toward human cloning. The bill stated that "Congress finds that the Federal Government has a moral obligation to the nation to prohibit the cloning of human beings."[16]

Another approach used in the Senate was to criminalize human cloning. The Human Cloning Prohibition Act proposed to amend the federal criminal code to prohibit any person or entity from using human somatic cell nuclear transfer technology or from importing an embryo produced through such technology.[17] This highly restrictive bill would prohibit the use of somatic cell nuclear transfer technology for any purpose. Furthermore, the bill would create penalties of up to 10 years in prison, a fine, or both for violations, although the fine could not be more than twice the amount of any gross pecuniary gain derived from a violation. The bill would also establish a national commission within the Institute of Medicine to promote a national dialogue on bioethics and expresses the sense of Congress that the federal government should advocate for and join an international effort to prohibit the use of human somatic cell nuclear transfer technology to produce a human embryo.

Much controversy has surrounded the language in the highly restrictive Human Cloning Prohibition Act, described earlier, and The Prohibition on Cloning of Human Beings Act of 1998.[18] The Prohibition on Cloning of Human Beings Act proposed to amend the Public Health Service Act to make it unlawful for any person to implant or attempt to implant the product of somatic cell nuclear transfer into a woman's uterus, to ship the product of somatic cell nuclear transfer in interstate or foreign commerce for the purpose of implanting such product into a woman's uterus, or to use government funds for an activity prohibited by the bill. This main controversy involves the use of somatic cell nuclear transfer technology for research purposes other than to create a human being. The Prohibition on Cloning of Human Beings Act would not restrict areas of biomedical and agricultural research or practices not expressly prohibited by the Act, including research or practices involving the use of somatic cell nuclear transfer or other cloning technologies to clone molecules, DNA, cells, and tissues; of mitochondrial, cytoplasmic, or gene therapy; or of somatic cell nuclear transfer techniques to create non-human animals.

The proposed Act would also require the NBAC to submit another report to the President and Congress in the future and would extend the life of the NBAC for 10 years. It would also provide for civil penalties, civil actions, and the forfeiture of certain property. Furthermore, it would give the Attorney General enforcement authority under the Act and the ability to render binding advisory opinions. This bill also suggests that the President should cooperate with foreign countries regarding the uses of cloning technology. Finally, the bill would preempt any state or local law that prohibits cloning-related research.

The bills introduced in the House of Representatives in 1998 were similar to the Senate proposals. The Human Cloning Research Prohibition Act combined different aspects of the Senate bills.[19] This proposed legislation would prohibit the expenditure of federal funds to conduct or support any research on the cloning of humans. The amended bill expressly states that the Act does not restrict other areas of scientific research, such as the use of somatic cell nuclear transfer or other cloning technologies to clone molecules, DNA, cells other than human embryo cells or tissues, or non-human animals. Next, the Human Cloning Prohibition Act proposes that "it shall be unlawful for any person to use a human somatic cell for the process of producing a human clone" and sets forth a civil monetary penalty not to exceed $5000. Finally, the Human Cloning Research Prohibition Act would prohibit the expenditure of federal funds to conduct or support research on the cloning of humans but expressly states that other "important and promising" scientific research using cloning technology would not be prohibited.[20] The bill further encourages other countries to establish substantially equivalent restrictions. The two bills proposed in 1999 in the House of Representatives both prohibit the expenditure of federal funds to conduct or support research on human cloning.[21]

Although none of the federal bills described above were passed into law, the different methods proposed are all examples of how the federal government exercises its power to promote or discourage an activity. A limitation on federal funds used for the purpose of cloning a human being is not the most effective method to prohibit human cloning throughout the entire country. If federal funds are restricted, and even if the private sector is asked to voluntarily comply, private researchers and companies can attempt to clone a human without penalty. Much research in this country is, however, supported by monies from governmental entities such as The National Institutes of Health or The National Science Foundation, and therefore much human cloning research would be effectively stopped. The prohibition of federal funds tactic could be made more effective by combining it with other methods of regulating cloning. Such a strategy would effectively ban the cloning of a human being from any federally funded agencies along with regulating the private sector through criminal or civil penalties. These types of congressional attempts at prohibiting cloning include either criminalizing human cloning or making the practice unlawful by imposing a civil monetary fine on violators. Both of these methods offer some deterrent, which may be more or less threatening to particular groups or individuals. Large companies or research institutions that have the funds and facilities to develop human cloning may not be effectively deterred with a civil fine.

In addition, Congress included in its different legislative proposals mandates or suggestions regarding its collective beliefs about several issues related to human cloning. Some proposed bills included attempts by Congress to promote a particular moral stance, others included statements about the promoting discourse on the subject, and yet others included recommendations for United States participation in international agreements. These types of suggestions are Congress' method of expressing its collective voice on an issue and offer insight into the reasoning behind the proposed legislation. For example, the promotion of a national discourse serves as an acknowledgment that cloning is a novel issue that deserves public attention before binding decisions are made. Along the same lines, another feature in many of the bills is what is termed a *sunset* clause. Legislation that includes a *sunset* clause has an expiration period. For instance, human cloning could be outlawed for 5 or 10 years during which time the public and national commissions could discuss the benefits and harms of cloning humans, and then the legislation would "sunset" and expire so new legislation could be passed.

The last major difference between the proposed federal bills was whether to prohibit the cloning of human beings and allow the use of cloning technology to continue for other purposes or whether to just prohibit the use of somatic cell nuclear transfer cloning technology for any purpose. While the use of somatic cell nuclear transfer technology is discussed in this country and around the world, it seems prudent only to outlaw the cloning of human beings and to allow somatic cell nuclear transfer technology to progress. Based on the numerous potential medical benefits, many legislators, scientists, President Clinton, and the NBAC thought that cloning technology itself should proceed. The concern with allowing the technology to develop, however, is based on a slippery slope argument about the eventuality of the creation of cloned humans. The cloning of human beings remains morally suspect, and is discussed later.

The State Level

Even before the NBAC convened, both federal and state legislation addressing the prohibition of human cloning and human cloning research were proposed. Following President Clinton's actions at the federal level, states continued to take steps to regulate human cloning. The proposed state bills vary in their specific prohibitions regarding human cloning. The state legislators chose mainly the same methods to prohibit human cloning as their federal counterparts. The main categories of types of prohibitions include banning the use of state funds for any research using cloned cells or tissue; prohibiting the use of state funds for cloning an entire individual; banning any research using cloned cells or tissue; and banning cloning of an entire individual. Like the federal proposals, some states criminalize human cloning by making the practice a felony, and others provide high civil monetary fines. Several bills would also require the creation of panels to analyze issues associated with human cloning, which would serve to advise state legislatures. In addition, the states have another punishment tactic at their disposal. Several states in their legislative proposals threaten to revoke the medical license of any statutory violators. Finally, several states proposed joint resolutions to urge Congress to prohibit human cloning.

Twenty-eight states introduced bills to regulate human cloning in their 1997 or 1998 legislative sessions. In addition, 10 states introduced human cloning bills in 1999 and 1 state has introduced a bill in 2000. Most of the 1999 bills were not carried over for the next session or are still in committee. As of March 2000, only 5 states have passed laws banning human cloning.[22] A few of these laws are described as representative examples.

California is among the few states that have enacted legislation that outlaws human cloning.[23] The prohibition became effective on January 1, 1998, and lasts for 5 years. The legislation addresses a number of issues surrounding human cloning. First, the legislation requires California to set up a panel of experts to study the ramifications of human cloning.[24] The panel is to report its recommendations to both the governor and the legislature so that issues surrounding human cloning may be further studied before the 5 year ban ends. The law also prohibits a person from cloning a human being and from purchasing or selling an ovum, zygote, embryo, or fetus for the purpose of human cloning. The California measure punishes violators with a civil monetary fine. The state health director has the authority to fine corporations, clinics, firms, hospitals, laboratories, or research facilities up to $1,000,000 for violating the ban. The state health director may fine individuals who violate the ban the greater of *(1)* up to $250,000 or *(2)* double the profit made off their efforts. Additionally, if any profit results from human cloning, the state health director may double the amount of the fines. The law also includes provisions for the revocation of licenses issued to individuals who or business that violate the ban on human cloning.

The state of Missouri chose a different tactic to regulate human cloning. The Missouri law prohibits state funds from being used for human cloning research.[25] In contrast, Rhode Island's law bans the creation of a human being through somatic cell nuclear transfer and imposes administrative penalties.[26] The statute indicates that this ban does not apply to the cloning of human genes, cells, tissues, or organs that would not result in the replication of an entire individual. Penalties for violating the law are in the form of civil fines similar to those imposed by the California statute. The legislature also included a statement of its intent and purpose for passing the legislation. The law states that it is intended "to protect the citizens of the state from potential abuse deriving from cloning technologies." In addition, the stature sunsets in July 2003, 5 years from its passage.

In yet another example, the state of Michigan employed several different tactics in its effort to ban human cloning.[27] Its law prohibits individuals from engaging in or attempting to engage in human cloning, but it exempts other uses of cloning technology. Furthermore, violators are guilty of a felony punishable by imprisonment for not more than 10 years or a fine of not more than $10,000,000, or both. In addition, state funds are prohibited for the purpose of cloning a human being.

Despite the large number of bills proposed throughout the states in the last several years, only five were actually signed into law. The fervor to regulate human cloning died down in the state legislatures between 1997 and 1999, as the number of states with cloning bills dropped from 28 to 10. Many bills died in committee; others were not carried over to the next legislative session. Several bills are described here to illustrate the different policy approaches to human cloning regulation chosen by the states.

The bill introduced in Connecticut is an interesting example. The Connecticut House introduced a bill in 1998 that would ban the cloning of human beings in an effort to address the threat to human dignity posed by genetic engineering.[28] The bill would prohibit a person from intentionally growing or creating a human being by replacing the nucleus of a human oocyte cell with the nucleus of a differentiated somatic cell of any person for implantation and gestation of the resultant embryo. The prohibition against cloning a human being would not include *(1)* research for the purposes of scientific investigation of disease or cure of disease or illness provided that such research does not result in the cloning of a human or *(2)* in vitro fertilization. A person whose gamete material is used without such person's knowledge for the purpose of human cloning in violation of this bill could bring a civil action and recover treble damages, punitive damages, court costs, and reasonable attorney fees. Additionally, a person who was conceived by cloning in violation of the bill could take the same legal action. Finally, a commission could revoke the license or permit of a practitioner who violates the bill. This proposal is noteworthy because it gives standing to sue in civil court to people whose genetic material is used for cloning and to the person created through the cloning process and because it provides for license revocation. The 1999 version of this bill failed and was not carried over to the next legislative session.

The Delaware bill is fairly standard in its prohibition of the cloning of a human being, with exemptions for other biomedical research. The Delaware Senate introduced a bill that would create a ban on human cloning using the somatic cell nuclear transfer technique.[29] The bill includes a sunset clause that would terminate the ban on January 1, 2003, unless reauthorized. The bill would allow biomedical and agricultural research, including, but not limited to, the use of somatic cell nuclear transfer or other cloning technologies to clone molecules, DNA, cells, and tissues or to develop animals. The penalty for an intentional violation of these provisions would be a fine of the greater of $250,000 or two times the gross gain or loss from the offense.

Two bills from Illinois serve as examples of criminal statutes in the effort to ban human cloning along with the restriction on the use of state monies for cloning a person. The Illinois House introduced two bills in March 1997 titled the Human Cloning Prohibition Act.[30] The House bills would prohibit human cloning and forbid the use of public funds or property for human cloning. The proposed Illinois legislation would make an intentional violation a Class Four felony. The Illinois Senate also introduced two bills in the 1997–1998 Regular Session titled the Human Cloning Prohibition Act.[31] The Senate bills would prohibit the cloning of human beings. The first bill would make an intentional violation of the provisions a Class Three felony. This bill would also amend the State Finance Act to provide that any appropriation act shall not be construed to authorize the expenditure of public funds for human cloning or for the support of any project or institution that engages in human cloning. Finally, this first bill would amend the Unified Code of Corrections to make a person who intentionally violates the provisions ineligible for parole. The second bill would prohibit a person from purchasing or selling an ovum, zygote, embryo, or fetus for the purpose of cloning a human being. Under this bill, various licenses could be revoked for the violation of its provisions. Also, it would forbid a person from engaging in an activity that involves the use of a human somatic cell for the process of producing a human clone, and violations would constitute a Class Four felony. The 1999 versions of the Illinois bills ended the year in committee.

Minnesota proposed another interesting statute. Its bill combines criminal sanctions with license revocations. Similar to other state proposals, the Minnesota bill exempts other reproductive technologies from the statutory understanding of human cloning. The first section of the proposal would make it unlawful for any person to engage in human cloning.[32] The penalty for such a violation would constitute a felony. The second section of the bill would make it unlawful to purchase or sell an ovum, zygote, embryo, or fetus for the purpose of human cloning. The penalty for a violation of the second section would constitute a gross misdemeanor. The bill also provides that human cloning be distinguished from currently allowable assisted reproductive technologies, as long as the pregnancy is not intended to result in a child who is genetically identical to another human being or results in two or more natural identical twins. The bill would also allow a health-related licensing board to revoke the license of a regulated person who violates the provisions.

The New Jersey bill combines a criminal penalty with a declaration that genetic information belongs to the person from whom it is obtained. In 1997, 1998, and 1999 the New Jersey Assembly introduced bills that would make the cloning of a human being a first-degree crime.[33] A violation of the New Jersey bill would result in a fine of $100,000 to $200,000 or a prison term of 10 to 20 years, or both. The New Jersey bill would also provide that an individual's genetic information is the property of that individual. The 2000 version of this bill criminalizing human cloning is still in committee.

Finally, the New York proposals are an attempt to combine many different approaches to regulating cloning. In February and March 1997, Senator John Marchi introduced two complex and detailed bills.[34] The New York bills define cloning as the growing or creating of a human from a single cell of a genetically identical being by means of asexual reproduction. The New York bills would prohibit anyone from extracting the nucleus from an unfertilized human egg and implanting DNA from another cell into the egg. Additionally, the bills would give the New York State Department of Health regulatory authority over animal cloning research. The New York bills would create a new crime of "cloning of a human being." The new crime would be a Class D felony. The New York Senate introduced another bill that would create a Temporary State Commission on Cloning and Genetic Engineering.[35]

In 1998, the New York Assembly introduced two bills regarding human cloning. The first Assembly bill would prohibit a person from cloning a human being and from purchasing or selling an ovum, zygote, embryo, or fetus for the purpose of cloning a human being.[36] This bill would also establish civil penalties for violation of the provisions. The second Assembly bill would prohibit human cloning and the use of public funds, resources, property, employees, or those of political subdivisions or public corporations for the purpose of human cloning.[37] A violation of this bill would constitute a felony and provide grounds for license revocation.

The New York Senate introduced three bills in 1998. The first bill would prohibit a person from cloning a human being and from purchasing or selling an ovum, zygote, embryo, or fetus for the purpose of cloning a human being.[38] This bill would also establish civil penalties for violation of its provisions. The second Senate bill was titled the Cloning Prohibition and Research Protection Act. It would prohibit the cloning of human beings while permitting scientific research and experimentation, including, but not limited to, the use of somatic cell nuclear transfer and other cloning technologies to clone molecules, DNA, cells, and tissues and to develop non-human animals.[39] The penalty for a violation of this bill would be a civil fine of $250,000. The third Senate bill would create a temporary state commission on cloning and genetic engineering to examine and make responses to the scientific, technological, moral, and ethical issues raised by human cloning research and development.[40] The purpose of the commission would be to study such issues and advise the governor and the legislature of its findings, including the possible scientific and medical benefits of human cloning research, the feasibility of human cloning, and the possible scientific and medical circumstances under which human cloning should or should not be sanctioned. The eight bills introduced in 1999 are very similar to those described earlier.

These various laws and bills serve as representative examples of the many attempts to regulate human cloning at the state level. Much of the proposed state legislation is similar to the federal attempts, but, as matters of health and family are typically reserved to the states, the states have additional tactics available. For example, the states can revoke state medical licenses and can regulate assisted reproductive technologies, along with the more common approaches like the prohibition of government monies and civil and criminal penalties. Aside from the legislative efforts within the United States, the international community and several individual countries are concerned with enacting human cloning laws and are preparing declarations prohibiting human cloning.

The International Level

One of the NBAC's policy options was cooperation among nations to enforce common policies regarding the prohibition of human cloning. The NBAC suggested that countries agree to enforce each other's prohibitory legislation. Some of the federal and state bills described earlier also included the suggestion that the United States cooperate in a multinational effort to regulate or ban human cloning or at least to recognize the current international proposals. The Council for Responsible Genetics has called for a worldwide ban on human cloning, in addition to increased public discussion about biotechnology.[41] UNESCO and the Human Genome Organization (HUGO), two international bodies with ethics committees, are also involved in exploring the ethical and legal implications of human cloning.[42]

Many individuals have advised that international guidelines should be enacted. Ian Wilmut, for example, has recommended the passage of international guidelines regarding human cloning. Having informed the United States Senate Committee of Public Health and Safety that human cloning can and should be controlled, Wilmut specifically endorsed an international ban on human cloning.[43] Wilmut and other scientists agree that while animal cloning has numerous potential benefits, such as new medicines or new disease treatments, human cloning research is unethical. Yet others claim that halting human cloning research entirely is the sole means of supporting an international prohibition of human cloning.[44] Following President Clinton's instructions to the NBAC, several other countries asked commissions to review issues relating to human cloning.

On January 12, 1998, 19 countries signed the Council of Europe Protocol,[45] which prohibits the cloning of human beings.[46] The 40 member countries of the Council of Europe, plus Australia, Canada, the United States, Japan, Holy See, and the European Community, were invited to sign the Protocol. This document is the first binding international treaty on human cloning. The Protocol prohibits "any intervention seeking to create a human being genetically identical to another human being, whether living or dead," without exception.[47] In developing the Protocol, the Council of Europe considered the "serious difficulties of a medical, psychological, and social nature that such a deliberate biomedical practice might imply for all the individuals involved."[48] The Protocol took effect May 1, 1998. The United States did not sign the Protocol.

Jacques Chirac, the President of France, Jacques Santer, the President of the European Commission, and Federico Mayor, the Director General of UNESCO, had all previously asked their own bioethics advisory committees to make recommendations on human cloning.[49] Santer had informed the chair of the Group of Advisors on the Ethical Implications of Biotechnology (GAEIB) that the commission would adhere to the GAEIB's recommendations on both animal and human cloning.[50] The GAEIB submitted its advice to the European Commission on May 30, 1997. The GAEIB suggested to the European Commission that reproductive human cloning by nuclear transfer should be banned, but that the cloning of human parts for organ and skin replacement should remain legal. At that time, it remained unclear how the human cloning legislation in Europe would be shaped.

Other countries are also considering the human cloning issue. In China, scientist delegates at the annual meeting of China's parliament agreed that new legislation was necessary to ban human cloning.[51] Additionally, two Japanese groups, the Committee for Basic Plans for Life Sciences and the Committee for Life Sciences, plan to present the Japanese government with a report and recommendations. Kanji Fujiki, the Director of the Life Sciences Division of the Science and Technology Agency in Tokyo, believes that the two Japanese committees will make reports and recommendations similar to those produced in both Europe and the United States. Because Japan does not have any embryology legislation, Fujiki thinks it will be difficult to implement a human cloning ban into legislation.

In addition to the Council of Europe Protocol, some signatories had previously enacted human cloning legislation. Denmark and Spain have legislation against the cloning of humans. The Danish law forbids experiments "whose purpose is to enable the production of genetically equal human beings."[52] The law in Spain includes "creating human beings by cloning or other procedures directed to selection of traits; creating human beings by cloning in any of its variants, or any other procedure capable of yielding several identical human beings . . ." under the category of "very serious offenses."[53] France has vowed to enact legislation against human cloning if someone attempts a "monstrous" experiment.[54]

Germany has also attempted to address the human cloning issue. Human cloning is purportedly prohibited under Germany's 1990 Embryo Protection Act.[55] Although some argue that this law is broad enough to include a prohibition on the cloning of human beings, others believe that Germany's current law on human experimentation may contain a loophole that permits human cloning. Ernst Benda, a former President of the German Constitutional Court, has disapproved of UNESCO's draft convention on bioethics for its failure to explicitly prohibit the cloning of human beings.

Britain's Human Fertilization and Embryology Act of 1990 states that an embryo cannot be created outside of the human body without authorization.[56] According to David Shapiro of the Nuffield Council on Bioethics, the 1990 Act provides a legal framework to forbid human application of the technology used to clone Dolly.[57] Conversely, others think that the 1990 Act may contain loopholes and allow human cloning. The British House of Commons Select Committee on Science and Technology has decided to convene and discuss whether the current British legislation includes loopholes that might actually permit human cloning.[58] Although the 1990 legislation prohibited the transplant of nuclei into embryos, it may not explicitly forbid the transfer of nuclei into eggs, which is somatic cell nuclear transfer. British law may need to specifically state that such experimental cloning on humans is prohibited in order to close any loopholes.

As these countries attempt to settle their own ethical and legal issues surrounding human cloning, and as the United States decides whether to pass its own legislation or become a signatory on an international initiative, one main issue unique to the United States revolves around whether statutory cloning prohibitions would be constitutional.

Cloning-related constitutional challenges for United States legislation

All legislation enacted in the United States must pass constitutional challenge. Finding clear guidance from the United States Constitution or judicial interpretations about whether human cloning restrictions are constitutional is extremely difficult. In the cloning discussion, the main constitutional issue is whether the concept of procreative liberty exists and, if so, whether it is broad enough to encompass human cloning. If recognized, a right to procreative liberty could be contained within the right of privacy, or it could be considered part of a broader substantive due process liberty interest. Furthermore, other "constitutional values," such as the protection of the freedom of scientific inquiry and the potential right to one's own uniqueness and individuality, will be considered. The last constitutional issue addressed will be whether regulation of human cloning should occur at the federal level or be reserved to the individual states.

In the United States, there is a "presumption in favor of individual freedom of action. . . ."[59] Absent specific prohibitions, people have the freedom and liberty to act as they wish; however, this freedom is constrained "to ensure the good order of society."[60] At the same time, certain fundamental rights are carefully protected under the Constitution.[61] Fundamental rights are those rights "so deeply rooted in our culture and history . . . [that they] are necessary to a system of ordered liberty."[62] Our fundamental rights include the right to vote, the right to travel, and the right of privacy. Various privacy rights, including marriage, sexual relations, abortion, and childrearing, are also deemed fundamental.

The standard that courts use to review the legitimacy of governmental acts that restrict or impinge on fundamental rights is strict scrutiny. Under the strict scrutiny standard, any government action restricting such fundamental rights must be necessary to protect a compelling governmental interest, and the means must be narrowly tailored to achieve that end; thus, there must be no less restrictive means to achieve the governmental goal. Therefore, it must be decided whether individuals have rights to avail themselves of human cloning technology for use with in vitro fertilization, whether this right is protected and fundamental, and whether governmental action to restrict human cloning is necessary to protect a compelling governmental interest. An individual's choice to reproduce using a cloning technique or a scientist's choice to continue with cloning research may be constitutionally restricted based on the potential harms associated with the cloning of human beings if those harms rise to the level of a compelling government interest.

Reproductive Liberty

Human cloning technology may eventually be used to assist in bringing children into the world. Whether to interpret the Constitution to provide protection for a right to create children through the cloning process involves a debate about the scope and meaning of procreative liberty. Certain aspects of childbearing do fall within the penumbra of privacy rights embedded in the Constitution and are generally grounded in a right to bodily integrity.[63] In more recent years, rights associated with childbearing have been grounded in the constitutional doctrine of substantive due process.[64] The modern substantive due process analysis is based on the Due Process Clause of the Fourteenth Amendment. Substantive due process analysis reflects a court's interpretation of what rights are encompassed within the term *liberty*. Basically the analysis entails determining whether a particular activity is so crucial to individual liberty, dignity, and autonomy that, even though the right to that activity is not explicitly granted in the Constitution (such as creating a child using somatic cell nuclear transfer technology) the court may determine the extent to which it can be regulated. The issue becomes whether different aspects of procreative liberty fall within the freedoms guaranteed by the Fourteenth Amendment. A broad view of the constitutionally protected rights related to reproduction is that an individual possesses the "right to submit to a medical procedure that may bring about . . . pregnancy."[65] Furthermore, the Fourteenth Amendment generally is interpreted to protect "freedom of personal choice in matters of marriage and family,"[66] which could potentially encompass the right to clone a child.

On one side of this debate, proponents of human cloning argue that access to cloning should be protected by individuals' "legal right to reproductive freedom."[67] The concept of reproductive freedom is the idea "that we have a right to reproduce the way we choose. . . ."[68] Reproductive freedom protects one's bodily integrity from direct governmental interference so that the law does "not unduly burden women's choices."[69] These proponents suggest that "[c]loning opponents need to come up with a 'compelling reason to overcome that right' [to reproductive freedom]."[70] Commentators such as John Robertson and Ruth Macklin suggest that "a commitment to individual liberty requires that individuals be left free to create children using somatic cell nuclear transfer if they so choose. . . ."[71] Robertson has stated that "[a]s long as the interests of couples and offspring are well served [by human cloning], there will be no need for governmental restrictions on the decisions made by medical professionals and their patients."[72]

This argument is bolstered with an analogy to current medical technologies employed to assist infertile couples. Other types of assisted reproductive technologies, such as in vitro fertilization (IVF), are currently practiced without constitutional challenges. Because IVF technology is widely available and legally permissible, one may argue that the implantation of an embryo created from somatic cell nuclear transfer should be permissible as well. Therefore, it must be determined whether procreation through cloning is distinguishable from currently allowed reproductive technologies. Proponents argue that the right to reproductive freedom includes access to new assisted reproductive technologies. Testifying at the NBAC hearings, Robertson "unequivocally defended the right to reproductive liberty and argued that Dolly marked just one more perfectly acceptable step on a continuum of artificial reproduction methods that help infertile couples have children."[73]

On the other hand, opponents of human cloning believe governmental interference is reasonable and even necessary. They argue that "individuals [are not guaranteed] unfettered access to assisted reproductive technologies."[74] Opponents accede that, in general, a couple's reproductive choices are considered private affairs. The "ongoing controversies regarding the moral standing of human genetic material" have, however, necessitated governmental intervention. When the government has compelling reasons to curtail individual liberty, society allows curtailment with minimal limitations. It is clear that "[g]overnment in our constitutional, democratic society has the authority and obligation to make and enforce reasonable regulations to manage the new reproductive market in order to protect the interests of the public, prospective parents, and their future children."[75] Bonnie Steinbock claims that "[e]ven if the Supreme Court has held procreation, in some contexts, to be a fundamental liberty, it does not follow that it is protected in every context, nor that individuals have a constitutional right to procreate 'by any means necessary.' "[76]

The main argument that opponents to human cloning assert is that cloning does not fall within our previously recognized Constitutional liberties because cloning is distinguishable from currently practiced reproductive technologies. Opponents to human cloning thus claim that previously acknowledged reproductive rights are significantly different from somatic cell nuclear transfer because these other rights involve embryos created from a male and a female gamete donor. Traditional reproductive technologies have resulted from combining the genes of two genetic parents of a child and involve the "transmission of genes vertically across a generation."[77] Although the new cloning technology has the ultimate effect of transmitting genes, the "child" produced will be genetically identical to a single "parent."

This essential difference has led some to question whether human cloning is even "procreation" at all. These critics view cloning as "an entirely new means of creating persons, more a means of manufacturing a person than reproducing."[78] In this view, cloning correlates with " 'replication' not 'reproduction,' and is not constitutionally protected."[79] Steinbock argues that "[i]t is virtually inconceivable that the present Court—or any Court in the near future—would deem SCNT [somatic cell nuclear transfer] cloning to be a fundamental constitutional right."[80] Steinbock bases her argument on the following facts: Most Americans do not assume that cloning is a basic right; cloning is not part of our country's history and tradition; and access to cloning is not essential to ordered liberty.[81]

In sum, it is unclear whether the somatic cell nuclear transfer technique will be considered "procreation" akin to currently accepted reproductive techniques and the corresponding, recognized rights. According to the NBAC, past United States Supreme Court decisions have not yet decided this issue. Previous interpretations of reproductive liberties by the United States Supreme Court offer only partial guidance as to whether cloning is procreation or something entirely new. If the right to create children using a cloning method is considered a fundamental right or found to be part of our liberty guarantees, any government regulation will need to satisfy the strict scrutiny standard, that is, the government must have a compelling interest and must choose narrowly tailored means to achieve the governmental purpose. The speculative and potential psychological and social harms that could occur must be evaluated using this strict scrutiny standard. The main argument on which the NBAC based its recommendation that the moratorium should continue was that the somatic cell nuclear transfer technique would not be safe to attempt on children.[82] The American Medical Association has stated that using nuclear transfer cloning to treat infertility is uncertain and unsafe.[83] The NBAC report states that "the direct physical harms to the children who may result . . . is sufficient to justify a prohibition at this time, even if such efforts were to be characterized as the exercise of a fundamental right to procreate."[84] Thus, the potential psychological and social harms thought to be associated with human cloning may be sufficiently compelling or legitimate to justify a prohibition even if cloning is found to fall within procreative liberty.

Is There a Constitutionally Protected Freedom of Scientific Inquiry?

One of our "constitutional values" is to promote the freedom of scientific inquiry. Our society has long valued and encouraged scientific research and advances.[85]

Although scientific inquiry is considered an important value, neither statutes nor case law specifically recognizes such a protected right under the Constitution. Initially, we must determine whether this "scientific liberty" interest is a constitutionally protected right. Also, we must determine whether the government's interest in banning or regulating such a right (i.e., banning scientists from developing or offering human cloning technology) would be strong enough to withstand the test associated with the appropriate level of scrutiny.

Proponents of human cloning research claim that a "prohibition of somatic cell nuclear transfer with the wrong intent and its unavoidable chilling effect on research may infringe freedom of scientific inquiry. . . ."[86] Many scientific societies oppose a legal ban because they fear that an " 'ambiguous definition of cloning' could shut down a lot of uncontroversial, ongoing research."[87] They believe that anti-cloning laws could prohibit or stifle tremendous opportunities that derive from the application of the cloning technique to animal biotechnology.[88]

Conversely, because scientific developments and applications can have profound social implications, the freedom of scientific inquiry is not absolute. Many governmental regulations restrict types of scientific research based on moral constraints and safety concerns, such as human embryo research. Even if scientific inquiry were determined to be constitutionally protected, "the government could regulate to protect against compelling harms. . . ."[89] Robertson claims:

[I]f the government can show that restrictions on cloning and cloning technology are sufficiently important to the general well being of individuals or society, such restrictions are likely to be upheld as legitimate, constitutional governmental actions, even if scientists were held to have a First Amendment right of scientific inquiry.[90]

A logical argument that would justify governmental restriction is that cloning is simply too harmful and morally distasteful.

Assuming a right to scientific inquiry exists, any restriction on cloning research must be narrowly drawn. The NBAC recommends that any "regulatory or legislative actions . . . should be carefully written so as not to interfere with other important areas of scientific research."[91] The Commission warns against regulating the cloning of human DNA sequences and cell lines because "neither activity raises the scientific and ethical issues that arise from"[92] cloning human beings. The NBAC also suggests that the cloning of animals by the somatic cell nuclear transfer technique should continue subject to regulations requiring the humane treatment of animals.

A Right to Individuality?

Within the human cloning discussion, some commentators argue that United States citizens have constitutional rights to their own individuality and uniqueness.[93] Because of the novelty of somatic cell nuclear transfer, society has not yet fully considered the issue of the right to genetic individuality. Cloning technology may infringe on this "moral or human right" to individuality if such a right exists.[94] Cloning technology has the potential to lead to "excessive control of children and their characteristics."[95] Such uses of the cloning technology will decrease the genetic uniqueness of each human being. According to Husted and Husted,

The individual rights of a human being are the most concrete of ethical facts. . . . This is a right that supersedes every other right. Individuals have the right to be who they are simply because they are who they are. Their right to their own life, liberty, and the pursuit of their happiness is identical to their right to be who they are. . . . Cloning violates this right and violates one's destiny.[96]

Conversely, opponents of the view that cloning will violate a right to individuality first claim that such a right does not exist. There is little grounding for such a right in the Constitution or in judicial interpretations. In addition, proponents of human cloning claim that even if such a right exists, "our uniqueness comes not just from our genes, but as well from our environment, personal history, human relationships, and choices through which we create our own biographies. Cloning would not deny anyone a unique human identity."[97]

Federalism

The last constitutional concern related to regulating human cloning regards the concept of federalism. Federalism involves the idea that all powers not delegated to the federal government are reserved to the states. A federal ban on human cloning may exceed the limits of federal power, especially when one considers that "the regulation of health and clinical practice has traditionally fallen to the states."[98] The United States has a tradition of state regulation governing certain areas such as family affairs and medical practice. Furthermore, a federal ban "could stifle the diverse policy responses of the states, should some states wish to be more liberal in permitting nuclear transfer to create a child."[99] The individual states are often described as "laboratories" where different legislative approaches and judge-made law serve as experiments from which other states and the federal government may watch and learn. Any broad federal ban would quash such legal experimentation of the best methods of regulating human cloning and cloning technology.

On the other hand, federal powers are often given an expansive interpretation. More and more frequently, federal legislators and federal regulatory bodies pass laws and regulations that affect matters traditionally reserved for the states. The challenge by the federal government would be to regulate cloning or cloning technology and withstand constitutional scrutiny. In addition, there may be some advantages to federal as opposed to state legislation such as comprehensive coverage and clarity, an assurance against state inconsistency, and prevention against forum shopping.

Discussion

When legislation is drafted and its constitutionality assessed, several related concerns factor into the decision-making process. In general, our legislators are utilitarian in practice. In broad terms, they aim to legislate to protect the largest number of people from harm and to promote the good of the greatest number. This aim is achieved through a balancing process in which the harms and benefits of a particular proposal are weighed. Generally speaking, the benefits afforded by any legislation must outweigh the burdens imposed. The considerations involved in the human cloning discussion are whether the conduct legislatively prohibited is ethical, scientifically sound, moral, and accepted by religious teachings. To ensure that the enactment of constitutionally valid cloning legislation will receive public support, the discussion of human cloning must include several components.

On one side of the balancing equation, the burdens created by human cloning are strongly evidenced by the danger of and moral repugnance to the practice. The proposed bills in federal and state legislatures outlawing or banning human cloning are the result of the public reaction to the prospect of human cloning. Initially fearful public reaction varied from images of "Mary Shelley's Frankenstein, armies of drones, and clone farms to produce spare parts"[100] to dreadful images of organs grown from headless human clones.[101] Upon further consideration, the public became alarmed with the possibility that human cloning could interfere with "traditional notions of family, kinship, procreation, and human power over nature."[102] The prospect of utilizing human cloning to adjust the genetic make-up of society could alter the future of all humankind. The widespread public outcry against human cloning, along with the general fear of and aversion to it, has provoked and fueled the current public policy discussions.

Yet others focus on the benefits of human cloning and advocate for the use of the somatic cell nuclear transfer cloning technique. Human cloning could provide a viable option to couples unable to have their own children. In addition, the unknown possibilities associated with the somatic cell nuclear transfer technique could offer both life-saving and life-enhancing technologies. Furthermore, the protection of human cloning would promote the right to autonomy of scientists and safeguard the freedom to investigate. Finally, there are several potentially useful plant and animal technologies yet to be created from the use of somatic cell nuclear transfer technology that could also have vast human advantages.

Balancing these divergent interests and creating public policy are onerous tasks. Even a cursory glance at the tremendous volumes of legislative history warrants an appreciation of the difficulty of establishing widespread, acceptable public policy. Because the United States is a composite of divergent traditions, values, religions, and morals, any attempt to accommodate the various interests is an arduous undertaking. Regulating human cloning is especially challenging because the prospect of human cloning provokes such a distasteful "gut reaction" and a diversity of opinions. To create sound cloning public policy, legislatures are striving to harmonize individual interests and beliefs while promoting the good and general welfare of the greater public.

Both the NBAC recommendations and the proposed legislation are examples of the attempt to balance the interests involved. The NBAC acknowledges that the creation of public policy regarding human cloning encompasses more than a simple analysis of the benefits and harms of cloning. The NBAC suggests that enacting cloning public policy also entails the complex consideration of "traditions, customs, and principles of constitutional law."[103] In its effort to make public policy recommendations, the NBAC struggled to incorporate the multitude of public opinions. During their 90 day assessment, the NBAC relied on hired contractors to document the science underlying cloning, as well as the main religious and ethical arguments raised by the prospect of cloning human beings. The NBAC ultimately rested its conclusion to temporarily ban human cloning on safety and ethical concerns.

The recommendations of the NBAC are the product of a broad and quick analysis of cloning-related issues and a balancing of the benefits and harms at stake. The NBAC offered several justifications for a federal legal ban on research related to the cloning of human beings. The recommendations "reflect[ed] the Commission's best judgments about the ethics of attempting such an experiment and [its] view of traditions regarding limitations on individual actions in the name of the common good."[104] The NBAC determined that the fetuses and children resulting from cloning would be exposed to ethically unacceptable physical, psychological, and social risks and harms. Based on current public and academic perception, the NBAC deemed these risks and harms to outweigh the benefits of human cloning. Therefore, the NBAC advocated a prohibition on human cloning.

Some commentators have suggested a different assessment of the harms and benefits. A notable representative of such a view is Andrea Bonnicksen. She cautions against a premature legislative ban because human cloning is a "speculative technique" and because legislators are acting under "a false sense of urgency."[105] Bonnicksen suggests creating a cloning policy that "combines private and public oversight and that incorporates two other potential methods of replicating genomes: twinning and embryo cell nuclear transfer."[106] Another commentator, Susan Wolf, also criticizes the NBAC's recommendation for a ban. She thinks cloning warrants regulation, but not a ban. She suggests "extend[ing] human subjects protection in the private sphere and regulat[ing] reproductive technologies efficiently, with a central advisory body for" such novel issues.[107] John Robertson also criticizes the NBAC's recommendation of a federal criminal ban, stating that "[the NBAC] has not shown that the risks are so great or so likely to occur as to justify criminal law at the federal level, nor is it sufficiently sensitive to the procreative liberty and federalism costs of such an approach."[108]

The different policy considerations and recommendations and the resulting leg- islation will inevitably face constitutional challenge. The prospect of human cloning forces a re-examination of basic constitutional values and guarantees. As the Constitution is interpreted over time, the protections afforded evolve. The Framers of the Constitution intended to develop a flexible document capable of varying interpretations. Judges and policy makers attempt to create law that re- sponds to new scientific developments and emerging public attitudes. The Supreme Court has recognized rights embedded within the meaning of the Constitution. For example, while not explicitly stated in the text of the Constitution, the right to privacy has been acknowledged as a fundamental right, but the limits of this right are challenged on a continual basis. Whether human cloning is included in the penumbra of recognized privacy rights or falls within the liberties guaranteed by the Fourteenth Amendment will be determined by and reflective of our moral, cultural, and religious values. Determining whether human cloning falls within the spirit of our Constitution is the essence of the current controversy.

Conclusion

The differing opinions expressed regarding the prospect of human cloning em- phasize our current vague understanding of its implications. Federal and state legislatures are presently assessing the morality and legality of human cloning research. Similarly, international initiatives are exploring the vast ramifications of the new technology. In the Unites States, the human cloning discussion is in- evitably intertwined with considerations regarding the constitutional validity of prohibitive legislation. A discussion of the scope of our protected liberty inter- ests and the countervailing governmental interests is necessitated by the somatic cell nuclear transfer technique and its applicability to human cloning. The cur- rent NBAC recommendations and the federal and state proposals reflect a bal- ancing of the divergent interests at stake and are an attempt at responsible pub- lic policy regarding human cloning.

The opinions expressed here are the authors' and do not represent the views of the State of Michigan, the National Institutes of Health, or the United States Department of Health and Human Services.

Notes

Introduction

1. The text of the President's letter along with the commission's report can be found in National Bioethics Advisory Commission, *Cloning Human Beings: Report and Recommendations of the National Bioethics Advisory Commission* (Rockille, MD: National Bioethics Advisory Commission, June 1997).

2. For a helpful summary of the history of cloning research, see Gina Kolata, *Clone: The Road to Dolly, and the Path Ahead* (New York: William Morrow and Company, 1998).

3. J. B. S. Haldane, "Biological Possibilities for the Human Species in the Next Ten Thousand Years" in *Man and His Future*, ed. Gordon Wolstenholme (Edinburg: J & A Churchill Ltd., 1963). Lederberg's speculations can be found in a column he wrote for the *Washington Post*, September 30, 1967.

4. See, for example, Paul Ramsey, "Shall We Reproduce?" *Journal of the American Medical Association* 220/11 (1972).

5. Leon Kass, *Toward a More Natural Science* (New York: The Free Press, 1985), p. 126. Kass's more recent reflections on cloning can be found in the article "The Wisdom of Repugnance: Why We Should Ban the Cloning of Humans," *The New Republic* 216 (June 1997): 17–26.

6. National Institutes of Health, *Report of the Human Embryo Research Panel* (Bethesda, MD: National Institutes of Health, September 1994).

7. For a brief review of the history and politics of embryo research, see Bonnie Steinbock, *Life Before Birth: The Moral and Legal Status of Embryos and Fetuses* (New York: Oxford University Press, 1992), esp. ch. 5.

8. For a good discussion of recent debates on the use of human stem cells, see the "Symposium: Human Primordial Stem Cells," *Hastings Center Report* 29/2 (March–April 1999): 30–48.

9. "Researchers Join in Effort on Cloning Repair Tissue," *The New York Times*, May 5, 1999, Sec. A, p. 22.

10. This is a point that Lee Silver makes in is book *Remaking Eden* (New York: Avon Books, 1997). According to Silver, it is the development of IVF that represents "a singular moment in human evolution." It does so, he says, because "the development of IVF marks the point in history when human beings gained the power to seize control of their own evolutionary destiny" (pp. 74–5).

11. Lori B. Andrews and Nanette Elster, "Cross-Cultural Analysis of Policies Regarding Embryo Research," in *Papers Commissioned for the NIH Human Embryo Research Panel* (Washington, DC: NIH Publication No. 95-3916, September, 1994).

12. For a discussion of the controversy surrounding the panel by one of its members, see Ronald M. Green, "At the Vortex of Controversy: Developing Guidelines for Human Embryo Research," *Kennedy Institute of Ethics Journal* 4/4 (1994): 345–56.

13. The President moved to block one recommendation made by the HERP, namely, that embryos could be created solely for research purposes "when the research by its very nature cannot otherwise be validly conducted" and when doing so is "necessary for the validity of a study that is potentially of outstanding scientific and therapeutic value."

14. See Appendix 2 in this volume.

15. For a discussion of the George Washington University experiment, see the essays devoted to this topic in the *Kennedy Institute of Ethics Journal* 4/3 (1994). See also Andrea Bonnicksen, "Ethical and Policy Issues in Human Embryo Twinning," *Cambridge Quarterly of Healthcare Ethics* 4 (1995): 268–84.

16. George Annas, Arthur Caplan, and Sherman Elias. "The Politics of Human-Embryo Research—Avoiding Ethical Gridlock," *New England Journal of Medicine* 334 (1996): 1330.

Chapter 1

1. Mary Anne Warren, "On the Moral and Legal Status of Abortion," *The Monist* 57 (1973): 43–61.

2. Not everyone agrees that patients in a persistent vegetative state are alive. See Robert Veatch, "The Whole-Brain-Oriented Concept of Death: An Outmoded Philosophical Formulation," *Journal of Thanatology* 3 (1975): 13–30; and Michael Green and Daniel Wikler, "Brain Death and Personal Identity," *Philosophy and Public Affairs* 9, no 2 (1980): 105–33.

3. See, for example, Joel Feinberg, "The Mistreatment of Dead Bodies," *Hastings Center Report* 15/1 (1985): 31–37, and J. Feinberg, "Sentiment and Sentimentality in Practical Ethics," in *Freedom and Fulfillment* (Princeton, NJ: Princeton University Press, 1992), pp. 98–123.

4. See my *Life Before Birth: The Moral and Legal Status of Embryos and Fetuses* (New York: Oxford University Press, 1992), pp. 54–55.

5. Mary Anne Warren, *Moral Status* (Oxford: Clarendon Press, 1997), p. 50.

6. See Steinbock, *Life Before Birth*, ch. 1, "The Interest View."

7. The interest view is based on Joel Feinberg's "interest principle," which he elaborated in "The Rights of Animals and Unborn Generations," *Philosophy and Environmental*

Crisis, ed. William T. Blackstone (Athens, GA: University of Georgia Press, 1974), pp. 43–68.

8. The distinction between biological life (being alive) and biographical life (having a life) is drawn by James Rachels in *The End of Life: Euthanasia and Morality* (New York: Oxford University Press, 1985), p. 25.

9. Don Marquis, "Why Abortion Is Immoral," *Journal of Philosophy* 86, no. 4 (1989): 183–202.

10. I shift here from talking about the moral status of embryos to talking about the moral status of fetuses, because Marquis talks about fetuses. This is because he is concerned to show the wrongness of abortion, which invariably involves killing fetuses rather than embryos. Everything I say about embryos applies (at least) to first-trimester fetuses, however, and everything Marquis says about fetuses applies to embryos, at least after implantation. To my knowledge, he has not yet discussed in print the moral status of extracorporeal embryos.

11. Actually, even at the end of fertilization, there may not yet be a new genome, as recent studies suggest that a new genome is not expressed until the four-cell to eight-cell stage of development. See John Robertson, *Children of Choice* (Princeton, NJ: Princeton University Press, 1994), p. 251, n. 14). Moreover, until implantation, there is the possibility of twinning, so that before implantation a single individual cannot be said to exist, as Marquis acknowledges (Marquis, "Why Abortion is Immoral," p. 194). Therefore, contraceptives that prevent implantation (like the IUD) would not be seriously wrong on the "future like ours," (FLO) account.

12. A notable exception is R. M. Hare, who holds that abortion, contraception, and abstaining from procreation are all *prima facie* morally wrong and all easily justifiable. See Hare, "Abortion and the Golden Rule," *Philosophy and Public Affairs* 4 (1975): 3.

13. Some people who support women's rights to have abortions hate the term "pro-life" because they believe this suggests that they are "anti-life." Similarly, some people who oppose legalized abortion hate the term "pro-choice" because they think it suggests that they are generally opposed to women making their own choices, when it is only the choice of abortion they oppose. In my view, it is impossible to find neutral terms that will make everyone happy. Therefore I use the terms by which members of the two groups identify themselves.

14. See my "Why Most Abortions are not Wrong," in *Bioethics for Medical Education*, eds. Rem B. Edwards and Edward Bittar, (Stamford, CT: JAI Press, 1999), pp. 245–267.

15. See Steinbock, "Why Most Abortions are not Wrong" and *Life Before Birth*, ch. 2.

16. The topic of abortion is so heated and so emotional because it raises questions of the proper place of sexuality, the correct ideal of motherhood, the appropriate role of women, and so forth. Entire world views are contained in the labels "pro-life" and "pro-choice," and each side feels threatened by the other. See Kristin Luker's perceptive and convincing *Abortion and the Politics of Motherhood* (Berkeley: University of California Press, 1984).

17. I put to one side embryos that will become people. There are clearly limits on what may be done to embryos that are going to become people because their interests can be set back or thwarted by what happens at the embryonic stage. The harm or wrong is not to the embryo, but rather to the person who has developed out of the embryo. See Steinbock, *Life Before Birth*, chs. 3 and 4, where I am concerned only with moral limits to the treatment of embryos not intended for implantation.

18. Ethics Advisory Board, Department of Health, Education and Welfare [HEW], *Report and Conclusions: HEW Support of Research Involving Human In Vitro Fertilization and Embryo Transfer* (Washington, DC: U.S. Government Printing Office, May 4, 1979).

19. Mary Warnock, *A Question of Life: The Warnock Report on Human Fertilisation and Embryology* (New York: Basil Blackwell, 1985).

20. John A. Robertson, "Symbolic Issues in Embryo Research," *Hastings Center Report* 25, no. 1 (1995): 37–38.

21. Ronald Dworkin, *Life's Dominion* (New York: Knopf, 1993), pp. 71–84.

22. Different cultures display respect for the dead in different ways. In one culture, burying the dead is mandatory and cremation forbidden; in another, exactly the opposite is mandatory. The point is that every culture demands some ritual treatment of dead bodies in order to show proper respect.

23. Feinberg, *Freedom and Fulfillment*, p. 53.

24. Robertson, "Symbolic Issues in Embryo Research," p. 37.

25. *Ibid.*, p. 38.

26. Daniel Callahan, "The Puzzle of Profound Respect," *Hastings Center Report* 25, no. 1 (1995): 39–40.

27. Gina Kolata, "Medicine's Troubling Bonus: Surplus of Human Embryos," *New York Times*, March 16, 1997, p. A1.

28. "British Clinics, Obeying Law, End Embryos By Thousands," *New York Times*, August 2, 1996, p. A3.

29. Youssef M. Ibrahim, "Ethical Furor Erupts in Britain: Should Unclaimed Embryos Die?" *New York Times*, August 1, 1996, p. A1.

30. Annabel Ferriman, "2,500 'orphan embryos' to be destroyed within days" *Independent on Sunday*, July 7, 1996, p. 1.

31. See Dworkin, *Life's Dominion*, p. 84.

32. *Cloning Human Beings: Report and Recommendations of the National Bioethics Advisory Commission* (Rockville, MD: National Bioethics Advisory Commission, June 1997).

33. See John Robertson, "Liberty, Identity, and Human Cloning," *Texas Law Review* 76, no. 6 (1998): 1371–456, esp. pp. 1405–09.

34. Leon Kass, "The Wisdom of Repugnance: Why We Should Ban the Cloning of Humans," *The New Republic*, June 2, 1997. Excerpted and reprinted in John D. Arras and Bonnie Steinbock, eds., *Ethical Issues in Modern Medicine*, 5th Ed. (Mountain View, CA: Mayfield Publishing Company, 1998), pp. 496–510.

35. For an illuminating account of how the Human Embryo Research Panel conducted its deliberations and suggestions for a more explicitly political and pragmatic approach, see R. Alta Charo, "The Hunting of the Snark: The Moral Status of Embryos, Right-to-Lifers, and Third World Women," *Stanford Law and Policy Review* 6, no. 2 (1995): 11–37.

Chapter 2

1. Throughout this essay, I often use the phrase "human embryo" as shorthand for embryos up to 14 days after fertilization that may be considered for biomedical research. In *Body, Soul, and Bioethics*, (Notre Dame: University of Notre Dame Press, 1995), Gilbert Meilaender has persuasively argued that it is misleading to refer to such em-

bryos as "pre-implantation" because there is no intent in a research protocol to implant the embryo for gestation. Thus, I follow his language of "unimplanted" embryo as more scientifically and ethically honest.

2. Peter Singer, *Embryo Experimentation* (Cambridge: Cambridge University Press, 1990).

3. National Institutes of Health, *Report of the Human Embryo Research Panel* (Bethesda, MD: September 1994).

4. Gregory Pence, *Who's Afraid of Human Cloning* (New York: Rowman and Littlefield, 1998), p. 88.

5. National Institutes of Health, *Report of the Human Embryo Research Panel*, p. 2.

6. John Ziman, "Is Science Losing Its Objectivity?" *Nature* 382 (August 1996): 751–54.

7. National Institutes of Health, *Report of the Human Embryo Research Panel*, p. 2.

8. National Academy of Sciences, *On Being a Scientist* (Washington, DC: National Academy Press, 1989), pp. 6–8.

9. Max Weber, "Science as a Vocation," in *From Max Weber: Essays in Sociology*, eds. H. H. Gerth and C. Wright Mills (New York: Oxford University Press, 1958), p. 144.

10. National Institutes of Health, *Report of the Human Embryo Research Panel*, pp. 20–21.

11. Paul Lauritzen, "What Price Parenthood?" *Hastings Center Report* 20 (March/April 1990): 38–46.

12. Richard Gold, *Body Parts: Property Rights and the Ownership of Human Biological Materials* (Washington, DC: Georgetown University Press, 1996), p. 149.

13. Mary Rosner and T. R. Johnson, "Telling Stories: Metaphors of the Human Genome Project," *Hypatia* 10 (1995): 104–29.

14. Albert Einstein, "Strange Is Our Situation Here Upon Earth," in *The World Treasury of Modern Religious Thought* ed. J. Pelikan (Boston: Little, Brown, and Company, 1990), pp. 202–05.

15. Evelyn Fox Keller, *A Feeling for the Organism* (San Francisco: W. H. Freeman Press, 1983).

16. R. D. Land and L. A. Moore, eds. *Life at Risk: The Crises in Medical Ethics* (Nashville, TN: Broadman and Holman Publishers, 1995).

17. Russell Belk, "Me and Thee Versus Mine and Thine," in *Organ Donation and Transplantation: Psychological and Behavioral Factors*, eds. J. Shanteau and R. J. Harris (Washington, DC: American Psychological Association, 1990, p. 144.

Chapter 3

1. "The Inhuman Use of Human Beings: A Statement on Embryo Research by the Ramsey Colloquium," *First Things* (January 1995): 17–21; Daniel Callahan, "The Puzzle of Profound Respect," *Hastings Center Report* 25, no. 1 (1995): 39–40.

2. "Embryos: Drawing the Line," *The Washington Post*, October 2, 1994, p. C6.

3. Dena S. Davis, "Embryos Created for Research Purposes," *Kennedy Institute of Ethics Journal* (December 1995): 343–54, 343.

4. Bonnie Steinbock, *Life Before Birth: The Moral and Legal Status of Embryos and Fetuses* (New York: Oxford University Press, 1992).

5. See also Bonnie Steinbock, "Ethical Issues in Human Embryo Research," in National Institutes of Health, *Report of the Human Embryo Research Panel*, vol. II (Bethesda, MD: National Institutes of Health, September, 1994), pp. 27–50.

6. Citations for Steinbock's *Life Before Birth* throughout this section are given in parentheses within the body of the text.

7. Here Steinbock is quoting John Harris, "Embryos and Hedgehogs: On the Moral Status of the Embryo," in *Experiments on Embryos* eds. Anthony Dyson and John Harris (London: Routledge, 1990), pp. 65–81.

8. John A. Robertson, "Symbolic Issues in Embryo Research," *Hastings Center Report* 25, no. 1 (January–February 1995): 37–38.

9. Gilbert C. Meilaender, *Body, Soul and Bioethics* (Notre Dame, IN: University of Notre Dame Press, 1995), p. 87.

10. Robertson, "Symbolic Issues in Embryo Research," p. 38; Davis, "Embryos Created for Research Purposes," p. 352.

11. See John A. Robertson, *Children of Choice: Freedom and the New Reproductive Technologies* (Princeton, NJ: Princeton University Press, 1994), esp. pp. 22–42.

12. National Institutes of Health, *Report of the Human Embryo Research Panel*, p. 43.

13. Callahan, "The Puzzle of Profound Respect," p. 39.

14. Ibid., p. 40; National Institutes of Health, *Report of the Human Embryo Research Panel*, pp. 41–42.

15. Sheldon Krimsky and Ruth Hubbard, "The Business of Research," *Hastings Center Report* 25, no. 1 (1995): 41–43.

16. Mary Briody Mahowald, *Women and Children in Health Care: An Unequal Majority* (New York: Oxford University Press, 1993), p. 119.

17. Stanley K. Henshaw and Margaret Terry Orr, "The Need and Unmet Need for Infertility Services in the United States," *Family Planning Perspectives* 19, no. 4 (July/August, 1987), p. 183.

18. See David S. Broder, "The Real Issue Ought To Be Family Planning," in *South Bend Tribune*, June 9, 1997, p. B10.

19. Krimsky and Hubbard, "The Business of Research," p. 42.

20. Other permissible sources of research gametes identified by the Human Embryo Research Panel include women undergoing scheduled pelvic surgery or diagnostic procedures and women who have died. Until techniques for oocyte maturation are well developed, it is likely that living oocyte donors would agree to undergo hormonal stimulation similar to that used to generate multiple ova for fertilization in assisted reproduction. See National Institutes of Health, *Report of the Human Embryo Research Panel*, pp. 56–60.

21. Lee M. Silver, *Remaking Eden: Cloning and Beyond in a Brave New World* (New York: Avon Books, 1997), p. 75.

22. Ibid.

23. See Maura A. Ryan, "The Argument for Unlimited Procreative Liberty: A Feminist Critique," in *Hastings Center Report*, 20, no. 4 (July/August 1990): 6–12; also, "The New Reproductive Technologies: Defying God's Dominion?" *Journal of Medicine and Philosophy* (February 1995): 419–38.

24. GIFT (gamete intrafallopian transfer) and ZIFT (zygote intrafallopian transfer) are forms of IVF.

25. Margaret A. Farley, "Feminist Theology and Bioethics," in *Women's Consciousness, Women's Conscience*, eds. Barbara Hilkert Andolsen, Christine E. Gudorf, and Mary D. Pellauer (Minneapolis, MN: Winston Press, 1985), pp. 285–305.

26. Patricia Spallone, *Beyond Conception: The New Politics of Reproduction* (Granby, MA: Bergin and Garvey Publishers, Inc., 1989), p. 183. See also Gina Corea, *The Mother Machine* (New York: Harper and Row, 1985).

27. Lisa Sowle Cahill, "Women, Marriage, Parenthood: What Are Their 'Natures'?" *Logos* 9 (1988): 31.

28. Ibid.

29. Ibid.

30. National Institutes of Health, *Report of the Human Embryo Research Panel*, p. 59. It is interesting to note that the panel does not raise the same degree of concern about exposing donors undergoing pelvic surgery to the long-term risks of hormonal stimulation. When possible, the panel argues, the risk of hyperstimulation should be avoided. The question of whether donors not already undergoing assisted reproduction should be exposed to ovarian stimulation drugs in the first place is not, however, raised.

31. I thank Paul Lauritzen for pressing me on this question.

32. Even if we want to argue that cloning by nuclear transfer is merely "replication" rather than "reproduction," insofar as the aim is to produce offspring, it is reasonable to ask whether it honors the moral character of reproduction. We might say that cloning violates that character *precisely because* it is replication rather than procreation (understood as biological as well as relational partnership).

33. In a private communication (January 2, 1998), Paul Lauritzen has suggested that if I agree that parthenogenesis (at least as described in the report of the Human Embryo Research Panel) need not be held to the moral ideals governing procreation in this analysis then I must also agree that the creation of embryos for research in which implantation is not planned cannot be held to those ideals. The unimplanted embryo, he argues, has no more chance of developing into a human person than the parthenote. There is, however, an important difference between a case in which the entity lacks the intrinsic potentiality for development (i.e., consists of human cells but is not a human embryo) and a case in which it is the decision not to attempt implantation that poses the obstacle to development. I assume, joining panel member Patricia King, that fertilization represents an important stage in the trajectory of human development and a point at which concerns about our obligations to respect human embryos properly arise. I have argued that decisions about the manipulation of gametes, fertilization in vitro, and implantation ought to be integrally related to intentions to create a child. When attempt at implantation does not serve the goal of responsible reproduction and the embryos would otherwise be destroyed, donation for research can be justified.

34. National Institutes of Health, *Report of the Human Embryo Research Panel*, p. A3.

35. Lisa Sowle Cahill, *Sex, Gender and Christian Ethics* (Cambridge: Cambridge University Press, 1996), p. 254.

Chapter 4

1. Albert Jonsen and Stephen Toulmin, *The Abuse of Casuistry: A History of Moral Reasoning* (Berkeley: University of California Press, 1988).

2. Donald Evans, ed., *Conceiving the Embryo: Ethics, Law and Practice in Human Embryology* (Boston: Martinus Nijhoff, 1996).

3. Arlene Klotzko "The Regulation of Embryo Research Under the Human Fertilisation and Embryology Act of 1990." In Evans, *Conceiving the Embryo*, pp. 303–314.

4. For instance, Alex Mauron, "The Human Embryo and the Relativity of Biological Individuality," in Evans, *Conceiving the Embryo*, pp. 55–74; Martyn Evans, "Human Individuation and Moral Justification," in Evans, *Conceiving the Embryo*, pp. 75–87; Zbigniew Szawarski, "Talking About Embryos," in Evans, *Conceiving the Embryo*, pp. 119–34.

5. Donald Evans, "Pro-attitudes to Pre-embryos," in *Conceiving the Embryo*, pp. 27–46.

6. Maurizio Mori, "Is the Human Embryo a Person? No," in Evans, *Conceiving the Embryo*, pp. 151–63; see also Mori, "Genetic Selection and the Status of the Embryo," *Bioethics* 7 (1993): 141–48.

7. On the one hand, see the excellent essay by Soren Holm, "The Moral Status of the Pre-personal Human Being: The Argument from Potential Reconsidered," in Evans, *Conceiving the Embryo*, pp. 193–220; on the other hand, see the excellent essay by Massimo Reichlin, "The Argument From Potential," *Bioethics* 11 (1997): 1–23. See also Christopher Belshaw, "Abortion, Value and the Sanctity of Life," *Bioethics* 11 (1997): 130–50; and John Crosby, "The Personhood of the Human Embryo," *Journal of Medicine and Philosophy* 18 (1993): 399–417.

8. Here then is the call to understand ourselves as related to embryonic life; see Lisa Cahill, "The Embryo and the Fetus: New Moral Contexts," *Theological Studies* 54 (1993): 142–59; James Keenan, "Genetic Research and the Elusive Body," in *Embodiment, Medicine and Morality*, eds. M. Farley and L. S. Cahill (Dordrecht: Kluwer Academics, 1995), pp. 59–73; Paul Lauritzen, "Whose Bodies? Which Selves? Appeals to Embodiment in Assessments of Reproductive Technology," in Farley and Cahill, *Embodiment, Medicine and Morality*, pp. 113–26.

9. See Jean-Marie Thevoz, "The Status of the Embryo—More Place for Moral Intuitions," in Evans, *Conceiving the Embryo*, pp. 47–54.

10. See Ruyter, "Embryos as Moral Subjects and the Limits of Responsibility," in Evans, *Conceiving the Embryo*, pp. 173–91.

11. An analysis of this case appears in Louis Vereecke, "L'assurance maritime chez les theologiens des XVe et XVIe siecles," *Studia Moralia* 8 (1970): 347–85. See a broader discussion of it in James Keenan, "The Casuistry of John Major, Nominalist Professor of Paris," in *The Context of Casuistry*, eds. James Keenan and Thomas Shannon (Washington, DC: Georgetown University Press, 1995), pp. 85–102.

12. Precisely the argument of Thomas Kopfensteiner, "Science, Metaphor, and Casuistry," in Keenan and Shannon, *The Context of Casuistry*, pp. 207–20.

13. John Connery, *Abortion: The Development of the Roman Catholic Perspective* (Chicago: Loyola University Press, 1977), pp. 124–129; Navarre makes the case in *De ablatorum restitutione*, b. 2, c. 3. (Brescia, 1605).

14. Connery, *Abortion*, pp. 129–31; Vasquez, *De restitutione*, c. 2, dub. 7., nn. 27–28 (Lyons, 1631).

15. Connery, *Abortion*, pp. 133; Ioannes Azor, *Institutiones morales*, Pars 3, b. 2., c. 3. (Rome, 1610).

16. Connery, *Abortion*, pp. 134–41; Sanchez, *De matrimonio*, b. 9, d. 17, n. 15; d. 20, n. 6 (Antwerp, 1620).

17. Jonsen and Toulmin, *The Abuse of Casuistry*, pp. 251–59. See Richard Miller's use of the just war paradigm in order to analyze the issues concerning the use of cadaverous tissue in "On Transplanting Human Fetal Tissue: Presumptive Duties and the Task of Casuistry," *Journal of Medicine and Philosophy* 14 (1989): 617–40. See also his more recent important work, *Casuistry and Modern Ethics: A Poetics of Practical Reasoning* (Chicago: University of Chicago, 1996).

18. For further discussion, see James Kennan, "The Function of the Principle of Double Effect," *Theological Studies* 54 (1993): 294–315.

19. For further discussion, see James Keenan, "The Return of Casuistry," *Theological Studies* 57 (1996): 123–29.

20. Bonnie Steinbock, "Ethical Issues in Human Embryo Research," in *Papers Commissioned for the NIH Human Embryo Research Panel* (Bethesda, MD: National Institutes of Health, 1994), pp. 27–50.

21. Dena Davis, "Embryos Created for Research Purposes," *Kennedy Institute of Ethics Journal* 5 (1995): 343–54.

22. David Heyd, "Experimenting with Embryos: Can Philosophy Help?" *Bioethics* 10 (1996): 292–309.

23. See Bonnie Steinbock, *Life Before Birth: The Moral and Legal Status of Embryos and Fetuses* (New York: Oxford University Press, 1992).

24. Steinbock, "Ethical Issues in Human Embryo Research," p. 43.

25. This is proven fairly definitively by Bruno Schueller in "The Double Effect in Catholic Thought: A Reevaluation," in *Doing Evil to Achieve Good*, eds. Richard McCormick and Paul Ramsey (Chicago: Loyola University Press, 1978), pp. 165–91. In support of Schueller, see James Keenan, "Taking Aim at the Principle of Double Effect," *International Philosophical Quarterly* 28 (1988): 201–06; Richard McCormick, *Notes on Moral Theology: 1965 through 1980* (Washington, DC: University Press of America, 1981), pp. 751–56; and Joseph Selling, "The Problem of Reinterpreting the Principle of Double Effect," *Louvain Studies* 8 (1980): 47–62. The most definitive study of its meaning and use is Lucius Ugorji, *The Principle of Double Effect* (Frankfurt am Main: Peter Lang, 1985).

26. Carol Tauer, "Bringing Embryos into Existence for Research Purposes," in *Contingent Future Persons: Philosophical and Theological Challenges*, eds. Nick Fotion and Jan Heller (Boston: Kluwer, 1997), pp. 171–89.

27. Davis, "Embryos Created for Research Purposes," p. 349.

28. Steinbock, "Ethical Issues in Human Embryo Research," p. 43.

29. James Keenan, "What's Your Worst Moral Argument?" *America* 164 (1993): 17–18, 28–30.

30. Thomas Kuhn, *The Structure of Scientific Revolutions* (Chicago: University of Chicago Press, 1973).

31. Tauer, "Bringing Embryos into Existence for Research Purposes," p. 176.

32. Davis, "Embryos Created for Research Purposes," p. 344.

33. Ibid., p. 350.

34. John Robertson, "Symbolic Issues in Embryo Research," *Hastings Center Report* 25, no. 1 (1995): 37–38.

35. Tauer, "Bringing Embryos into Existence for Research Purposes," 176. Tauer, like others, relies on a similar argument from Nicholas Gerrand, "Creating Embryos for Research," *Journal of Applied Philosophy* 10 (1993): 175–87.

36. National Institutes of Health, *Report of the Human Embryo Research Panel* (Bethesda, MD: National Institutes of Health, September 1994), p. 42.

37. Ibid.

38. Ibid. To dissolve the difference, they cite Gerrand, "Creating Embryos for Research," 175–187.

39. See Bernadine Healy and Lynn Sargent Berner, "A Position Against Federal Funding for Human Embryo Research: Words of Caution for Women, for Science, and for Society," *Journal of Women's Health* 4 (1995): 609–13.

40. Callahan, "Response to Hogan and Green," *Hastings Center Report* 25, no. 3 (1995): 5–6.

41. David Heyd acknowledges that comparing the produced embryos to spare embryos offers no ethical standard. He suggests that being born is not considered an *in se* benefit and therefore argues that there is no moral difference between whether the "embryo exists 'anyway' or is intentionally created." To make the case, he uses some taxonomic casuistry and compares these two cases with the difference between forcing

a child to donate bone marrow to a sibling versus producing a child with the purpose of eventually making it donate the organ to its sibling. These parallel sets of cases are congruent with one another, he claims; what distinguishes each set is really the status of the moral agents. Then, however, Heyd acknowledges the difficulty of determining the status of the embryo: Because the status determines the cut-off point for experimentation, he notes that doctors may want to have a later cut-off point, whereas philosophers would simply disagree among themselves (as they do) about the status, drawing lines at conception, 14 days, or brain activity. The philosophers' lines, remarks Heyd, "would be made on the basis of a principle" (Heyd, "Experimenting with Embryos," p. 308). After all is said and done, Heyd, like the other proponents, provides us with no standard for the nature of the human embryo. If he were to abandon the conundrum and provide us instead with a paradigm that could arbitrate the rightness or wrongness of both sets of activities, we might have grounds for moral positions and standards.

42. Ramsey Colloquium, "The Inhuman Use of Human Beings: A Statement on Embryo Research by the Ramsey Colloquium," *First Things* (January 1995): 17–21.

43. Daniel Callahan, "The Puzzle of Profound Respect," *Hastings Center Report* 25, no 1 (1995): 39–40.

44. R. Alta Charo, "The Hunting of the Snark: The Moral Status of Embryos, Right-to-Lifers, and Third World Women," *Stanford Law and Policy Review* 6 (1995): 11–37.

45. Ibid., p. 18.

46. Robertson, "Symbolic Issues in Embryo Research," p. 38.

47. Ibid.

48. Davis, "Embryos Created for Research Purposes," pp. 350–53.

49. Courtney Campbell, "Awe Diminished," *Hastings Center* 25, no. 1 (1995): 44–46.

50. Campbell, "Response to Hogan and Green," p. 5.

51. Callahan, "The Puzzle of Profound Respect," p. 40.

52. Davis, "Embryos Created for Research Purposes," p. 349.

53. Gina Kolata, "Medicine's Troubling Bonus: Surplus of Human Embryos," *The New York Times*, March 16, 1997, pp. 1, 32.

54. National Institutes of Health, *Report of the Human Embryo Research Panel*, p. 44.

55. Brigid Hogan and Ronald Green, "Embryo Research Revisited," *Hastings Center Report* 25, no. 3 (1995): 2–4.

56. Callahan responded, "Perhaps what I'm asking for could not be developed by a commission: a moral theory to make such distinctions. Yet without such a theory the decisions reached seem arbitrary, and the word 'respect' is rendered vacuous" (Callahan, "Response to Hogan and Green," p. 6).

57. Charo, "The Hunting of the Snark," p. 18.

58. Keenan, "What's Your Worst Moral Argument?"

59. Patricia King, "Statement of Patricia King," *Report*, A-3–4, at 3. Likewise, Carol Tauer expresses her disagreement with the panel's decision to recommend for further review "embryonic stem cell research that uses deliberately fertilized oocytes." Tauer argues that the recommendation goes against "the Panel's desire to maintain clear limitation on the fertilization of oocytes for research purposes" (Tauer, "Statement of Carol Tauer," *Report*, B-3).

60. Charo, "The Hunting of the Snark," p. 14.

61. I explored our self-understanding in human genetics in "What Is Morally New in Genetic Engineering?" *Human Gene Therapy* 1 (1990): 289–98.

62. See Cahill, "The Embryo and the Fetus," pp. 142–59; Keenan, "Genetic Research and the Elusive Body," pp. 59–73; and Lauritzen, "Whose Bodies?" pp. 113–26.

63. See, for instance, Earl Shelp, ed., *Virtue and Medicine* (Boston: Reidel, 1984). Also James Drane, "Character and the Moral Life: A Virtue Approach in Biomedical Ethics," in *A Matter of Principles?* eds. Edwin DuBose et al. (Park Ridge: Trinity Press, 1994), pp. 284–309; Charles Henry, "The Place of Prudence in Moral Decision-Making," *Journal of Religion and Health* 32 (1993): 27–37; Leon Kass, "Practicing Ethics: Where's the Action?" *Hastings Center Report* 20, no. 1 (1990): 5–12; and Dorothy Wertz and George Fletcher, "Privacy and Disclosure in Medical Genetics Examined in an Ethics of Care," *Bioethics* 5 (1991): 212–27.

64. I use it in "Genetic Research and the Elusive Body," and in "What is Morally New in Genetic Engineering?"

65. See his "Development in Moral Doctrine," in Keenan and Shannon, *The Context of Casuistry*, pp. 188–203. For concrete instance, see his *The Scholastic Analysis of Usury* (Cambridge: Harvard University, 1957), pp. 171–92, 194–95, 199–201.

Chapter 5

1. "Every Sperm Is Sacred." Lyrics by Michael Palin and Terry Jones; composed by David Howman and Andre Jacquemin.

2. A review of the science, ethics, and policy questions surrounding cloning may be found in National Bioethics Advisory Commission (NBAC), *Cloning Human Beings: Report and Recommendations of the National Bioethics Advisory Commission* (Rockville, MD: NBAC, June 1997); available online at http://www.bioethics.gov or in print from the NBAC office, 6100 Executive Boulevard, Rockville, MD 20892-7508. Tel: 301-402-4242; Fax: 301-480-6900.

3. I. Wilmut, A. E. Schienke, J. McWhir, A. J. Kind, and K. H. Campbell, "Viable Offspring Derived From Fetal and Adult Mammalian Cells," *Nature* 385 (1997): 810–13.

4. See, for example, John Noonan, Jr., "An Absolute Value in History," in *The Morality of Abortion: Legal and Historical Approaches* (Cambridge: Harvard University Press, 1970) ed. John T. Noonan, Jr. (ed.) pp. 51–59. See also Massimo Reichlin, "The Argument from Potential: A Reappraisal," *Bioethics* 11, no. 1 (1997): 1–23; and R. E. Joyce, Personhood and the Conception Event, in *What is a Person?* ed. Michael Goodman, p. 199. Note that the "moment of fertilization" is actually more complex a concept than it would appear at first blush. It could mean the moment the sperm first penetrates the egg wall, the moment the chromosomes of the sperm and egg begin to mingle, or the moment the chromosomes of the egg and sperm have completed their sorting process. The distinction is important in theory for determining whether experimentation designed to look solely at the process of sperm penetration through the egg wall (such as research on "zona drilling" to help relieve certain forms of male infertility) would entail research on a "fertilized" egg and thus be impermissible according to those who believe that all research on fertilized eggs is immoral. For a description of possible avenues for infertility research, including zona drilling, see generally United States Congress, Office of Technology Assessment, *Infertility: Medical and Social Choices* (Washington, DC: United States Government Printing Office, 1988).

5. See, for example, Noonan, "An Absolute Value in History," p. 57.

6. See Ronald Dworkin, *Life's Dominion* (New York: Knopf, 1993), pp. 41–46.
7. Consider the following example: Assume an eight-cell embryo is an individual whom we will call "Isaac." While in the womb, the embryo divides in two. Each of the resulting four-cell embryos will continue on to develop into a baby. Are both of the babies "Isaac"? They are genetically identical, but they have separate bodies and minds. If they are not both Isaac, however, where is he? Did he vanish, leaving two new individuals, Jacob and Esau? Or is one of them Isaac and the other a new individual? If so, where did that new individual come from?

   Now assume there are two embryos in a womb, Ruth and Naomi, who are fraternal twins. If they should combine into a mosaic, who is the resulting individual? Ruth? Naomi? Neither? Both?

   For critiques of the argument from individuation, see, for example, Karen Dawson, "Fertilization and Moral Status: A Scientific Perspective," *Embryo Experimentation: Ethical, Legal, and Social Issues*, eds. Peter Singer and Karen Dawson (Cambridge: Cambridge University Press, 1990), pp. 43–52; Richard A. McCormick, "Who or What Is a Pre-Embryo?" *Kennedy Institute of Ethics Journal* 1, (1991): 1–15.
8. See British Royal College of Physicians (RCOG), *Report of the RCOG Ethics Committee on In Vitro Fertilisation and Embryo Replacement or Transfer* (London: RCOG, 1983).
9. Ibid., p. 47.
10. One commentator describes with meticulous precision the dilemma of characterizing the destruction of potential as a wrong to the being with the potential if that being at the time it is "wronged" has no ability to perceive itself as wronged. *See* Michael Tooley, "In Defense of Abortion and Infanticide" in *What Is a Person*, ed. Michael Goodman (Totowa, NJ: Humana Press, 1988), pp. 83–114. This does not answer the question, of course, as to whether such destruction is a wrong to someone other than the being with the potential, such as already born people who are saddened by the loss of potential or an omniscient presence such as a god that has an interest in the development of that potential to fruition. The claim that destroying potential babies is a wrong visited upon those who wish to see them develop is one this author takes seriously and is discussed *infra*.
11. Joel Feinberg, "Potentiality, Development and Rights," in *The Problem of Abortion*, ed. Joel Feinberg (Belmont, CA: Wadsworth, 1984), pp. 145–150.
12. "Brain activity" encompasses the most rudimentary electrical signaling among small clumps of cells (about the sixth or seventh week of development) to the fully functioning nervous system, capable of supporting sentience, awareness, or pain. At its earliest stages, the presence of rudimentary electrical activity does not indicate a developmental maturity that could encompass a current (as opposed to still potential) interest in continued existence because a current interest requires some prior or contemporaneous preferences, which in turn requires some rudimentary awareness. Thus, at this stage, one has nothing more than another application of the argument from potentiality. See, for example, Bonnie Steinbock, *Life Before Birth: The Moral and Legal Status of Embryos and Fetuses* (New York: Oxford University Press, 1992).
13. John T. Noonan, "An Almost Absolute Value in History," in Feinberg, *The Problem of Abortion*, pp. 12–13.
14. See, for example, Edmund Husserl, *Allgemeine Einführing in die reine Phänomenologie*; vol. 1 of *Ideen zu einer reinen Phänomenologie und phänomenologischen Philosophie*; and vol. 3 of *Husserliana: Gesammelte Werke* (The Hague: Martinus Nijhoff, 1952). Translated by Fred Kersten under the title *Ideas Pertaining*

to a Pure Phenomenology and to a Phenomenological Philosophy: First Book: General Introduction to a Pure Phenomenology. (The Hague: Martinus Nijhoff, 1982).

15. Massimo Reichlin, "The Argument from Potential: A Reappraisal," *Bioethics* 11, no. 1 (1997): 1–23.
16. Peter Singer and Deane Wells, *The Reproduction Revolution: New Ways of Making Babies* (Oxford: Oxford University Press, 1984), p. 91.
17. Jonathan Glover, *Causing Death and Saving Lives* (Hammondsworth: Penguin, 1977) p. 122.
18. Reichlin, "The Argument from Potential," pp. 1–23.
19. Announcements concerning the ability to retrieve and immortalize embryonic stem cells raise an analogous point. These stem cells are genetically complete and, left alone to divide, are capable of forming any kind of cell found in the body. In this sense they are "totipotent," just as are the other cells of an embryo or the fertilized egg itself. The stem cells will not, however, organize themselves in a fashion that permits a viable fetus to develop; rather, they can divide into all the necessary cells, but in the form of a disorganized mass of tissue. For this reason, some researchers refer to them as "pluripotent" rather than "totipotent." Nonetheless, researchers again raise the question of why stem cells should not be considered as sacred as an embryo itself in light of their innate tendency to divide into all the cells of the body and not merely into one kind of cell, as is the case with an adult somatic skin cell, for example. In a related example, scientists in a Massachusetts company claimed to have cloned a human somatic cell by fusing it with an enucleated cow egg and growing it up to the blastocyst stage, at which point stem cells would be retrievable. If the fused cell were incapable of developing into a viable fetus, for example, due to mitochondrial incompatibilities, then it would be a virtual human embryo that nonetheless lacked the capability of developing into a child. See, generally, J. A. Thomson et al., "Human Embryonic Stem Cells," *Science*, 282 (November 6, 1998): 1145–47; Eugene Russo, "Hearing Sets Stage for Stem Cell Funding Debate," *The Scientist*, 13, no. 1 (January 4, 1999): 3; Eugene Russo, Cow–Human Cell News Raises Ethical Issues," *The Scientist*, 12, no. 23 (November 23, 1998): 1.
20. National Institutes of Health, *Report of the Human Embryo Research Panel* (Bethesda, MD: National Institutes of Health, September 1994).
21. Public Law 104-91; Public Law 104-208.
22. Robert Larmer, "Abortion, Personhood, and the Potential for Consciousness," *Journal of Applied Philosophy* 12 (1995): 241–51.
23. National Institutes of Health, *Report of the Human Embryo Research Panel.*

Chapter 6

1. I. Wilmut, et al., "Viable Offspring Derived From Fetal and Adult Mammalian Cells" *Nature* 385 (1997): 810–13.
2. World Health Organization [WHO] Press Office, *WHO Director General Condemns Human Cloning* (Geneva, Switzerland: World Health Organization, March 11, 1997).
3. Council of Europe, Parliamentary Assembly, *Recommendation 1046 (1988): on the Use of Human Embryos and Foetuses for Diagnostic, Therapeutic, Scientific, Industrial and Commercial Purposes*, in *Human Reproduction* 2 (1987): 67–75.
4. J. Cohen and G. Tomkin, "The Science Fiction and Reality of Embryo Cloning," *Kennedy Institute of Ethics Journal* 4 (1994): 193–204.
5. R. Dworkin, *Taking Rights Seriously* (London: Duckworth, 1978).

6. J. S. Mill, *On Liberty* (Indianapolis: Bobbs-Merrill Publishing, 1859); and R. Rhodes, "Clones, Harms, and Rights," *Cambridge Quarterly of Healthcare Ethics* 4 (1995): 285–90.

7. J. A. Robertson, *Children of Choice: Freedom and the New Reproductive Technologies* (Princeton, NJ: Princeton University Press, 1994); and D. W. Brock, "Reproductive Freedom: Its Nature, Bases and Limits," in *Health Care Ethics: Critical Issues for Health Professionals*, eds. D. Thomasma and J. Monagle (Gaithersburg, MD: Aspen Publishers, 1994), pp. 43–61.

8. G. J. Annas, "Regulatory Models for Human Embryo Cloning: The Free Market, Professional Guidelines, and Government Restrictions," *Kennedy Institute of Ethics Journal* 4, no. 3 (1994): 235–49.

9. L. Eisenberg, "The Outcome as Cause: Predestination and Human Cloning," *The Journal of Medicine and Philosophy* 1 (1976): 318–31; J. A. Robertson, "The Question of Human Cloning," *Hastings Center Report* 24 (1994): 6–14; J. A. Robertson, "A Ban on Cloning and Cloning Research Is Unjustified," testimony presented to the National Bioethics Advisory Commission (March 1997); and M. LaBar, "The Pros and Cons of Human Cloning" *Thought* 57 (1984): 318–33.

10. National Advisory Board on Ethics in Reproduction, *Report on Human Cloning Through Embryo Splitting: An Amber Light, Kennedy Institute of Ethics Journal* 4 (1994): 251–82.

11. Robertson, "The Question of Human Cloning," pp. 6–14.

12. Ibid.; Robertson, "A Ban on Cloning and Cloning Research is Unjustified," March 1997; C. Kahn, "Can We Achieve Immortality?" *Free Inquiry* 9 (1989): 14–18; and J. Harris, *Wonderwoman and Superman: The Ethics of Biotechnology* (Oxford: Oxford University Press, 1992).

13. Kahn, "Can We Achieve Immortality?", pp. 14–18.

14. Robertson, "The Question of Human Cloning," pp. 6–14.

15. L. Thomas, "Notes of a Biology Watcher: On Cloning a Human Being" *New England Journal of Medicine* 291 (1974): 1296–97.

16. J. Lederberg, "Experimental Genetics and Human Evolution" *The American Naturalist* 100 (1966): 519–31; and R. McKinnell, *Cloning: A Biologist Reports*. (Minneapolis: University of Minnesota Press, 1979).

17. W. A. W. Walters, "Cloning, Ectogenesis, and Hybrids: Things to Come?" in *Test-Tube Babies*, eds. W. A. W. Walters and P. Singer (Melbourne: Oxford University Press, 1982) pp. 110–18; and G. P. Smith, "Intimations of Immortality: Clones, Cyrons and the Law" *University of New South Wales Law Journal* 6 (1983): 119–32.

18. P. Ramsey, *Fabricated Man: The Ethics of Genetic Control* (New Haven CT: Yale University Press, 1970).

19. L. Kass, *Toward a More Natural Science* (New York: The Free Press, 1985); and National Advisory Board on Ethics and Reproduction, "Report on Human Cloning Through Embryo Splitting: An Amber Light," 1994.

20. R. Macklin, "Splitting Embryos on the Slippery Slope: Ethics and Public Policy," *Kennedy Institute of Ethics Journal* 4 (1994): 209–26; and R. F. Chadwick, "Cloning," *Philosophy* 57 (1982): 201–09.

21. H. Jonas, *Philosophical Essays: From Ancient Creed to Technological Man* (Englewood Cliffs, NJ: Prentice-Hall, 1974); and J. Feinberg, "The Child's Right to an Open Future," in *Whose Child? Children's Rights, Parental Authority, and State Power*, eds. W. Aiken and H. LaFollette (Totowa, NJ: Rowman and Littlefield, 1980).

22. D. Callahan, "Perspective on Cloning: A Threat to Individual Uniqueness," *Los Angeles Times*, November 12, 1993, p. B7; LaBar, "The Pros and Cons of Human

Cloning," pp. 318–33; Macklin, "Splitting Embryos on the Slippery Slope," pp. 209–26; R. McCormick, "Should We Clone Humans?" *Christian Century* 110 (1993): 1148–49; A. Studdard, "The Lone Clone," *Man and Medicine: The Journal of Values and Ethics in Health Care* 3 (1978): 109–14; J. D. Rainer, "Commentary," *Man and Medicine: The Journal of Values and Ethics in Health Care* 3 (1978): 115–17; and A. D. Verhey, "Cloning: Revisiting an Old Debate," *Kennedy Institute of Ethics Journal* 4 (1994): 227–34.

23. Rainer, "Commentary," pp. 115–17.
24. LaBar, "The Pros and Cons of Human Cloning," pp. 318–33.
25. Robertson, "The Question of Human Cloning," pp. 6–14.
26. J. L. Hall, et al., *Experimental Cloning of Human Polypoid Embryos Using an Artificial Zona Pellucida*, The American Fertility Society conjointly with the Canadian Fertility and Andrology Society, Program Supplement, 1993, Abstracts of the Scientific Oral and Poster Sessions, Abstract 0-001, S1.
27. Verhey, "Cloning," pp. 201–209; Robertson, "The Question of Human Cloning," pp. 6–14; and Macklin, "Splitting Embryos on the Slippery Slope," pp. 209–26.
28. D. Parfit, *Reasons and Persons* (Oxford: Oxford University Press, 1984).
29. D. Brock, "The Non-Identity Problem and Genetic Harm," *Bioethics* 9 (1995): 269–75.
30. R. Pollack, "Beyond Cloning," *New York Times*, November 17, 1993, p. A27.
31. R. Weiss, "Cloning Suddenly Has Government's Attention," *International Herald Tribune*, March 4, 1997.
32. Macklin, "Splitting Embryos on the Slippery Slope," pp. 209–26.
33. LaBar, "The Pros and Cons of Human Cloning," pp. 318–33; and Callahan "Perspective on Cloning: A Threat to Individual Uniqueness," p. B7.
34. P. O. Turner, "Love's Labor Lost: Legal and Ethical Implications in Artificial Human Procreation," *University of Detriot Journal of Urban Law* 58 (1981): 459–87.
35. A. Huxley, *Brave New World* (London: Chalto and Winders, 1932).
36. Ira Levin, *The Boys From Brazil*, (New York: Dell, 1977).
37. Eisenberg, "The Outcome as Cause," pp. 318–31.
38. M. Adams, ed., *The Well-Born Science* (Oxford: Oxford University Press, 1990).

Chapter 7

1. National Bioethics Advisory Commission, *Cloning Human Beings: Report and Recommendations of the National Bioethics Advisory Commission* (Rockville, MD: National Bioethics Advisory Commission, June 1997).
2. The experience of some lesbian couples in this regard is reported by Annette Baran and Reuben Pannor in their book *Lethal Secrets: The Psychology of Donor Insemination, Problems and Solutions* (New York: Amistad/Penguin, 1993).
3. The mother of a child born with a serious genetic disease expressed to me her interest in cloning as a way of avoiding the recurrence of this genetic disease in her family.
4. It can be argued that cloning and other assisted reproductive technologies can help us address world population problems through research leading to improved contraception, delayed childbearing, and greater parental control over reproduction generally.
5. For a discussion of this, see Rosa Beddington, *Mill Hill Essays* (London: National Institute for Medical Research, 1997). Available at *http://www.nimr.mrc.ac.uk/ mhe97/cloning.htm*.

6. Aldous Huxley's *Brave New World* (1932) exerts a major influence on all our think-
ing about genetics and reproductive technologies, including cloning (which takes form
in the World State's use of the "Bokanovsky" method, a technology involving not
SCNT but blastomere twinning and multiplication). For a good review of some lesser
known science fiction works on cloning, see Gregory E. Pence, *Who's Afraid of Human
Cloning?* (Lanham, MD: Rowman & Littlefield, 1998), pp. 39–43; see also Ursula
LeGuin, "Nine Lives," reprinted in *The Science Fiction Research Association
Anthology*, eds. Patricia S. Warrick, Charles G. Waugh, Martin H. Greenberg (New
York: Harper Collins, 1988), pp. 391–410.

7. Richard Barlow, "Hoping For Extra-Brainy Offspring, Some Seek Eggs of Ivy
Women," *Valley News* (W. Lebanon, NH), January 24, 1999, p. A1.

8. Derek Parfit, *Reasons and Persons* (Oxford: Clarendon Press, 1984); and David Heyd,
Genethics: Moral Issues in the Creation of People (Berkeley, CA: University of
California Press, 1992). Related treatments of this issue include Mary Anne Warren,
"Do Potential People Have Moral Rights?" *Canadian Journal of Philosophy* 7 (1977):
275–89; Gregory Kavka, "The Paradox of Future Individuals," *Philosophy and Public
Affairs* 11 (1982): 93–112; J. Woodward, "The Non-identity Problem," *Ethics* 96
(1986): 804–31; M. Hanser, "Harming Future People," *Philosophy and Public Affairs*
19 (1990): 47–70; Ruth Faden, "Reproductive Genetic Testing and the Ethics of
Parenting," *Fetal Diagnosis and Therapy* 8, suppl. 1 (1993): 142–47; Bonnie Steinbock
and Ron McClamrock, "When Is Birth Unfair to the Child?" *Hastings Center Report*
244 (1994): 15–21; Dan Brock, "The Non-identity Problem and Genetic Harms—The
Case of Wrongful Handicaps," *Bioethics* 9 (1995): 269–75; J. C. Heller, *Human
Genome Research & The Challenge of Contingent Future Persons* (Omaha, NE:
Creighton University Press, 1996); Melinda Roberts, "Human Cloning: A Case of No
Harm?" *Journal of Medicine and Philosophy* 21 (1996): 337–554.

9. John Robertson, *The Children of Choice* (Princeton, NJ: Princeton University Press,
1994); "Wrongful Life, Federalism, and Procreative Liberty: A Critique of the NBAC
Cloning Report," *Jurimetrics* 38 (February 1997), 69–82; and "Liberty, Identity, and
Human Cloning," *Texas Law Review* 76, no. 6 (May 1998): 1371–456.

10. See my "Parental Autonomy and the Obligation Not to Genetically Harm One's Child:
Implications for Clinical Genetics," *Journal of Law, Medicine & Ethics* 25, no. 1
(1997): 5–15.

11. Michael B. Kelly, "The Rightful Position in 'Wrongful Life' Actions," *Hasting Law
Journal* 42 (1991): 505–90, esp. n. 203.

12. Ibid., pp. 549–56. This kind of comparison can also be applied to reproductive decision making.

13. In some cases it may also be true that the parents have been harmed in terms of their
reasonable expectations. It is probably, however, worth preserving the ability to say
that the children themselves have been harmed because, in some cases, parents may
be responsible for inflicting the injury. See my "Parental Autonomy and the Obligation
Not to Genetically Harm One's Child."

14. John D. Arras, "Having Children in Fear and Trembling," *Milbank Quarterly* 68
(1990): 53–82; W. R. Cohen, "Maternal–Fetal Conflict, I," in *Ethics and Perinatology*,
eds. Aaron Goldworth, William Silverman, D. K. Stevenson, and E. W. D. Young (New
York: Oxford University Press, 1995), pp. 10–28; P. H. Jos, Mary F. Marshall, and
M. Perlmutter, "The Charleston Policy on Cocaine Use During Pregnancy: A
Cautionary Tale," *Journal of Law, Medicine & Ethics* 23 (1995): 120–28; and Ruth

Macklin, "Maternal–Fetal Conflict, II," in Goldworth et al., *Ethics and Perinatology*, pp. 29–46.

15. W. D. Ross makes a distinction here between *prima facie* duties, as separated components or individual vectors within a larger moral conclusion, which he terms *duty proper*. See his *Foundations of Ethics* (Oxford: The Clarendon Press, 1939).

16. See my "Parental Autonomy and The Obligation Not to Genetically Harm One's Child."

17. Ibid. There are, however, limits to the harms that parents can knowingly inflict on a child.

18. I. Wilmut, A. E. Schnieke, J. McWhir, A. J. Kind, and Keith H. Campbell, "Viable Offspring Derived from Fetal and Adult Mammalian Cells," *Nature* 385 (1997): 810–13.

19. An effort to get around this problem was announced by researchers at Advanced Cell Technologies in Worcester, MA, who inserted nuclei from human somatic cells into cow eggs and produced embryonic cells resembling early human stem cells. See Nicholas Wade, "Human Cells Revert to Embryo State, Scientists State," *New York Times*, November 12, 1998, pp. A1, A24.

20. There would be reason for concern here, however, if this loss rate signaled possible genetic anomalies and other unknown factors jeopardizing the born child.

21. Peter Singer and Deane Wells, *The Reproductive Revolution: New Ways of Making Babies* (New York: Oxford University Press, 1984), p. 161.

22. Incest concerns have been mentioned in this respect. See Timothy M. Renick, "A Cabbit in Sheep's Clothing: Exploring the Sources of our Moral Disquiet About Cloning," *Annual of the Society of Christian Ethics* 1998. (Washington, DC: Georgetown University Press, 1998), pp. 243–74.

23. Richard Lewontin, "The Confusion Over Cloning," *The New York Review of Books* (October, 1997): 18–23, p. 18.

24. Dena S. Davis, "What's Wrong with Cloning?" *Jurimetrics* 38 (February 1997): 83–89.

25. Ibid., pp. 87–88.

26. Andrea L. Bonnicksen, "Creating a Clone in Ninety Days: In Search of a Cloning Policy," *Jurimetrics* 38 (February 1997): 23–31.

27. This point is made by Jeffrey P. Kahn, "A Temporary Halt: National Bioethics Commission's and NBAC's Cloning Report," *Jurimetrics* 38 (February 1997): 33–34.

28. Alta Charo, "Dealing with Dolly: Cloning and the National Bioethics Advisory Commission," *Jurimetrics* 38 (February 1997): 11–22, See also her remarks quoted by Gina Kolata in "Little-Known Panel Challenged To Make Quick Cloning Study," *New York Times*, March 18, 1997, p. C9.

29. John A. Robertson, "Liberty, Identity, and Human Cloning" *Texas Law Review* 76, no. 6 (May 1998): 1436–37.

30. National Bioethics Advisory Commission, *Cloning Human Beings*, p. 109.

31. In House hearings on proposed cloning legislation, Alison Taunton-Rigby noted that one of the prohibitory bills being proposed requires confiscation of "any property . . . used to commit a violation." She asks whether this bill would permit confiscation of the entire university, certainly a chilling consideration for any research bordering on cloning. See "Testimony of Alison Taunton-Rigby, Ph.D., President and CEO, Aquila Biopharmaceuticals, Worcester, Massachusetts, On Behalf of the Biotechnology Industry Organization (BIO) Before the Subcommittee on Technology, Committee on

Science." United States House of Representatives, *Legislative Proposals Regarding Cloning Human Beings* (July 22, 1997): 82 (Appendix C, p. 8).

32. See Alta Charo, "Dealing with Dolly," pp. 16–17.

Chapter 8

1. An earlier draft of this project was a paper delivered at the American Academy of Religion's national meeting, Ethics Section, San Francisco, November 1997.
2. H. Freeman et al., eds. *Midrash Rabbah.* (Soncino Press). This midrash is found linked to several places, in Genesis and Job. The midrash, in an amended form, is also found in the *Tzenah Erenah* (trans. Miriam S. Zakan, Mesorah Publications, 1983), a traditional Yiddish text that retells and elaborates on the midrash, authored by Yaakov ben Yitzchah Ashkenasi, 1726.
3. *San Francisco Chronicle*, (November 1997), sect. B. This ad appears every week.
4. *The Book of Job* (Philadelphia: Jewish Publication Society, 1971).
5. "Who is the Mother?," a panel at the American Association for Bioethics and The Society for Health and Human Values, Baltimore Joint National Meeting, November 1997.
6. Freeman et al., *Midrash Rabbah*; Midrash on Babel.
7. Talmud Balui, Soncino Press, 1956. Discussion in Zoloth, "Mapping the Normal Human Self," in *Genetics*, edited by Peter Pilgrim Press, 1996.
8. Carl Djerassi, in an interview on the CBS network affiliate, San Francisco. This panel on reproductive technology was a feature of the program on Religion and Public Life, October 1997.

Chapter 9

1. The "preimplantation human embryo" that results from IVF is defined by the HERP as "a fertilized ovum in vitro that has never been transferred to or implanted in the uterus." It may possibly be sustained beyond the stage where it would normally implant in the uterus.
2. Alexander Capron, "Slow the Rush to Human Cloning," *Los Angeles Times*, February 13, 1998, p. B9.
3. See Keenan (Chapter 4) and Ryan (Chapter 3), this volume.
4. J. A. Thomson et al., "Embryonic Stem Cell Lines Derived From Human Blastocysts," *Science* 282 (1988): 1145–47.
5. See Carol Tauer, "Preimplantation Embryos, Research Ethics, and Public Policy," *Bioethics Forum* 11, no. 3 (1995): 30–37.
6. R. Weiss, "NIH to Fund Controversial Research," *Washington Post*, January 20, 1999, p. A2.
7. See Forster and Ramsey (Chapter 12), this volume, for a discussion of federal and state efforts to regulate cloning.
8. Cynthia Cohen, "Unmanaged Care: The Need to Regulate New Reproductive Technologies in the United States," *Bioethics* 11 (1997): 348–65.
9. Daniel Callahan, "The Puzzle of Profound Respect," *Hastings Center Report* 25, no. 1 (1995): 39–40.
10. See Keenan (Chapter 4), this volume.
11. Many authors distinguish between the two concepts of human being and person, setting higher criteria for personhood such as consciousness, rationality, or self-

consciousness. The terms are used interchangeably in this chapter, however, because the status of either human being or person would be sufficient to qualify an embryo for full protection as a human subject, both morally and legally.

12. John Ladd, "Are Science and Ethics Compatible?" in *Science, Ethics, and Medicine*, eds. H. T. Engelhardt, Jr., and D. Callahan (Hastings-on-Hudson, New York: The Hastings Institute, 1976), pp. 49–78.

13. Some moral theories do not allow for morally neutral or morally indifferent acts. For example, utilitarianism holds that one is always morally required to perform the act that is expected to achieve the greatest good of the greatest number or the greatest balance of (non-moral) good over (non-moral) evil.

14. See, for example, N. M. Ford, *When Did I Begin* (Cambridge: Cambridge University Press, 1989); Richard McCormick, "Who or What Is the Preembryo?" *Kennedy Institute of Ethics Journal* 1 (1991): 1–15; and M. Mori, "Is the Human Embryo a Person? No," in *Conceiving the Embryo*, eds. D. Evans and N. Pickering (The Hague: Martinus Nijhoff, 1996), pp. 151–63.

15. In its *Declaration on Abortion* (Washington, DC: United States Catholic Conference, 1975), the Sacred Congregation for the Doctrine of the Faith states: "This declaration expressly leaves aside the question of the moment when the spiritual soul is infused [i.e., the time when the embryo becomes a human person]. There is not a unanimous tradition on this point and authors are as yet in disagreement."

16. Mori, "Is the Human Embryo a Person? No," p. 146.

17. In a detailed study of this issue, I considered three possible reasons that might ground a prohibition of embryo research and showed that these arguments were unpersuasive. See Carol A. Tauer, *The Moral Status of the Prenatal Human Subject of Research* (Ann Arbor, MI: University Microfilms International, 1982).

18. Carol A. Tauer, "Bringing Embryos into Existence for Research Purposes," in *Contingent Future Persons*, eds. Nick Fotion and Jan C. Heller (Dordrecht: Kluwer Academic Publishers, 1997), pp. 171–89.

19. "Statement of Patricia King" in National Institutes of Health, *Report of the Human Embryo Research Panel* (Bethesda, MD: National Institutes of Health, September 1994).

20. See Arthur Caplan, ed. *When Medicine Went Mad* (Totowa, NJ: Humana Press, 1992).

21. Sacred Congregation for the Doctrine of the Faith, *Donum Vitae* in *Origins* 16 (1987): 697–711.

22. See Robert Edwards and Patrick Steptoe, *A Matter of Life: The Story of a Medical Breakthrough* (New York: William Morrow, 1980), pp. 40–52.

23. Although surgical patients had probably signed a standard consent form agreeing that their tissues could be used for study, the use of their eggs for the possible creation of embryos without their specific knowledge and explicit consent would be considered unethical today.

24. Edwards and Steptoe, *A Matter of Life*, pp. 82–83.

25. R. G. Edwards, P. C. Steptoe, and J. M. Purdy, "Fertilization and Cleaving In Vitro of Preovulator Human Oocytes," *Nature* 227 (1970): 1307–09.

26. Ethics Advisory Board, *Report and Conclusions: HEW Support of Research Involving Human In Vitro Fertilization and Embryo Transfer* (Washington, DC: United States Government Printing Office, 1979).

27. V. Cohn, "Test-Tube Baby Study Debated by HEW Panel," *Washington Post*, February 3, 1979, p. A7.

28. The scientific chapter of the HERP report devoted 19 pages to describing research on reproduction and reproductive technologies (pp. 11–26 and 28–30) and two pages to other possible types of research (pp. 26–27). No author I am aware of, however, differentiates the morality of creating research embryos from the research use of surplus embryos based on whether the research project studies an aspect of reproduction or has other goals.

29. Cohen, "Unmanaged Care," pp. 350–51.

30. Jonathan Van Blerkom, "The History, Current Status and Future Direction of Research Involving Human Embryos," in *Papers Commissioned by the Human Embryo Research Panel* (Washington, DC: National Institutes of Health, 1994), pp. 1–25.

31. Cohen, "Unmanaged Care," p. 359.

32. Centers for Disease Control and Prevention, "1997 Assisted Reproductive Technology Success Rates." Available at *http://www.cdc.gov/nccdphp/drh/art.htm*, February 1, 2000.

33. M. J. Seller, "The Human Embryo: A Scientist's Point of View," *Bioethics* 7 (1993): 135–140.

34. J. A. Martin and M. M. Park, "Trends in Twin and Triplet Births: 1980–97," *National Vital Statistics Reports* 47, no. 24 (September 14, 1999). Available at *http://www.cdc.gov/nchs.releases/99facts/99sheets/multiple.htm*, February 1, 2000.

35. National Center for Health Statistics, "Multiple Births Multiply During the Past Two Decades," 1997 Fact Sheets, November 13, 1997.

36. J. A. Martin and M. M. Park, "Trends."

37. Cynthia Cohen, "Give Me Children or I Shall Die!" *Hastings Center Report* 26, no. 2 (1996): 19–27.

38. Alan Trounson, "Why Do Research on Human Pre-embryos?" in *Embryo Experimentation* eds. Peter Singer et al. (Cambridge: Cambridge University Press, 1990), pp. 14–25.

39. "For the First Time in United States, Infertility Researchers Report Success from Using Frozen Eggs," *Star Tribune*, October 17, 1997, p. A4. (Reprinted from the *Washington Post*.)

40. Helen Rumbelow, "Ban on Thawing Frozen Human Eggs to be Lifted," *The Times* (London), January 26, 2000. Available at *http://www.the-times.co.uk/news/pages/tim/2000/01/26/timnwsnws01017.html*, March 28, 2000.

41. Trounson, "Why Do Research?" p. 16.

42. G. D. Palermo et al., "Evolution of Pregnancies and Initial Follow-Up of Newborns Delivered After Intracytoplasmic Sperm Injection" *JAMA* 276 (1996): 1893–1897.

43. A. Van Steirteghem, "Outcome of Assisted Reproductive Technology," *New England Journal of Medicine* 338 (1998): 194–95.

44. Van Blerkom, "The History," p. 10.

45. Gina Kolata, "On Cloning Humans, 'Never' Turns Swiftly Into 'Why Not,'" *New York Times*, December 2, 1997, pp. A1, A4.

46. B. Gaze and K. Dawson, "Who Is the Subject of Research?" in *Embryo Experimentation* eds. Peter Singer et al. (Cambridge: Cambridge University Press, 1990), p. 122.

47. The recent United States Supreme Court decision that the Americans with Disabilities Act (ADA) applies to persons with human immunodeficiency virus infection reinforces skepticism that infertility treatment could be legally curtailed in the United States. The court's decision in this case rests mainly on the plaintiff's claim that she was unable to bear children because of her infection, hence was reproductively im-

paired. The court majority held that having children qualified as a "major life activity" under the ADA's definition of disability and hence the plaintiff was disabled (*Bragdon v. Abbott* 118 S.Ct. 1206 1998). It is only a short step to a future case in which a person or couple experiencing infertility will be found to be protected by the ADA. What rights and specific protections will be enunciated remains to be seen, but it is unlikely that the federal government will raise the issue by enacting laws that restrict the provision of infertility treatments.

48. Cohen, "Unmanaged Care," p. 363. See also the New York State Task Force on Life and the Law, *Assisted Reproductive Technologies: Analysis and Recommendations for Public Policy* (New York: New York State Task Force, 1998). This report also called for sweeping changes in the regulation of reproductive technologies.

49. Lori Andrews, "Human Cloning: Assessing the Ethical and Legal Quandaries," *Chronicle of Higher Education* 44, no. 23 (February 1998), pp. B4–B5.

Chapter 10

1. Here, and throughout the following, we refer to "public" bioethics groups and committees to distinguish the practical orientation of governmental and professional policy-making bodies from the more theoretical or philosophical concerns of what we might call "academic" bioethics. This is not to suggest that there is no room for theory of philosophy in governmental and professional policy-making bodies. It is simply meant to provide a rough way of distinguishing two different contexts in which bioethical concerns are commonly addressed.

2. Jonathan D. Moreno, *Deciding Together: Bioethics and Moral Consensus* (New York: Oxford University Press, 1995).

3. Ronald Bayer, "Ethics, Politics, and Access to Health Care: A Critical Analysis of the President's Commission for the Study of Ethical Problems in Medicine and Biomedical and Behavioral Research," *Cardozo Law Review* 6, no. 2 (1984): 303–20.

4. Ibid., pp. 84–86.

5. H. Tristram Engelhardt, Jr., *The Foundations of Bioethics* (New York: Oxford University Press, 1986).

6. Martin Benjamin, *Splitting the Difference: Compromise and Integrity in Ethics and Politics* (Lawrence: University Press of Kansas, 1990).

7. Martin Benjamin, "Review of *Deciding Together*," *Hastings Center Report* 26, no. 1, 1996: 39–40.

8. This is an issue on which the authors of this paper differ. One of us (J.D.M.) has defended a version of the latter view, called *ethical naturalism*. The other (A.J.L.) has more sympathy for a kind of hybrid view that gives significant weight to a version of the former view while incorporating aspects of the latter.

9. Ad Hoc Group of Consultants to the Advisory Committee to the Director, National Institutes of Health, *Report of the Human Embryo Research Panel* (Bethesda, MD: National Institutes of Health, 1994). (Further citations to this report in the text are given in parentheses.) Other recommendations related to the way federally funded embryo research should be reviewed include, for example, that the research is necessary to provide important scientific knowledge or clinical benefit; that the research is approved by an Institutional Review Board; that gametes and embryos not be purchased or sold; that no research be conducted more than 14 days after fertilization; and that informed consent be obtained from gamete donors.

10. George J. Annas, Arthur Caplan, and Sherman Elias, "The Politics of Human-Embryo Research—Avoiding Ethical Gridlock," *New England Journal of Medicine* 334, no. 20 1329–1332, 1997. It is well and good to call, as do Annas et al., for a moral analysis that will settle the problem of the pre-embryo's moral status, but the HERP should not be chastised for falling somewhat short of the wisdom of Solomon. Considering the proximity of this problem to the notoriously recalcitrant and highly politicized abortion quagmire, authority of near-Biblical proportions might be needed to meet the challenge Annas and his colleagues set for the panel. Notice that they did not provide one.

11. National Bioethics Advisory Commission, *Cloning Human Beings: Report and Recommendations of the National Bioethics Advisory Commission* (Rockville, MD: National Bioethics Advisory Commission, June 1997).

12. Ibid., p. 65.

13. Erik Parens expresses these views in "Tools from and for Democratic Deliberations," *Hastings Center Report* 27, no. 5 (September–October 1997): 20–22.

14. National Bioethics Advisory Commission, *Cloning Human Beings*, p. 8.

15. Ibid., p. 93.

16. James F. Childress, "The Challenges of Public Ethics: Reflections on NBAC's Report" *Hastings Center Report* 27, no. 5 (September–October, 1997): 10.

17. National Bioethics Advisory Commission, *Cloning Human Beings*, p. 49.

18. This sort of objection is elaborated at length by Susan M. Wolf in "Ban Cloning? Why NBAC Is Wrong," *Hastings Center Report* 27, no. 5 (September–October, 1997): 12–15.

19. George Johnson, "Ethical Fears Aside, Science Plunges On," *The New York Times*, December 7, 1997, p. 6, Sec. 4. At one point Johnson claims that it is as though society wants its scientists to surprise them with technological wonders, and the piece itself exemplifies the way we have come to look to expect science to dash our "old moral mindset" asunder.

20. Laurence Tribe, "Second Thoughts on Cloning," *The New York Times*, Sec. A, p. 31, December 5, 1997.

Chapter 11

1. In the context of bioethics, a public ethics body has been defined as "a group convened to deliberate about social and ethical issues stemming from developments in biomedicine. Such groups may exist at the level of the institution, professional society, community, state, federal agency, or federal government. Generally, these groups address public policy issues that involve moral ideas such as dignity, freedom rights, fairness, respect, equality, solidarity, responsibility, justice, and integrity." Ruth Ellen Bulger, Elizabeth Meyer Bobby, and Harvey V. Fineburg, eds., "Executive Summary," *Society's Choices: Social and Ethical Decision Making in Biomedicine* (Washington, DC: National Academy Press, 1995), p. 9, n.

2. Ad Hoc Group of Consultants to the Advisory Committee to the Director, National Institutes of Health, *Report of the Human Embryo Research Panel* (Bethesda, MD: National Institutes of Health, September 1994), vol. 1, p. ix.

3. Ibid., pp. 3–4.

4. Ibid., p. 4.

5. Ibid., pp. x, 65.

6. Daniel Callahan makes a similar point about the issues not discussed in the NBAC report: "Cloning: The Work Not Done," *Hastings Center Report* 27, no. 5 (1997): 18–20.

7. National Institutes of Health, *Report*, pp. 35–38.

8. Ibid., p. 38.

9. Ibid., p. 48. Other considerations were that the 14 day limit coheres with protocols established or recommended by other commissions and countries and that a firm time limit will guard against a slippery slope in embryo research and the public perception of such. The rationale for this limit, and the advantages and disadvantages of setting it, are discussed in the report on pp. 47–50.

10. Ibid., pp. 39–40. In the course of this paragraph, the report cites John Rawls's discussion of public reason in *Political Liberalism* (New York: Columbia University Press, 1993), pp. 212–54.

11. National Institutes of Health, *Report*, pp. vi, ix.

12. R. Alta Charo, "The Hunting of the Snark: The Moral Status of Embryos, Right-to-Lifers, and Third World Women," *Stanford Law and Policy Review* 6, no. 2 (1995): p. 12.

13. Ibid., p. 19.

14. Ibid., p. 21.

15. George Annas, Arthur Caplan, and Sherman Elias, "The Politics of Human-Embryo Research—Avoiding Ethical Gridlock," *New England Journal of Medicine* 334, no. 20 (May 16, 1996), 1329–30.

16. Ibid., p. 1330.

17. Ibid. The internal quotation is a reference to John A. Robertson, "Symbolic Issues in Embryo Research," *Hastings Center Report* 25, no. 1 (1995): 37–38.

18. National Bioethics Advisory Commission, *Cloning Human Beings: Report and Recommendations of the National Bioethics Advisory Commission* (Rockville, MD: National Bioethics Advisory Commission, June 1997).

19. Ibid., pp. 39–40.

20. Ibid., pp. 57–58.

21. Ibid., p. 57.

22. Ibid., pp. 49–51.

23. Ibid., p. 56.

24. Ibid., pp. 45–46, 57.

25. Ibid., p. 57.

26. Courtney S. Campbell, "Prophecy and Policy," *Hastings Center Report* 27, no. 5 (1997): p. 17.

27. I defend this claim at length in *Religion and the Common Good* (Lanham, MD: Rowman & Littlefield, 1999).

28. Quoted in Gina Kolata, "On Cloning Humans, 'Never' Turns Swiftly into 'Why Not,'" *New York Times*, December 2, 1997, p. A1.

29. Susan Cohen, "A House Divided," *The Washington Post Magazine*, October 12, 1997, p. 27. This article reports on the NBAC's public hearings and the process by which it came to its recommendations. Cohen had access to the commissioners' electronic mail messages, from which she characterizes Murray's position but does not quote it.

30. The way the legitimacy of such reliance on religious beliefs is characterized ranges from the minimal position that citizens have the liberty to rely on their religious beliefs even though it is ideal that they use publicly accessible discourse whenever possible, to the maximal position that there is no reason to restrict, even by an ideal stan-

dard, what language citizens use. See, for example, the instructive debate between Robert Audi and Nicholas Wolterstorff in their book, *Religion in the Public Square: The Place of Religious Convictions in Political Debate* (Lanham, MD: Rowman & Littlefield, 1997).

31. Michael Walzer, *Thick and Thin: Moral Argument at Home and Abroad* (South Bend, IN: University of Notre Dame, 1994), pp. 11–12.

32. Ibid., 12.

33. Annette C. Baier, "Claims, Rights, and Responsibilities," in *Prospects for a Common Morality*, eds. Gene Outka and John P. Reeder, Jr. (Princeton, NJ: Princeton University Press, 1993), p. 168.

34. Ah, but there's the rub: which interpretation of liberalism? For the theoretical issues, see the works cited in this chapter by Audi and Wolterstorff, Stiltner, and Walzer, as well as Michael Sandel, *Democracy's Discontent: America in Search of a Public Philosophy* (Cambridge, MA: Belknap Press of Harvard University, 1996).

35. National Bioethics Advisory Commission, *Cloning Human Beings*, p. 39.

36. The religious scholars who testified before the NBAC on March 13 and 14, 1997, were Lisa Cahill (Boston College), Rabbi Elliot Dorff (University of Judaism, Los Angeles), Nancy Duff (Princeton Theological Seminary), Gilbert C. Meilaender, Jr. (Valparaiso University), Father Albert S. Moraczewski (National Conference of Catholic Bishops), Abdulaziz Sachedina (University of Virginia), and Rabbi Moshe Tendler (Yeshiva University).

37. Campbell, "Prophesy and Policy," pp. 16–17.

38. This picture of religion's contributions to the common good is explicated and defended in my *Religion and the Common Good*, especially ch. 4.

39. Campbell, "Prophecy and Policy," p. 16.

40. See ch. 10 in this volume by Jonathan D. Moreno and Alex John London.

41. Before the United States House Science Subcommittee on Technology, the NBAC's chairman Harold T. Shapiro said that the commission strongly supports the idea of public education about cloning and related issues, but did not have the time to develop a program, even though many commissioners wanted to. He said that much could be done within existing government-funded programs (such as high school science curricula), and perhaps more money could be targeted to public education about cloning. See Congress, House, Committee on Science, *Review of the President's Commission's Recommendations on Cloning: Hearing before the Subcommittee on Technology*. 105th Congress, First Session, June 12, 1997, pp. 221–22.

42. A selection of statements from Christian churches in 1997 can be found in Ronald Cole-Turner, ed., *Human Cloning: Religious Responses* (Louisville, KY: Westminister/ John Knox, 1997), Appendix II.

43. American Life League director John Cavanaugh-O'Keefe attended all the NBAC public sessions and told the commission, "We'll be watching you." (Reported in Cohen, "A House Divided," p. 24.) Yet the expert testimony before the NBAC was much calmer than the testimony and public hearings before the HERP, in which a number of professionals and members of the public expressed their strong opposition to all or most human embryo research.

44. This is Campbell's phrase ("Prophecy and Policy, p. 16), mirroring the NBAC's call for improved scientific literacy among the public.

45. For an overview of the President's Initiative on Race, see its report, *One America in the 21st Century: Forging a New Future* (Washington, DC: The White House, September 1998).

46. This hearing is mentioned by NBAC member James F. Childress in "The Challenges of Public Ethics: Reflections on NBAC's Report," *Hastings Center Report* 27, no. 5 (1997): p. 11.

Chapter 12

1. This article has been revised from its original publication in *Valparaiso University Law Review*. See Heidi Forster and Emily Ramsey, "The Legal Responses to the Potential Cloning of Human Beings," *Valparaiso University Law Review* 32, no. 2 (1998): 433.
2. "Scientist Who Cloned Sheep: Cloning Humans Would Be 'Inhuman'" (CNN Interactive, March 12, 1997). Available at *http://www.cnn.com/Health/9703/12/nfm/ cloning/index.html.*
3. Ibid.
4. See Declan Butler and Meredith Wadman, "Calls for Cloning Ban Sell Science Short," *Nature* 386 (1997): 8.
5. S. 368, 105th Cong. (1997).
6. "President's Remarks Announcing the Prohibition on Federal Funding for Cloning of Human Beings and an Exchange with Reporters," *Weekly Compilation of Presidential Documents* 33 (March 10, 1997): 278–79.
7. H.R. 923, 105th Cong. (1997).
8. National Bioethics Advisory Commission, *Cloning Human Beings*, p. i.
9. "President's Message to the Congress Transmitting the Proposed 'Cloning Prohibition Act of 1997,'" *Weekly Compilation of Presidential Documents* 33 (June 16, 1997): 845–46.
10. Paul Recer, "Clinton Bill Section A Page 3 Would Ban Cloning of Humans," *The Columbian*, June 9, 1997 (quoting remarks made by President Clinton to Harold Shapiro, the chairman of the NBAC, during Rose Garden ceremony).
11. *Weekly Compilation of Presidential Documents* 33 (June 16, 1997): 844–45.
12. National Bioethics Advisory Commission, *Cloning Human Beings*, p. 87.
13. S. 368, 105th Cong. (1997).
14. Ibid.
15. S. 1574, 105th Cong. (1998).
16. Ibid.
17. S. 1601, 105th Cong. (1998).
18. S. 1602, 105th Cong. (1998).
19. H.R. 922, 105th Cong. (1997).
20. H.R. 3133, 105th Cong. (1998).
21. H.R. 2326, 106th Cong. (1999) and H.R. 571, 106th Cong. (1999).
22. California, Michigan, Missouri, Rhode Island, and Louisiana.
23. Cal. Health & Safety Code § 24185 (Deering 1997).
24. Cal. Health & Safety Code § prec. 24185 (Deering 1997). See also 1997 Cal. Stat. c. 688.
25. Mo. Ann. Stat § 1.217 (West 1999).
26. R. I. Gen. Laws. §§ 23-16.4–1 to 4–4 (1999).
27. Mich. Comp. Laws Ann. §§ 333.16274 to 333.16275; § 333.20197; §§ 333.26401 to 333.26406; and § 750.430a.
28. H.R. 5475, 1st Reg. Sess. (Conn. 1998).
29. S. 241, 139th Gen. Assembly, 2d Reg. Sess. (Del. 1998).

30. H.R. 1829, 90th Gen. Assembly, 1st Reg. Sess. (Ill. 1997); H.R. 2235, 90th Gen. Assembly, 1st Reg. Sess. (Ill. 1997).

31. S. 1230, 90th Gen. Assembly, 1st Reg. Sess. (Ill. 1997); S. 1243, 90th Gen. Assembly, 1st Reg. Sess. (Ill. 1997).

32. H.R. 2730, 80th Reg. Sess. (Minn. 1998).

33. A.B. 2849, 207th Leg., 1st Reg. Sess. (N.J. 1997); A.B. 329, 208th Leg., 1st Reg. Sess. (N.J. 1998).

34. S. 2877, 220th Leg., 1st Reg. Sess. (N.Y. 1997); A.B. 5383, 220th Leg., 1st Reg. Sess. (N.Y. 1997).

35. S. 5503, 221st Leg., 1st Reg. Sess. (N.Y. 1997).

36. A.B. 9116, 221st Leg., 1st Reg. Sess. (N.Y. 1998).

37. A.B. 9183, 221st Leg., 1st Reg. Sess. (N.Y. 1998).

38. S. 5993, 221st Leg., 1st Reg. Sess. (N.Y. 1998).

39. S. 6071, 221st Leg., 1st Reg. Sess. (N.Y. 1998).

40. S. 5503, 221st Leg., 1st Reg. Sess. (N.Y. 1998).

41. "Council for Responsible Genetics, Position Statement on Cloning" (last accessed June 4, 1998). Available at *http://www.essential.org/crg/cloning.html*.

42. National Bioethics Advisory Commission, *Cloning Human Beings*, pp. 102–03. Both of these organizations are committed to protecting human rights and dignity. UNESCO particularly is dedicated to preserving human rights based on international agreements.

43. "Scientist Who Cloned Sheep." Others at the Roslin Institute agree with Wilmut. Aside from believing it to be unethical, the scientists also believe that the sheep cloning technique would not be clinically useful if applied to humans. K. H. S. Campbell et al., "Implications of Cloning," *Nature* 380 (1996): 383.

44. See Editorial, "One Lamb, Much Fuss," *Lancet* 349 (1997): 661 (advocating stopping any research aimed at cloning humans but recognizing that research involving farm-animal breeding and medicine is acceptable).

45. The "Council of Europe Protocol" is distinct from the "Additional Protocol" to the Convention for the Protection of Human Rights and Dignity of the Human Being with regard to the Application of Biology and Medicine, on the Prohibition of Cloning Human Beings, ETS No. 168 (January 12, 1998). Available at *http://www.coe.fr/eng/legaltxt/168e.htm*.

46. Christiane Dennemeyer, "Europe Takes a Stand Against Human Cloning," *Council of Europe Press Service* (January 12, 1998). Available at *http://www.coe.fr/cp/98/6a(98).htm*. The Council of Europe was founded in 1949 and is the oldest European Organization. The 19 signing countries were Denmark, Estonia, Finland, France, Greece, Iceland, Italy, Latvia, Luxembourg, Moldova, Norway, Portugal, Romania, San Marino, Slovenia, Spain, Sweden, "the Former Yugoslav Republic of Macedonia," and Turkey. See Ibid.

47. Council of Europe, "Additional Protocol."

48. Ibid.

49. Butler and Wadman, "Calls for Cloning Ban Sell Science Short," p. 8. See also Adam Michael, "Europe/Japan Face up to Legal Hurdles to Cloning," *Nature Biotechnology*. 15 (1997): 609–10 (discussing the GAEIB report and its consequences).

50. Michael, "Europe/Japan Face Up to Legal Hurdles," p. 610.

51. See Nigel Williams, "Cloning Sparks Calls for New Laws," *Science* 275 (1997): 1415.

52. See Law no. 68 of 12 June 1987 on artificial fertilization. *International Digest of Health Legislation* 38 (1987): 782–85.

53. Law no. 35 of 22 November 1988 on assisted reproduction procedures. *International Digest of Health Legislation* 90 (1989): 82–93.

54. Editorial, "One Lamb, Much Fuss," p. 661.

55. Declan Butler and Meredith Wadman, "Putting a Lid on Pandora's Box of Genetics," *Nature* 386 (1997): 9.

56. See Ehsan Masood, "Cloning Technique 'Reveals Legal Loophole,' " *Nature* 385 (1997): 757. Note that Baroness Mary Warnock, chair of the government's advisory committee on human fertilization and embryology, stated that the act only included research current at that time and that the act probably should be amended to ban human cloning. See Ibid.

57. See Jacqui Wise, "Sheep Cloned from Mammary Gland Cells," *British Medical Journal* 314 (1997): 623. See also Owen Dyer, "Sheep Cloned by Nuclear Transfer," *British Medical Journal* 314 (1997): 623.

58. See Butler and Wadman, "Putting a Lid on Pandora's Box of Genetics," p. 9. See also Masood, "Cloning Technique 'Reveals Legal Loophole,' " (noting that some believe the Human Fertilization and Embryology Act of 1990, which was intended to ban human cloning, may not include the technique used to clone Dolly).

59. National Bioethics Advisory Commission, *Cloning Human Beings*, p. 92.

60. Ibid.

61. Other ordinary individual liberties can be limited if the government has a rational reason to do so. The more important the liberty at stake, the stronger the reasons must be for its limitation or restriction.

62. National Bioethics Advisory Commission, *Cloning Human Beings*, p. 94. See *Palko v. Connecticut*, 302 U.S. 319, 325–26 (1937); *Moore v. City of East Cleveland*, 431 U.S. 494, 503 (1977).

63. *Griswold v. Connecticut*, 381 U.S. 479 (1965); *Eisenstadt v. Baird*, 405 U.S. 438 (1972); *Planned Parenthood v. Casey*, 505 U.S. 833 (1992). See *Cleveland Bd. of Educ. v. LaFleur*, 414 U.S. 632, 639–40 (1974) (stating that "[f]reedom of personal choice in matters of marriage and family life is one of the liberties protected by the Due Process Clause of the Fourteenth Amendment"). See generally Debra Feuerberg Duffy, "To Be or Not To Be: The Legal Ramifications of the Cloning of Human Embryos," *Rutgers Computer & Technology Law Journal* 21 (1995): 189, 194–95.

64. For a discussion of modern substantive due process and related case law, see D. Lively, et al., *Constitutional Law: Cases, History, and Dialogues* (Cincinnati, Ohio, 1996), pp. 98–185.

65. *Lifchez v. Hartigan*, 735 F. Supp. 1361, 1377 (N.D. Ill.), aff'd without opinion, sub nom., *Scholberg v. Lifchez*, 914 F.2d 260 (7th Cir. 1990), cert. denied, 498 U.S. 1068 (1991).

66. John A. Robertson, "Embryos, Families, and Procreative Liberty: The Legal Structure of the New Reproduction," *Southern California Law Review* 59 (1986): 939, 958 (citing *Cleveland Bd. of Educ. v. LaFleur*, 414 U.S. 632, 639–40 [1973]).

67. Dan W. Brock, "Cloning Human Beings," *Medical Ethics Newsletter* (Lahey Hitchcock Clinic, Burlington, MA, Fall 1997), p. 1.

68. Susan Cohen, "What Is a Baby? Inside America's Unresolved Debate About the Ethics of Cloning," *Washington Post*, October 12, 1997, Magazine, p. W12.

69. See *Planned Parenthood of Southeastern Pennsylvania v. Casey*, 505 U.S. 833, 112 S. Ct. 2791, (1992).

70. See Cohen, "What is a Baby?" p. W25.
71. National Bioethics Advisory Commission, *Cloning Human Beings*, p. 76.
72. John A. Robertson, "The Question of Human Cloning," *Hastings Center Report* 24 (March–April 1994): 6, 13. Note that Robertson made this statement before the development of somatic cell nuclear transfer.
73. Cohen, "What is a Baby?"
74. National Bioethics Advisory Commission, *Cloning Human Beings*, p. 95.
75. George J. Annas, "Regulatory Models for Human Embryo Cloning: The Free Market, Professional Guidelines, and Government Restrictions," *Kennedy Institute of Ethics Journal* 4 (1994): 235.
76. Bonnie Steinbock, "The NBAC Report on Cloning Human Beings: What It Did— And Did Not—Do," *Jurimetrics* 38 (1997): 39, 46.
77. Ibid., 45.
78. Brock, "Cloning Human Beings."
79. See Steinbock, "The NBAC Report," p. 45.
80. Ibid., pp. 45–46.
81. Ibid., See generally *Bowers v. Hardwick*, 478 U.S. 186 (1986); *Moore v. City of East Cleveland*, 431 U.S. 494 (1977); *Palko v. Connecticut*, 302 U.S. 319 (1937).
82. For a related discussion, see Melinda A. Roberts, "Human Cloning: A Case of No Harm Done?" *Journal of Medicine & Philosophy* 21: (1996): 537. Roberts challenges Robertson's argument that offspring from cloning are not harmed because they owe their very existence to the cloning procedure. Roberts argues that cloning does place human offspring of cloning at risk of genuine harm. Ibid.
83. Cohen, "What is a Baby?" p. W26. Researchers used 277 embryos before succeeding with Dolly. "This failure rate was unacceptable in humans, and the failures showed evidence of lethal malformations." Ibid.
84. National Bioethics Advisory Commission, *Cloning Human Beings*, pp. 8–9.
85. National Bioethics Advisory Commission, *Cloning Human Beings*, pp. 78–79. Discussing the "value of intellectual freedom," the NBAC cites *Branzburg v. Hayes*, 408 U.S. 665, 705 (1972); *Meyer v. Nebraska*, 262 U.S. 390 (1923); and *Henley v. Wise*, 303 F. Supp 62 (N.D. Ind. 1969).
86. Susan M. Wolf, "Ban Cloning? Why NBAC Is Wrong," *Hastings Center Report* 27 (September–October 1997): 12, 13.
87. Cohen, "What Is a Baby?" p. W26.
88. Grahame Bulfield, "Roslin Unfunded," *Nature* 386 (1997): 12. Such opportunities include the production of valuable human proteins in animals for medical purposes and maintaining the competitiveness of the animal breeding industry. Ibid. See also "Companies Team up to Make Cloned Cattle, Human Milk" (Reuters, October 7, 1997), available at http://www.nando.net/newsroom/ntn/health/100797/health2_18393_noframes.html.
89. See generally June Coleman, "Playing God or Playing Scientist: A Constitutional Analysis of Laws Banning Embryological Procedures," *Pacific Law Journal* 27 (1996): 1331.
90. National Bioethics Advisory Commission, *Cloning Human Beings*, p. 79 (citing John Robertson, "The Scientist's Right to Research: A Constitutional Analysis," *Southern California Law Review* 51 (1977): 1203).
91. National Bioethics Advisory Commission, *Cloning Human Beings*, p. iv.
92. Ibid.

93. Mona S. Amer, Comment, "Breaking the Mold: Human Embryo Cloning and Its Implications for a Right to Individuality," *University of California Los Angeles Law Review* 43 (1996): 1659. See also Stephen A. Newman, "Human Cloning and the Family: Reflections on Cloning Existing Children," *New York Law School Journal of Human Rights* 13 (1997): 523.

94. Brock, "Cloning Human Beings." Perhaps this right is simply an ethical consideration and does not fall under constitutional purview, but will be discussed as a related concept.

95. Tom Murray, "Hello Dollies!" *CenterViews* (Center for Biomedical Ethics, Case Western Reserve University, Cleveland, Ohio, Fall 1997), p. 2.

96. Gladys L. Husted and James H. Husted, "An Ethical Examination of Cloning," *AORN Journal* 65 (1997): 1112–13.

97. Brock, "Cloning Human Beings," p. 2. See also Steinbock, "The NBAC Report," pp. 42–43 (explaining the "fallacy of 'genetic determinism'"); Dena S. Davis, "What's Wrong with Cloning?," *Jurimetrics* 38 (1997): 83.

98. See Wolf, "Ban Cloning?" p. 13.

99. National Bioethics Advisory Commission, *Cloning Human Beings*, p. 182.

100. Arlene J. Klotzko, "The Debate About Dolly," *Bioethics* 11 (1997): 427, 429.

101. The Associated Press, "Headless Human Clones Will Grow Organs in 10 Years," (October 19, 1997), available at http://www.globalchange.com/frogs.htm.

102. R. Alta Charo, "Dealing with Dolly: Cloning and the National Bioethics Advisory Commission," *Jurimetrics* 38 (1997): 11, 19.

103. National Bioethics Advisory Commission, *Cloning Human Beings*, p. 91.

104. Ibid., p. ii.

105. Andrea L. Bonnicksen, "Creating a Clone in Ninety Days: In Search of a Cloning Policy," *Jurimetrics* 38 (1997): 23.

106. Ibid., p. 24.

107. See Wolf, "Ban Cloning?" p. 12.

108. John A. Robertson, "Wrongful Life, Federalism, and Procreative Liberty: A Critique of the NBAC Cloning Report," *Jurimetrics* 38 (1997): 69, 81.

Appendix 1

Human Embryo Research Panel Report: Executive Summary

Charge to Panel

The mandate of the National Institutes of Health (NIH) Human Embryo Research Panel (the Panel) was to consider various areas of research involving the ex utero preimplantation human embryo and to provide advice as to those areas that *(1)* are acceptable for Federal funding, *(2)* warrant additional review, and *(3)* are unacceptable for Federal support. For those areas of research considered acceptable for Federal funding, the Panel was asked to recommend specific guidelines for the review and conduct of this research.

The Panel's charge encompasses only research that involves extracorporeal human embryos produced by in vitro fertilization or from other sources, or parthenogenetically activated oocytes. Research involving in utero human embryos, or fetuses, is not part of the charge, since guidelines for such research are embodied in Federal laws and regulations governing human subjects research. Research involving human germ-line gene modification also is not within the Panel's scope. Therapeutic human fetal tissue transplantation research is also not part of the Panel's mandate; guidelines are already in place to govern such research.

Throughout this report, "ex utero preimplantation embryo" or "preimplantation embryo" refers to a fertilized ovum in vitro that has never been transferred to or implanted in a uterus. This includes a fertilized ovum that has been flushed

251

from a woman before implantation in the uterus. This procedure, although infrequent and posing special risks, is included because it is one potential source of embryos.

Ethical considerations

Throughout its deliberations, the Panel considered the wide range of views held by American citizens on the moral status of preimplantation embryos. In recommending public policy, the Panel was not called upon to decide which of these views is correct. Rather, its task was to propose guidelines for preimplantation human embryo research that would be acceptable public policy based on reasoning that takes account of generally held public views regarding the beginning and development of human life. The Panel weighed arguments for and against Federal funding of this research in light of the best available information and scientific knowledge and conducted its deliberations in terms that were independent of a particular religious or philosophical perspective.

The Panel received a considerable volume of public input, which it carefully considered. The Panel heard from citizens who object to any research involving preimplantation embryos as well as those who support it and listened closely to the thinking underlying the various opinions expressed. In the process of receiving public input, the Panel realized that the scientific and policy issues involved in research on preimplantation embryos are complex and not easily comprehended. The Panel therefore recognizes that a special effort is required to enhance public understanding of the issues related to research involving the preimplantation embryo. It is the Panel's hope that this report will in some measure contribute to a process of increasing public awareness, discussion, and understanding of the issues.

From the perspective of public policy, the Panel concludes that sufficient arguments exist to support the permissibility of certain areas of research involving the preimplantation human embryo within a framework of stringent guidelines. This conclusion is based on an assessment of the moral status of the preimplantation embryo from various viewpoints and not solely on its location ex utero. In addition, the Panel weighed the important human benefits that might be achieved if preimplantation embryo research were federally funded under stringent guidelines.

The Panel believes that certain areas of research are permissible based on three primary considerations, which are listed below. Different members of the Panel may have accorded different weight to each of these considerations in reaching a conclusion about the permissibility of certain areas of research.

- The promise of human benefit from research is significant, carrying great potential benefit to infertile couples, families with genetic conditions, and individuals and families in need of effective therapies for a variety of diseases.

- Although the preimplantation human embryo warrants serious moral consideration as a developing form of human life, it does not have the same moral status as an infant or child. This is because of the absence of developmental individuation in the preimplantation embryo, the lack of even the possibility of sentience and most other qualities considered relevant to the moral status of persons, and the very high rate of natural mortality at this stage.
- In the continued absence of Federal funding and regulation in this area, preimplantation human embryo research that has been and is being conducted without Federal funding and regulation would continue, without consistent ethical and scientific review. It is in the public interest that the availability of Federal funding and regulation should provide consistent ethical and scientific review for this area of research. The Panel believes that because the preimplantation embryo possesses qualities requiring moral respect, research involving the ex utero preimplantation human embryo must be carefully regulated and consistently monitored.

Principles and guidelines for preimplantation embryo research

The Panel supports Federal funding of certain areas of preimplantation embryo research within the framework of the guidelines specified below. Any research conducted on the ex utero preimplantation human embryo or on gametes intended for fertilization should adhere to the following general principles as well as the more specific guidelines relevant to the nature of the particular research.

- The research must be conducted by scientifically qualified individuals in an appropriate research setting.
- The research must consist of a valid research design and promise significant scientific or clinical benefit.
- The research goals cannot be otherwise accomplished by using animals or unfertilized gametes. In addition, where applicable, adequate prior animal studies must have been conducted.
- The number of embryos required for the research must be kept to the minimum consistent with scientific criteria for validity.
- Donors of gametes or embryos must have given informed consent with regard to the nature and purpose of the specific research being undertaken.
- There must be no purchase or sale of gametes or embryos used in research. Reasonable compensation in clinical studies should be permissible to defray a subject's expenses, over and above the costs of drugs and procedures required for standard treatment, provided that no compensation or financial inducements of any sort are offered in exchange for the donation of gametes or embryos, and so long as the level of compensation is in accordance with Federal regulations governing human subjects research and that it is consistent with general compensation practice for other federally funded experimental protocols.

- Research protocols and consent forms must be reviewed and approved by an appropriate institutional review board (IRB) and, for the immediate future, an ad hoc review process that extends beyond the existing review process to be established by NIH and operated for at least 3 years.
- There must be equitable selection of donors of gametes and embryos, and efforts must be made to ensure that benefits and risks are fairly distributed among subgroups of the population.
- Out of respect for the special character of the preimplantation human embryo, research involving preimplantation embryos should be limited to the shortest time period consistent with the goals of each research proposal and, for the present, research involving human embryos should not be permitted beyond the time of the usual appearance of the primitive streak in vivo (14 days). An exception to this is made for research protocols with the goal of reliably identifying in the laboratory the appearance of the primitive streak.

Fertilization of oocytes expressly for research purposes

One of the most difficult issues the Panel had to consider was whether it is ethically permissible to fertilize donated oocytes expressly for research purposes or whether researchers should be restricted to the use of embryos remaining from infertility treatments that are donated by women or couples. In developing its recommendation concerning this issue, the Panel considered both the deeply held moral concerns about the fertilization of oocytes for research as well as the potential clinical benefits to be gained from such research. The Panel concludes that studies that require the fertilization of oocytes are needed to answer crucial questions in reproductive medicine and that it would therefore not be wise to prohibit altogether the fertilization and study of oocytes for research purposes. The Panel had to balance important issues regarding the health and safety of women, children, and men against the moral respect due the preimplantation embryo. Given the conclusions the Panel reached about the moral status of the preimplantation embryo, it concludes that the health needs of women, children, and men must be given priority.

The Panel recognizes, however, that the embryo merits respect as a developing form of human life and should be used in research only for the most serious and compelling reasons. There is also a possibility that if researchers had broad permission to develop embryos for research, more embryos might be created than is truly justified. The Panel believes that the use of oocytes fertilized expressly for research should be allowed only under two conditions. The first condition is when the research by its very nature cannot otherwise be validly conducted. Examples of studies that might meet this condition include *(1)* oocyte maturation or oocyte freezing followed by fertilization and examination for subsequent developmental viability and chromosomal normalcy and *(2)* investigations into the process of fertilization itself (including the efficacy of new contraceptives). If oocyte maturation techniques were improved, eggs could be obtained without reliance on stimulatory drugs, lessening some of the potential risks for both patients and egg donors.

The second condition under which the fertilization of oocytes would be allowed expressly for research is when a compelling case can be made that this is necessary for the validity of a study that is potentially of outstanding scientific and therapeutic value. One member of the Panel dissented from the Panel conclusion that under this condition oocytes may be fertilized expressly for research purposes.

Panel members believe that special attention is warranted for such research because of their concern that attempts might be made to create embryos for reasons that relate solely to the scarcity of embryos remaining from infertility programs and because of their interest in preventing the creation of embryos for any but the most compelling reasons. An example of studies that might meet this second condition is research to ensure that specific drugs used in reproductive medicine, such as those for inducing ovulation, have no harmful effect on oocytes and their developmental potential and do not compromise the future reproductive health of women.

In another case, future discoveries might provide strong evidence that some forms of infertility, birth defects, or childhood cancer are due to chromosomal abnormalities, DNA modifications, or metabolic defects in embryos from gametes of men and women of a particular category—for example, those exposed to specific environmental agents or carrying specific genetic traits. In order to test or validate such hypotheses, a compelling case might be made for comparing embryos from at-risk couples with control embryos from "normal" couples. While embryos from many infertile couples in in vitro fertilization (IVF) programs might be suitable for this control group, in specific cases a compelling argument might be made that gametes donated by fertile individuals carefully matched for age and ethnic background to those in the at-risk group are necessary for the most accurate and informative comparative scientific data.

Sources of gametes and embryos for research

Having concluded that Federal funding of certain areas of preimplantation embryo research is acceptable within stringent guidelines, the Panel went on to address another set of ethical dilemmas raised by the issue of acceptability of various sources of gametes and embryos. In considering these issues the Panel identified four concerns that require special vigilance: the need for informed consent, limits on commercialization, equitable selection of donors for research, and appropriate balancing of risks and benefits among subgroups of the population. These concerns parallel those addressed by well-established ethical guidelines for all human research. The selection of sources of gametes and embryos for research must be consistent with these established guidelines and in addition must show respect for the special qualities of the human gamete and embryo.

The Panel gave careful consideration to the two distinct means by which a preimplantation human embryo can become available for research. The first occurs when embryos already fertilized for infertility treatments are not used for that purpose but are donated by the progenitors for research (these embryos are sometimes referred to as "spare" embryos). The second occurs when an oocyte is fertilized expressly for the purpose of research. The Panel also considered the ethical acceptability of the various donor sources of oocytes for research involving transfer, research without transfer, and research involving parthenogenesis. These possible donor sources include women in IVF programs, healthy volunteers, women undergoing pelvic surgery, women and girls who have died, and aborted fetuses.

In analyzing the acceptability of donor sources of gametes and embryos for research, the Panel emphasized that the risks of the research, including the risks of gamete procurement, must be in proportion to the anticipated benefits. Risks that occur at various stages of research and in the context of diverse protocols restrict the acceptable sources of research gametes and embryos. For example, the need to consider the well-being of the future child when embryos are transferred to the uterus mandates particular attention to the acceptability of gamete and embryo sources, including a requirement that the gamete donors approve of the research as well as the transfer.

In general, the Panel concludes that, provided all conditions regarding consent and limits on commercialization are met, embryos donated by couples in IVF programs are acceptable sources for basic research that does not involve transfer, as well as for clinical studies that may involve transfer. Women undergoing IVF treatment may also donate oocytes not needed for their own treatment, provided other guidelines are met. In this regard, the Panel believes it is right for women and couples undergoing infertility treatment to assume a fair share of the burden of advancing research in this area given that they, as a class, stand to benefit most from the clinical applications that may result. However, the Panel also recognizes that infertility can cause great physical and psychological pain and that women and couples undergoing treatment may be more vulnerable as a result. For this reason one member of the Panel dissents from allowing women in IVF treatment the opportunity to donate oocytes for research that does not involve transfer. In order that women and couples in IVF programs are not made to feel compelled to donate, great care must be taken to ensure that there is no undue, or even subtle, pressure to donate. The voluntary nature of such donations is essential, and under no circumstances should individuals who do not wish to donate their gametes ever feel pressured to do so.

Donation of oocytes for research purposes without intent to transfer raises special concerns regarding risks to women. Some of the methods used to procure eggs, especially hyperstimulation, involve the use of powerful drugs and invasive procedures that could pose risks to the health of women. Women undergoing treatment for infertility consent to these risks in return for potential therapeutic benefit and are an acceptable source of oocytes for basic research that does not involve transfer, as well as for clinical studies that may involve transfer.

Women undergoing scheduled pelvic surgery are an additional permissible source of oocytes for research, provided that other guidelines are met and that no additional risks are imposed. Researchers must explain any changes from standard surgical procedures and, if hormonal stimulation is used, the risks of such drugs.

Women who are not scheduled to undergo a surgical procedure are not a permissible source of oocytes for embryos developed for research at this time, even if they wish to volunteer to donate their oocytes. The Panel, however, is willing to allow such volunteers to donate oocytes if the intent is to transfer the resulting embryo for the purpose of establishing a pregnancy. This is because the risks to the donor undergoing oocyte retrieval may be justified by the potential direct benefit to the infertile couple who hope to become parents as a result of the procedure. Absent the goal of establishing a pregnancy for an infertile couple, the lack of direct therapeutic benefit to the donor and the dangers of commercial exploitation do not justify exposing women to such risks.

Women who have died are a permissible source of oocytes for research without transfer, provided that the woman had not expressly objected to such use of her oocytes and that appropriate consent is obtained. If the woman had expressed no objection to such use of her oocytes, either she must have consented to donation before her death or, in the absence of explicit consent on her part, next of kin may give consent at the time of her death. One member of the Panel dissents from this recommendation based on the belief that consent must have been obtained from the woman before her death. Care must be taken to ensure that the consenting donors, or their next of kin who would be providing proxy consent, are clearly and specifically aware that the organ being donated is the ovary and that it might be used in research that could involve the fertilization of any oocytes derived from it. It should also be made clear to donors and next of kin that transfer of any embryo created from such material to the uterus is prohibited.

Because of strong concerns about the importance of parenthood and the orderly sequence of generations, as well as the need for detailed medical histories, the Panel concluded that research involving the transfer of embryos created from oocytes obtained from cadaveric sources, including aborted fetuses, should be unacceptable for Federal funding. The Panel also felt that it would be unwise public policy at this time to support, without additional review, research involving the fertilization of fetal oocytes, even if not intended for transfer to the uterus. Such research should not be supported until the ethical implications are more fully explored and addressed by a national advisory body.

Transfer of embryos to a uterus

In addition to these general guidelines, the Panel developed specific guidelines for research on preimplantation embryos intended for transfer and for those not intended for transfer, as well as guidelines for research involving parthenogenesis.

It is important to recognize that when transfer to a uterus is intended, research on the preimplantation embryo can result in harm to the child who could be born, a research subject whose treatment raises distinct ethical issues. In both law and ethics it is clear that fetuses who are brought to term are considered persons with full moral status and protectability. It would therefore be unacceptable to transfer an embryo if it is reasonable to believe that a child who might be born from these procedures will suffer harm as a result of the research. Even when research involves a diagnostic procedure, an embryo may not be transferred unless there is reasonable confidence that any child born as a result of these procedures has not been harmed by them. This distinction in treatment between embryos that will be transferred and those that will not is warranted by the need to avoid harm to the child who could be born.

Parthenogenesis

In keeping with its mandate, the Panel also considered the acceptability of Federal funding of research involving the parthenogenetic activation of eggs. Parthenogenesis is the activation of eggs to begin cleavage and development without fertilization. It has been shown in research involving parthenogenesis in mammals that when such parthenotes are transferred to the uterus, few reach the stage of implantation. The few that do reach implantation develop to various stages of early cell differentiation but then lose capacity for further development and die. Parthenotes fail to develop further because they lack expression of essential genes contributed by the sperm. All evidence therefore suggests that human parthenotes intrinsically are not developmentally viable human embryos. Thus, they do not represent a form of asexual reproduction.

Research of parthenotes, or activated eggs, might provide information on the specific role of the egg mechanisms in activating and sustaining early development, without generating a human embryo. Parthenotes may have research utility nearly identical to the normal embryo up to the blastocyst stage. In addition, a certain type of ovarian tumor originates from eggs that develop as parthenotes while still in the ovary. Research on parthenotes may shed light on problems arising during oocyte development that promote this type of tumor formation.

The Panel recommends that research proposals involving parthenogenesis be considered ethically acceptable on the conditions that they adhere to the general principles and that transfer of parthenogenetically activated oocytes not be permitted under any circumstances. The Panel wishes to allay fears expressed by members of the public who are concerned about the end point of research on parthenogenesis. To many, such research appears to represent a tampering with the natural order in unacceptable ways. Even though it is considered intrinsically impossible in humans, the Panel would preclude any attempts to develop a fetus or child without a paternal progenitor by prohibiting research involving the transfer of parthenotes.

Review and oversight of research

The Panel does not recommend that an Ethics Advisory Board (EAB) be reconstituted for the purpose of reviewing research protocols involving embryos and fertilized eggs. Although revisiting the EAB experience offers the potential for developing public consensus and a consistent application of the new guidelines, it nonetheless has significant disadvantages. These disadvantages include the creation of an additional standing government board, the likelihood of a significant delay before embryo research could be funded in order to meet legal requirements for new rulemaking prior to the official creation of the government body, and further possible delay if all proposals for embryo research were required to be considered individually by an EAB-type board, despite appearing to be consistent with a developed consensus at NIH about acceptability for funding.

The Panel wishes to retain the strengths of the old EAB—such as its assurance of consistent application of guidelines—without creating a new regulatory body. Therefore, the Panel recommends that all research proposals involving preimplantation human embryo research that are submitted to NIH for funding or that are proposed for conduct in the NIH intramural research program be subject to an additional review at the national level by an ad hoc body created with the discretionary authority of the Director of NIH. Two members of the Panel formally dissent from this recommendation, citing the adequacy of existing review through local IRBs and the possibility of such a review board being subject to undue pressures.

The purpose of the recommended review is to ensure that such research is conducted in accordance with guidelines established by NIH. This review is in addition to existing procedures and should occur after the standard reviews and approvals by the study section and council have been completed. The additional review process should continue for at least 3 years. If the NIH Director elects to dissolve this ad hoc review process after 3 years, a more decentralized review with certain additional oversight provisions, as specified further below, should begin.

When the ad hoc review body ceases to exist, the Panel recommends that all such research proposals continue to be specially monitored by the NIH councils and the NIH Office for Protection From Research Risks. This monitoring would include a commitment by the councils to pay particular attention to the protocols as they are presented for approval, in order to ensure that the local IRB and NIH study sections have correctly applied the guidelines adopted by the NIH Director.

Categories of research

Consistent with its mandate, the Panel considered specific areas of research in terms of acceptability for Federal funding. While it is clearly impossible to anticipate every type of research project that might be proposed, the Panel was charged to divide types of embryo research into three categories: *(1)* acceptable for Federal funding, *(2)* warranting additional review, and *(3)* unacceptable for Federal funding.

Acceptable for Federal Funding

A research proposal is presumed acceptable if it is in accordance with the guidelines described above and is not described below as warranting additional review or being unacceptable. A protocol not in the last two categories would be classified acceptable if it is scientifically valid and meritorious; relies on prior adequate animal studies and, where appropriate, studies on human embryos without transfer; uses a minimal number of embryos; documents that informed consent will be obtained from acceptable donor sources; involves no purchase or sale of gametes or embryos; does not continue beyond the time of the usual appearance of the primitive streak in vivo (14 days); and has passed the required review by a local IRB, appropriate NIH study section and council, and, for the immediate future, the additional ad hoc review body at the national level established at the discretion of the NIH Director.

Proposals in the acceptable category must also meet the specific guidelines set forth in this report concerning types of research (i.e., transfer, no transfer, parthenogenesis), and acceptable sources of gametes and embryos. Examples of such proposals include, but are not limited to the following:

- Studies aimed at improving the likelihood of a successful outcome for a pregnancy.
- Research on the process of fertilization.
- Studies on egg activation and the relative role of paternally derived and maternally derived genetic material in embryo development (parthenogenesis without transfer).
- Studies in oocyte maturation or freezing followed by fertilization to determine developmental and chromosomal normality.

- Research involving preimplantation genetic diagnosis with and without transfer.
- Research involving the development of embryonic stem cells, but only with embryos resulting from IVF for infertility treatment or clinical research that have been donated with the consent of the progenitors.
- Nuclear transplantation into an enucleated, fertilized or unfertilized (but activated) egg without transfer for research that aims to circumvent or correct an inherited cytoplasmic defect.

With regard to the last example, a narrow majority of the Panel believed such research should be acceptable for Federal funding. Nearly as many thought that the ethical implications of research involving the transplantation of a nucleus, whether transfer was contemplated or not, need further study before the research could be considered acceptable for Federal funding.

In addition to these examples, the Panel singled out two types of acceptable research for special consideration in the recommended ad hoc review process.

- Research involving the use of existing embryos where one of the progenitors was an anonymous gamete source who received monetary compensation. (This exception would apply only to embryos already in existence at the time at which this report is accepted by the Advisory Committee to the Director, NIH, should such acceptance occur.)
- A request to fertilize ova where this is necessary for the validity of a study that is potentially of outstanding scientific and therapeutic value.

In the first instance, for reasons explained in chapter 4 of this report, the Panel, with the exception of one member, would make an allowance for an interim period for research involving the use of existing embryos where one of the progenitors was anonymous and had received monetary compensation. However, the Panel believes that in order to determine whether the exception might apply, special attention must be given during the review process to ensure that payment has not been provided for the embryo itself and that all other proposed guidelines are met.

In the second instance, Panel members believe that special attention is warranted for such research because of concern that attempts might be made to create embryos for reasons that relate solely to the scarcity of embryos remaining from infertility programs and because of the Panel's interest in preventing the creation of embryos for any but the most compelling reasons.

Warrants Additional Review

The Panel places research of a particularly sensitive nature in this category. The Panel did not make a determination on the acceptability of these proposals and therefore recommends that there be a presumption against Federal funding of such research for the foreseeable future. This presumption could be overcome only by an extraordinary showing of scientific or therapeutic merit, together with explicit consideration of the ethical issues and social consequences. Such research proposals could be funded only after review by a broad-based ad hoc body created at the discretion of the Director, NIH, or by some other formal review process.

Research that the Panel determined should be placed in a category warranting additional review includes the following:

- Research between the appearance of the primitive streak and the beginning of neural tube closure.
- Cloning by blastomere separation or blastocyst splitting without transfer.
- Nuclear transplantation into an enucleated, fertilized or unfertilized (but activated) egg with transfer, with the aim of circumventing or correcting an inherited cytoplasmic defect.
- Research involving the development of embryonic stem cells from embryos fertilized expressly for this purpose. (One member of the Panel dissents from this categorization.)
- Research that uses fetal oocytes for fertilization without transfer.

The Panel wishes to note that it was extremely circumspect in its consideration of the appropriate classification of the last two research areas and that members were divided in their views about where to place the research. For research involving the development of embryonic stem cells from deliberately fertilized oocytes, a narrow majority of members agreed such research warranted further review. A number of other members, however, felt that the research was acceptable for Federal funding, while some believed that such research should be considered unacceptable for Federal funding. The Panel's deliberation about the use of fetal oocytes for research without transfer involved painstaking reflection about the ethical implications and public sensibilities. The decision to recommend that this research be placed in the further review category, rather than the unacceptable category, was made by a bare majority.

Unacceptable for Federal Funding

Four ethical considerations entered into the deliberations of the Panel as it determined what types of research were unacceptable for Federal funding: the potential adverse consequences of the research for children, women, and men; the respect due the preimplantation embryo; concern for public sensitivities about highly controversial research proposals; and concern for the meaning of humanness, parenthood, and the succession of generations.

Throughout its report, the Panel considered these concerns as well as the scientific promise and the clinical and therapeutic value of proposed research, particularly as it might contribute to the well-being of women, children, and men.

Regarding the types of research considered unacceptable, the Panel determined that the scientific and therapeutic value was low or questionable, or that animal studies did not warrant progressing to human research.

Research proposals in the unacceptable category should not be funded for the foreseeable future. Even if claims were made for their scientific or therapeutic value, serious ethical concerns counsel against supporting such research. Such research includes the following:

- Cloning of human preimplantation embryos by separating blastomeres or dividing blastocysts (induced twinning), followed by transfer in utero.
- Studies designed to transplant embryonic or adult nuclei into an enucleated egg, including nuclear cloning, in order to duplicate a genome or to increase the number of embryos with the same genotype with transfer.
- Research beyond the onset of closure of the neural tube.
- Research involving the fertilization of fetal oocytes with transfer.
- Preimplantation genetic diagnosis for sex selection, except for sex-linked genetic diseases.
- Development of human–nonhuman and human–human chimeras with or without transfer.
- Cross-species fertilization, except for clinical tests of the ability of sperm to penetrate eggs.
- Attempted transfer of parthenogenetically activated human eggs.
- Attempted transfer of human embryos into nonhuman animals for gestation.
- Transfer of human embryos for extrauterine or abdominal pregnancy.

Need for public education

Finally, the Panel believes that any successful efforts in preimplantation embryo research depend on improving public understanding of the nature of preimplantation embryo research and therefore recommends that NIH undertake efforts toward public education as it simultaneously educates the scientific community about guidelines for acceptable research.

Appendix 2

National Bioethics Advisory Commission Report on Cloning: Executive Summary

The idea that humans might someday be cloned—created from a single somatic cell without sexual reproduction—moved further away from science fiction and closer to a genuine scientific possibility on February 23, 1997. On that date, *The Observer* broke the news that Ian Wilmut, a Scottish scientist, and his colleagues at the Roslin Institute were about to announce the successful cloning of a sheep by a new technique which had never before been fully successful in mammals. The technique involved transplanting the genetic material of an adult sheep, apparently obtained from a differentiated somatic cell, into an egg from which the nucleus had been removed. The resulting birth of the sheep, named Dolly, on July 5, 1996, was different from prior attempts to create identical offspring since Dolly contained the genetic material of only one parent, and was, therefore, a "delayed" genetic twin of a single adult sheep.

This cloning technique is an extension of research that had been ongoing for over 40 years using nuclei derived from non-human embryonic and fetal cells. The demonstration that nuclei from cells derived from an adult animal could be "reprogrammed," or that the full genetic complement of such a cell could be re-activated well into the chronological life of the cell, is what sets the results of this experiment apart from prior work. In this report we refer to the technique, first described by Wilmut, of nuclear transplantation using nuclei derived from

264

somatic cells other than those of an embryo or fetus as "somatic cell nuclear transfer."

Within days of the published report of Dolly, President Clinton instituted a ban on federal funding related to attempts to clone human beings in this manner. In addition, the President asked the recently appointed National Bioethics Advisory Commission (NBAC) to address within ninety days the ethical and legal issues that surround the subject of cloning human beings. This provided a welcome opportunity for initiating a thoughtful analysis of the many dimensions of the issue, including a careful consideration of the potential risks and benefits. It also presented an occasion to review the current legal status of cloning and the potential constitutional challenges that might be raised if new legislation were enacted to restrict the creation of a child through somatic cell nuclear transfer cloning.

The Commission began its discussions fully recognizing that any effort in humans to transfer a somatic cell nucleus into an enucleated egg involves the creation of an embryo, with the apparent potential to be implanted in utero and developed to term. Ethical concerns surrounding issues of embryo research have recently received extensive analysis and deliberation in the United States. Indeed, federal funding for human embryo research is severely restricted, although there are few restrictions on human embryo research carried out in the private sector. Thus, under current law, the use of somatic cell nuclear transfer to create an embryo solely for research purposes is already restricted in cases involving federal funds. There are, however, no current federal regulations on the use of private funds for this purpose.

The unique prospect, vividly raised by Dolly, is the creation of a new individual genetically identical to an existing (or previously existing) person—a "delayed" genetic twin. This prospect has been the source of the overwhelming public concern about such cloning.

While the creation of embryos for research purposes alone always raises serious ethical questions, the use of somatic cell nuclear transfer to create embryos raises no new issues in this respect. The unique and distinctive ethical issues raised by the use of somatic cell nuclear transfer to create children relate to, for example, serious safety concerns, individuality, family integrity, and treating children as objects. Consequently, the Commission focused its attention on the use of such techniques for the purpose of creating an embryo which would then be implanted in a woman's uterus and brought to term. It also expanded its analysis of this particular issue to encompass activities in both the public and private sector.

In its deliberations, NBAC reviewed the scientific developments which preceded the Roslin announcement, as well as those likely to follow in its path. It also considered the many moral concerns raised by the possibility that this technique could be used to clone human beings. Much of the initial reaction to this possibility was negative. Careful assessment of that response revealed fears about harms to the children who may be created in this manner, particularly psychological harms associated with a possibly diminished sense of individuality and personal autonomy. Others expressed concern about a degradation in the quality of parenting and family life.

In addition to concerns about specific harms to children, people have frequently expressed fears that the widespread practice of somatic cell nuclear transfer cloning would undermine important social values by opening the door to a form of eugenics or by tempting some to manipulate others as if they were objects instead of persons. Arrayed against these concerns are other important social values, such as protecting the widest possible sphere of personal choice, particularly in matters pertaining to procreation and child rearing, maintaining privacy and the freedom of scientific inquiry, and encouraging the possible development of new biomedical breakthroughs.

To arrive at its recommendations concerning the use of somatic cell nuclear transfer techniques to create children, NBAC also examined long-standing religious traditions that guide many citizens' responses to new technologies and found that religious positions on human cloning are pluralistic in their premises, modes of argument, and conclusions. Some religious thinkers argue that the use of somatic cell nuclear transfer cloning to create a child would be intrinsically immoral and thus could never be morally justified. Other religious thinkers contend that human cloning to create a child could be morally justified under some circumstances, but hold that it should be strictly regulated in order to prevent abuses.

The public policies recommended with respect to the creation of a child using somatic cell nuclear transfer reflect the Commission's best judgments about both the ethics of attempting such an experiment and its view of traditions regarding limitations on individual actions in the name of the common good. At present, the use of this technique to create a child would be a premature experiment that would expose the fetus and the developing child to unacceptable risks. This in itself might be sufficient to justify a prohibition on cloning human beings at this time, even if such efforts were to be characterized as the exercise of a fundamental right to attempt to procreate.

Beyond the issue of the safety of the procedure, however, NBAC found that concerns relating to the potential psychological harms to children and effects on the moral, religious, and cultural values of society merited further reflection and deliberation. Whether upon such further deliberation our nation will conclude that the use of cloning techniques to create children should be allowed or permanently banned is, for the moment, an open question. Time is an ally in this regard, allowing for the accrual of further data from animal experimentation, enabling an assessment of the prospective safety and efficacy of the procedure in humans, as well as granting a period of fuller national debate on ethical and social concerns. The Commission therefore concluded that there should be imposed a period of time in which no attempt is made to create a child using somatic cell nuclear transfer.

Within this overall framework the Commission came to the following conclusions and recommendations:

I. The Commission concludes that at this time it is morally unacceptable for anyone in the public or private sector, whether in a research or clinical setting, to attempt to create a child using somatic cell nuclear transfer cloning. The Commission reached a consensus on this point because current scientific information indicates that this technique is not safe to use in humans at this point. Indeed, the Commission believes it would violate important ethical obligations were clinicians or researchers to attempt to create a child using these particular technologies, which are likely to involve unacceptable risks to the fetus and/or potential child. Moreover, in addition to safety concerns, many other serious ethical concerns have been identified, which require much more widespread and careful public deliberation before this technology may be used.

The Commission, therefore, recommends the following for immediate action:

* A continuation of the current moratorium on the use of federal funding in support of any attempt to create a child by somatic cell nuclear transfer.
* An immediate request to all firms, clinicians, investigators, and professional societies in the private and non-federally funded sectors to comply voluntarily with the intent of the federal moratorium. Professional and scientific societies should make clear that any attempt to create a child by somatic cell nuclear transfer and implantation into a woman's body would at this time be an irresponsible, unethical, and unprofessional act.

II. The Commission further recommends that:

* Federal legislation should be enacted to prohibit anyone from attempting, whether in a research or clinical setting, to create a child through somatic cell nuclear transfer cloning. It is critical, however, that such legislation include a sunset clause to ensure that Congress will review the issue after a specified time period (three to five years) in order to decide whether the prohibition continues to be needed. If state legislation is enacted, it should also contain such a sunset provision. Any such legislation or associated regulation also ought to require that at some point prior to the expiration of the sunset period, an appropriate oversight body will evaluate and report on the current status of somatic cell nuclear transfer technology and on the ethical and social issues that its potential use to create human beings would raise in light of public understandings at that time.

III. The Commission also concludes that:

* Any regulatory or legislative actions undertaken to effect the foregoing prohibition on creating a child by somatic cell nuclear transfer should be carefully written so as not to interfere with other important areas of scientific research. In particular, no new regulations are required regarding the cloning of human

DNA sequences and cell lines, since neither activity raises the scientific and ethical issues that arise from the attempt to create children through somatic cell nuclear transfer, and these fields of research have already provided important scientific and biomedical advances. Likewise, research on cloning animals by somatic cell nuclear transfer does not raise the issues implicated in attempting to use this technique for human cloning, and its continuation should only be subject to existing regulations regarding the humane use of animals and review by institution-based animal protection committees.

• If a legislative ban is not enacted, or if a legislative ban is ever lifted, clinical use of somatic cell nuclear transfer techniques to create a child should be preceded by research trials that are governed by the twin protections of independent review and informed consent, consistent with existing norms of human subjects protection.

• The United States Government should cooperate with other nations and international organizations to enforce any common aspects of their respective policies on the cloning of human beings.

IV. The Commission also concludes that different ethical and religious perspectives and traditions are divided on many of the important moral issues that surround any attempt to create a child using somatic cell nuclear transfer techniques. Therefore, the Commission recommends that:

• The federal government, and all interested and concerned parties, encourage widespread and continuing deliberation on these issues in order to further our understanding of the ethical and social implications of this technology and to enable society to produce appropriate long-term policies regarding this technology should the time come when present concerns about safety have been addressed.

V. Finally, because scientific knowledge is essential for all citizens to participate in a full and informed fashion in the governance of our complex society, the Commission recommends that:

• Federal departments and agencies concerned with science should cooperate in seeking out and supporting opportunities to provide information and education to the public in the area of genetics, and on other developments in the biomedical sciences, especially where these affect important cultural practices, values, and beliefs.

Appendix 2a

National Bioethics Advisory Commission Report on Cloning—Excerpts from Chapter 2, The Science and Application of Cloning

What is cloning?

The word *clone* is used in many different contexts in biological research but in its most simple and strict sense, it refers to a precise genetic copy of a molecule, cell, plant, animal, or human being. In some of these contexts, cloning refers to established technologies that have been part of agricultural practice for a very long time and currently form an important part of the foundations of modern biological research.

Indeed, genetically identical copies of whole organisms are commonplace in the plant breeding world and are commonly referred to as "varieties" rather than clones. Many valuable horticultural or agricultural strains are maintained solely by vegetative propagation from an original plant, reflecting the ease with which it is possible to regenerate a complete plant from a small cutting. The developmental process in animals does not usually permit cloning as easily as in plants. Many simpler invertebrate species, however, such as certain kinds of worms, are capable of regenerating a whole organism from a small piece, even though this is not necessarily their usual mode of reproduction. Vertebrates have lost this ability entirely, although regeneration of certain limbs, organs, or tissues can occur to varying degrees in some animals.

This work is derived in part from previously issued papers by Janet Rossant and Stuart Orkin.[1]

Although a single adult vertebrate cannot generate another whole organism, cloning of vertebrates does occur in nature, in a limited way, through multiple births, primarily with the formation of identical twins. However, twins occur by chance in humans and other mammals with the separation of a single embryo into halves at an early stage of development. The resulting offspring are genetically identical, having been derived from one zygote, which resulted from the fertilization of one egg by one sperm.

At the molecular and cellular level, scientists have been cloning human and animal cells and genes for several decades. The scientific justification for such cloning is that it provides greater quantities of identical cells or genes for study; each cell or molecule is identical to the others.

At the simplest level, molecular biologists routinely make clones of deoxyribonucleic acid (DNA), the molecular basis of genes. DNA fragments containing genes are copied and amplified in a host cell, usually a bacterium. The availability of large quantities of identical DNA makes possible many scientific experiments. This process, often called *molecular cloning*, is the mainstay of recombinant DNA technology and has led to the production of such important medicines as insulin to treat diabetes, tissue plasminogen activator (tPA) to dissolve clots after a heart attack, and erythropoietin (EPO) to treat anemia associated with dialysis for kidney disease.

Another type of cloning is conducted at the cellular level. In *cellular cloning* copies are made of cells derived from the soma, or body, by growing these cells in culture in a laboratory. The genetic makeup of the resulting cloned cells, called a cell line, is identical to that of the original cell. This, too, is a highly reliable procedure, which is also used to test and sometimes to produce new medicines such as those listed above. Since molecular and cellular cloning of this sort does not involve germ cells (eggs or sperm), the cloned cells are not capable of developing into a baby.

The third type of cloning aims to reproduce genetically identical animals. Cloning of animals can typically be divided into two distinct processes, blastomere separation and nuclear transplantation cloning.

In blastomere separation, the developing embryo is split very soon after fertilization when it is composed of two to eight cells. Each cell, called a blastomere, is able to produce a new individual organism. These blastomeres are considered to be totipotent, that is they possess the total potential to make an entire new organism. This totipotency allows scientists to split animal embryos into several cells to produce multiple organisms that are genetically identical. This capability has tremendous relevance to breeding cattle and other livestock.

In the early 1980s, a more sophisticated form of cloning animals was developed, known as nuclear transplantation cloning. The nucleus of somatic cells is diploid—that is, it contains one from the mother and one from the father. Germ cells, however, contain a haploid nucleus, with only the maternal or paternal genes. In nuclear transplantation cloning, the nucleus is removed from an egg and replaced with the diploid nucleus of a somatic cell. In such nuclear transplantation cloning there is a single genetic "parent," unlike sexual reproduction where a new organism is formed when the genetic material of the egg and sperm fuse. The first experiments of this type were successful only when the donor cell was derived from an early embryo. In theory, large numbers of genetically identical animals could be produced through such nuclear transplantation cloning. In practice, the nuclei from embryos which have developed beyond a certain number of cells seem to lose their totipotency, limiting the number of animals that can be produced in a given period of time from a single, originating embryo.

The new development in the experiments that Wilmut and colleagues carried out to produce Dolly was the use of much more developed somatic cells isolated from adult sheep as the source of the donor nuclei. This achievement of gestation and live birth of a sheep using an adult cell donor nucleus was stunning evidence that cell differentiation and specialization are reversible. Given the fact that cells develop and divide after fertilization and differentiate into specific tissue (e.g., muscle, bone, neurons), the development of a viable adult sheep from a differentiated adult cell nucleus provided surprising evidence that the pattern of gene expression can be reprogrammed. Until this experiment many biologists believed that reactivation of the genetic material of mammalian somatic cells would not be complete enough to allow for the production of a viable adult mammal from nuclear transfer cloning.

The science that led to Dolly

Until the birth of Dolly, developmental and molecular biologists focused their efforts on understanding the processes of cellular differentiation, the regulation of genes during this process, the factors that stimulate differentiation, and the reversibility of this process. Biologists have investigated whether, once cellular differentiation occurs, the process is reversible. These questions have by no means been fully answered by the appearance of Dolly. If anything, the existence of Dolly stimulates even more speculation and inquiry. This section describes the background of the science that led to the birth of the cloned sheep, including early studies of differentiation and development, research on regulation of gene expression, experiments using nuclear transfer in animals, and studies of cell programming and division.

Early Studies of Differentiation and Development

Nearly every cell contains a spheroid organelle called the nucleus which houses nearly all the genes of the organism. Genes are composed of DNA, which serve as a set of instructions to the cell to produce particular proteins. Although all somatic cells contain the same genes in the nucleus, the particular genes that are activated vary by the type of cell. For example, a differentiated somatic cell, such as a neuron, must keep a set of neural-specific genes active and silence those genes specific to the development and functioning of other types of cells such as muscle or liver cells.

Investigations which began over 40 years ago sought to determine whether a differentiated somatic cell still contained all genes, even those it did not express. Early experiments in frogs and toads by Gurdon (1962) and by Briggs and King (1952) provided strong evidence that the expression potential of the genes in differentiated cells is essentially unchanged from that of the early embryo.[2] Nuclei from donor differentiated cells were injected into recipient eggs in which the nucleus had been inactivated. The first series of experiments used cells from tadpoles as the source of donor nuclei and adult frogs were produced, albeit at a very low efficiency.[3] Although the cells used were highly specialized, they were not derived from the adult frog, so the cells might not have been fully differentiated.

In these experiments, because isolated nuclei were used, other cellular components were not transferred to the recipient egg. Among those other cellular components is an organelle called the mitochondrion, the energy-producing component of the cell. Although most of the genes specifying this cellular component reside in the nucleus, the mitochondrion itself houses some of its own genes. Thus, in somatic cell nuclear transfer, mitochondrial genes are not transferred to the enucleated egg along with the nuclear genes. Because there are some serious diseases associated with mitochondrial genes, nuclear transplantation could allow an embryo to develop with new, healthy mitochondria from a donor.

Gurdon and colleagues performed another carefully controlled series of experiments in which they used nuclei from adult frog skin cells for transfer to an enucleated egg.[4] Four percent of the nuclei transferred eventually gave rise to fully developed tadpoles. These experiments provided evidence that the genes contained in the nuclei of differentiated cells could be reactivated by the cytoplasm of the egg and thus direct normal development, but only up to a certain stage. No viable adult frog ever developed from these tadpoles and there was a decrease in the number of tadpoles born as the age of the transferred nucleus increased. This left open the possibility that complete reactivation of the adult nucleus was prevented by some irreversible change in the genetic material, and that there was a progressive decline in nuclear potential with age.

Careful analysis, however, suggested that the major reason for developmental failure of the transplanted embryos appeared to be chromosomal abnormalities that occurred during the process of nuclear transplantation itself. The rate of cell division of adult cells is much slower than that of the cells of the early frog embryo. Thus, in reality, for this technique to work it would be necessary that the transplanted adult nucleus reprogram its gene expression, replicate its DNA, and enter the normal embryonic cell division cycle within an hour of nuclear transfer. It is remarkable, given the mechanics and timing of the process, that *any* nuclei from adult somatic cells were successful in generating an embryo. Although they did not produce normal adult animals, the amphibian nuclear transfer experiments of Gurdon and others succeeded in demonstrating that the differentiated state of adult somatic cells do not involve major irreversible changes in their DNA.

Regulation of Gene Expression

In recent years, it has been determined that most patterns of differentiated gene expression are maintained by active control mechanisms, in which particular genes are turned on or off by regulatory proteins.[5] Further studies suggested that it might be possible to reprogram the gene expression of somatic cells so that they perform a different task. The role of a particular cell type (e.g., muscle, liver, or skin) depends on the combination of regulatory proteins it expresses. While in certain specialized cells, such as white blood cells, actual rearrangements and deletions of DNA occur, for the most part, however, gene expression is not regulated by the loss of DNA but by the turning off of specific genes. Thus, it should be possible to activate or inactivate almost any gene in a cell, given the right cellular environment containing the appropriate regulatory molecules.

To reprogram the gene expression of a somatic cell it is not essential to fuse it with an egg; in some cases re-programming can occur through fusion of two adult cells. Cell fusion experiments, in which different somatic cell types are fused, have demonstrated that extensive reprogramming of differentiated nuclei can occur. For example, when muscle cells are fused with non-muscle cells of various sorts, muscle-specific genes are activated in the non-muscle cells,[6] and, similarly, genes that code for hemoglobin can be activated in many cell types after fusion with red blood cells.[7] These and other kinds of experiments have led to the isolation of specific factors that regulate cell differentiation, such as the gene that regulates the formation of muscle cells.[8]

These studies have further demonstrated that the stability of the differentiated state is not absolute. Thus, given the appropriate regulatory molecules and enough time to reprogram an adult nucleus, somatic cells can re-initiate earlier programs of differentiation.

Nuclear Transfer in Mammals

Experiments in mammals have also suggested that it is possible to reprogram adult somatic cells. Following success in the nuclear transfer experiments in frogs, scientists attempted to repeat the experiments in mice. It was known that early development occurs at a considerably slower rate in mammals than amphibians, giving hope that reprogramming of the donor nucleus would occur more efficiently. For·example, the first cell division in mice occurs about a day after fertilization, giving ample time, it was thought, for the reprogramming of gene expression and adjustment of the cell division cycle. This proved not to be the case. Early experiments showed that nuclei from somatic cells fused with fertilized eggs did not undergo nuclear division.[9]

However, a series of experiments in mice in the mid 1980s showed that nuclei could be successfully exchanged between fertilized eggs, with 90 percent reaching the blastocyst stage of embryonic development and beyond.[10] Nuclei recovered and transplanted from embryos at the two-cell stage could direct development to the blastocyst stage. Nuclei transferred from embryos at later stages, however, could not successfully recapitulate development. In fact, in mice, nuclei show less totipotency than whole cells. Many experiments have shown that blastomeres up to the early blastocyst stage are still totipotent when combined with other embryonic cells.[11] This means that the failure of nuclear reprogramming has to be the result of something other than irreversible changes to the genetic material of the cells. In 1986, Willadsen reported experiments with sheep. Unlike the situation in mice, enucleated eggs from sheep could be fused with blastomeres taken from embryos at the eight-cell stage to provide donor nuclei and viable offspring were produced.[12]

Recent experiments have used nuclear transfer into enucleated unfertilized eggs. Using these very early stage eggs prolongs the period of possible reprogramming before the donor nucleus has to undergo the first division. And the advent in the last few years of electrofusion for both fusion of cells and activation of the egg has been another major advance, because activation and fusion occur simultaneously. Because these experiments use fusion of two cells and not simple injection of an isolated nucleus, all of the cellular components are transferred. Thus, the mitochondria, which contain some genes of their own, are transferred along with the nucleus. Because an enucleated egg also contains mitochondria, the result of a fusion experiment is a cell with a mixture of mitochondria from both the donor and the recipient. Since the mitochondrial genes represent an extremely small proportion of the total number of mammalian genes, mixing of mitochondria per se is not expected to have any major effects on the cell. However, if the nucleus donor suffers from a mitochondrial disease, and the egg donor does not, then mixture of the mitochondria may significantly alleviate the disease.

Over the past ten years or so there have been numerous reports of successful nuclear transfer experiments in mammals, nearly all of them using cells taken directly from early embryos. The oldest embryonic nucleus that can successfully support development differs among species. Four-cell blastomere nuclei have been successfully used in pigs.[13] In mice, no nucleus older than the eight-cell stage has been used successfully.[14] In rabbits, 32- to 64-cell early embryos can be used as nuclear donors.[15] In cows and sheep, cells from what is called the inner cell mass (ICM) or the 120-cell blastocyst stage have been used success-fully.[16] Indeed, in both cows and sheep, cell lines have been made from these ICM cells and nuclei from these cells have been used to reprogram development after transfer into enucleated unfertilized eggs.

In the first experiments of this sort by Sims and First (1994),[17] cow cells de-rived from embryos were grown in the laboratory for up to 28 days, and then used as nuclear donors, without any attempt at synchronization of the cell divi-sion cycle of the donor cells. Of those successfully fused with eggs, 24 percent developed to the blastocyst stage, and 4/34 (12 percent) of the blastocysts trans-ferred to recipient cows developed into normal calves. This success rate com-pares favorably with those seen using earlier blastomeres and suggests that it might be possible to achieve successful nuclear transfer from permanent cell lines established from early embryos.

Reprogramming of Nuclei and Synchronization of the Cell Division Cycle

There has been some study of the events that occur once a transferred nucleus is exposed to the cytoplasm of the egg and some, but not all, of the parameters that affect success of nuclear transfer are known.[18] Enucleated eggs used for fusion only proceed to division after activation by some artificial signal, such as the electrical current used in the electrofusion technique. When donor nuclei are in-troduced into the enucleated egg, they usually undergo DNA replication, nuclear envelope breakdown, and chromosome condensation. After activation of the egg the nuclear envelope is reformed around the donor chromosomes. The nucleus now takes on the appearance of a typical egg nucleus at this stage, which is large and swollen. It is assumed that this process begins the reprogramming of the transferred donor nucleus by exposing the chromosomes to the egg cytoplasm and beginning the exchange of egg-derived proteins for the donor nucleus' own proteins.[19]

It is not clear whether exposure to proteins found in the earliest stages of de-velopment and/or nuclear swelling is a prerequisite for reprogramming for later development. Experiments in a number of species have shown that, when nuclei are fused with eggs that have been activated some hours prior to fusion, no DNA replication, chromosome condensation, or nuclear swelling occurs, but normal development can transpire.[20]

Once again, it is not obvious which of the processes described above are re-quired for normal development. In rabbits, cows, sheep, and mice,[21] experiments have shown that nuclei from cells in the early phases of the cell division cycle do better than cells in later stages. In the first phase of the cell cycle, termed G1 (for Gap phase 1), cells contain only one complete set of chromosomes and are relatively quiescent. They then enter a period of DNA synthesis or replication, called S-phase, followed by a rest phase, called G2 (Gap phase 2), at which time they each have a duplicate copy of each chromosome. This doubling of the chromosomes is in preparation for cell division where an equal number will be divided between the two daughter cells. Because DNA replication is induced *after* nuclear transfer, any nucleus that has initiated replication *before* transfer will end up with too much DNA, which will likely result in chromosome anomalies. Thus, the need to transfer nuclei in the G1 phase before replication is initiated, is likely to be important to avoid chromosome damage that will prevent development of the embryo into a viable offspring.

Changes in technique that allowed for the birth of Dolly

In background work that preceded the birth of Dolly, Wilmut and colleagues established cell lines from sheep early embryos, or blastocysts, and used these cells as nuclear donors.[22] In an attempt to avoid the problems of nuclear transfer of non-G1 nuclei into activated eggs, they starved the donor cell line by removing all nutrients from the medium prior to nuclear transfer. Under these starvation conditions, the cells exit the cell cycle and enter the so-called "G0" state (Gap phase 0), similar to the G1 phase in which chromosomes have not replicated. Fusion of G0 nuclei with eggs ensures that the donor chromosomes have not initiated replication prior to fusion. It was also suggested that the G0 state might actually increase the capacity of the nucleus to be reprogrammed by the egg cytoplasm. However, there is currently no direct evidence to support this, nor to conclude that nuclei synchronized in the G0 stage are any better than nuclei synchronized in G1. For Wilmut and colleagues, approximately 14 percent of fusions resulted in development of blastocysts, and 4/34 (12 percent) embryos transferred developed into live lambs. Two died shortly after birth. The success rate in sheep and cow experiments was almost identical, and suggests that division of cells in culture for many days does not inhibit the ability of their nuclei to be reprogrammed by the egg environment. Could the same be true of nuclei from fully differentiated somatic cells?

All of this background work led up to Dolly.[23] Wilmut and colleagues took late embryo, fetal cell cultures, and cell cultures derived from the mammary gland of an adult sheep and applied the same approach of synchronizing the cells in the G0 stage prior to nuclear transfer. They reported successful production of live offspring from all three cell types, although only 29 of 277 (11 percent) of successful fusions between adult mammary gland nuclei and enucleated oocytes developed to the blastocyst stage, and only 1 of 29 (3 percent) blastocysts transferred developed into a live lamb. This experiment was, in fact, the first time any fully developed animal had been born following transfer of a somatic cell nucleus, since the earlier frog experiments only generated tadpoles.

It should be noted, however, that the amount of new information regarding the stability of the differentiated state derived from this experiment is small, as no attempt was made to document that the donor cells were fully differentiated cells, the genes of which expressed specialized mammary gland proteins. In the earlier experiments with frogs, the fact that the donor cells were fully differentiated was documented in such a manner. In the present case, Dolly could have been derived from a less-differentiated cell in the population, such as a mammary stem cell.

Remaining scientific uncertainties

Several important questions remain unanswered about the feasibility in mammals of nuclear transfer cloning using adult cells as the source of nuclei:

First, can the procedure that produced Dolly be carried out successfully in other cases? Only one animal has been produced to date. Thus, it is not clear that this technique is reproducible even in sheep.

Second, are there true species differences in the ability to achieve successful nuclear transfer? It has been shown that nuclear transfer in mice is much less successful than in larger domestic animals. Part of this difference may reflect the intensity of research in this area in the last ten years; agricultural interests have meant that more nuclear transfer work has been performed in domestic animals than in mice. But part of the species differences may be real and not simply reflect the greater recent effort in livestock. For example, in order for a differentiated nucleus to redirect development in the environment of the egg, its constellation of regulatory proteins must be replaced by those of the egg in time for the embryo to use the donor nucleus to direct normal development of the embryo. The species difference may be the result of the different times of embryonic gene activation.

In mammals, unlike many other species, the early embryo rapidly activates its genes and cannot survive on the components stored in the egg. The time at which embryonic gene activation occurs varies between species—the late 2-cell stage in mice,[24] the 4–8 cell stage in humans[25] and the 8–16 cell stage in sheep. The later onset of embryonic gene activation and transcription in sheep provides an additional round or two of cell divisions during which nuclear reprogramming can occur, unlike the rapid genome activation in the mouse. Further cross-species comparisons are needed to assess the importance of this difference in the time of genome activation for the success of nuclear transfer experiments. In humans, for example, the time period before gene activation is very short, which might not permit the proper reprogramming of genes after nuclear transfer to allow for subsequent normal development.

Third, will the phenomenon of genetic imprinting affect the ability of nuclei from later stages to reprogram development? In mammals imprinting refers to the fact that the genes inherited on the chromosomes from the father (paternal genes) and those from the mother (maternal genes) are not equivalent in their effects on the developing embryo.[26] Some heritable imprint is established on the chromosomes during the development of the egg and the sperm such that certain genes are expressed only when inherited from the father or mother. Imprinting explains why parthenogenetic embryos, with only maternally inherited genes, and androgenetic embryos, with only paternally inherited genes, fail to complete development.[27] Nuclei transferred from diploid cells, whether embryonic or adult, should contain maternal *and* paternal copies of the genome, and thus not have an imbalance between the maternally and paternally derived genes.

The successful generation of an adult sheep from a somatic cell nucleus suggests that the imprint can be stable, but it is possible that some instability of the imprint, particularly in cells in culture, could limit the efficiency of nuclear transfer from somatic cells. It is known that disturbances in imprinting lead to growth abnormalities in mice and are associated with cancer and rare genetic conditions in children.

Fourth, will cellular aging affect the ability of somatic cell nuclei to program normal development? As somatic cells divide they progressively age and there is normally a defined number of cell divisions that they can undergo before senescence. Part of this aging process involves the progressive shortening of the ends of the chromosomes, the telomeres, and other genetic changes. Germ cells (eggs and sperm) evade telomere shortening by expressing an enzyme, telomerase, that can keep telomeres full length. It seems likely that returning an adult mammalian nucleus to the egg environment will expose it to sufficient telomerase activity to reset telomere length, since oocytes have been found to be potent sources of telomerase activity.[28]

Fifth, will the mutations that accumulate in somatic cells affect nuclear transfer efficiency and lead to cancer and other diseases in the offspring? As cells divide and organisms age, mistakes and alterations (mutations) in the DNA will inevitably occur and will accumulate with time. If these mistakes occur in the sperm or the egg, the mutation will be inherited in the offspring. Normally mutations that occur in somatic cells affect only that cell and its descendants which are ultimately dispensable. Nevertheless, such mutations are not necessarily harmless. Sporadic somatic mutations in a variety of genes can predispose a cell to become cancerous. Transfer of a nucleus from a somatic cell carrying such a mutation into an egg would transform a sporadic somatic mutation into a germline mutation that is transmitted to all of the cells of the body. If this mutation were present in all cells it may lead to a genetic disease or cancer. The risks of such events occurring following nuclear transfer are difficult to estimate.

* * *

Potential therapeutic applications of nuclear transfer cloning

The demonstration that, in mammals as in frogs, the nucleus of a somatic cell can be reprogrammed by the egg environment provides further impetus to studies on how to reactivate embryonic programs of development in adult cells. These studies have exciting prospects for regeneration and repair of diseased or damaged human tissues and organs, and may provide clues as to how to reprogram adult differentiated cells directly without the need for oocyte fusion. In addition, the use of nuclear transfer has potential application in the field of assisted reproduction.

Potential applications in organ and tissue transplantation

Many human diseases, when they are severe enough, are treated effectively by organ or tissue transplantation, including some leukemias, liver failure, heart and kidney disease. In some instances the organ required is non-vital, that is, it can be taken from the donor without great risk (e.g., bone marrow, blood, kidney). In other cases, the organ is obviously vital and required for the survival of the individual, such as the heart. All transplantation is imperfect, with the exception of that which occurs between identical twins, because transplantation of organs between individuals requires genetic compatibility.

In principle, the application of nuclear transfer cloning to humans could provide a potential source of organs or tissues of a predetermined genetic background. The notion of using human cloning to produce individuals for use solely as organ donors is repugnant, almost unimaginable, and morally unacceptable. A morally more acceptable and potentially feasible approach is to direct differentiation along a specific path to produce specific tissues (e.g., muscle or nerve) for therapeutic transplantation rather than to produce an entire individual. Given current uncertainties about the feasibility of this, however, much research would be needed in animal systems before it would be scientifically sound, and therefore potentially morally acceptable, to go forward with this approach.

Potential applications in cell-based therapies

Another possibility raised by cloning is transplantation of cells or tissues not from an individual donor but from an early embryo or embryonic stem cells; the primitive, undifferentiated cells from the embryo that are still totipotent. This potential application would not require the generation and birth of a cloned individual. Embryonic stem cells provide an interesting model for such studies, since they represent the precursors of all cell lineages in the body. Mouse embryonic stem cells can be stimulated to differentiate in vitro into precursors of the blood, neuronal and muscle cell lineages, among others,[29] and they thus provide a potential source of stem cells for regeneration of all tissues of the body.

It might be possible to take a cell from an early blastomere and treat it in such a manner as to direct its differentiation along a specific path. By this procedure

it might be possible to generate in the laboratory sufficient numbers of specialized cells, for example bone marrow stem cells, liver cells, or pancreatic beta-
cells (which produce insulin) for transplantation. If even a single tissue type could
be generated from early embryonic cells by these methods and used clinically, it
would constitute a major advance in transplantation medicine by providing cells
that are genetically identical to the recipient.

One could imagine the prospect of nuclear transfer from a somatic cell to generate an early embryo and from it an embryonic stem cell line for each individual human, which would be ideally tissue-matched for later transplant purposes.
This might be a rather expensive and far-fetched scenario. An alternative scenario would involve the generation of a few, widely used and well characterized
human embryonic stem cell lines, genetically altered to prevent graft rejection in
all possible recipients.

The preceding scenarios depend on using cells of early human embryos, generated either by in vitro fertilization or nuclear transfer into an egg. Because of
ethical and moral concerns raised by the use of embryos for research purposes
it would be far more desirable to explore the direct use of human cells of adult
origin to produce specialized cells or tissues for transplantation into patients. It
may not be necessary to reprogram terminally differentiated cells but rather to
stimulate proliferation and differentiation of the quiescent stem cells which are
known to exist in many adult tissues, including even the nervous system.[30]
Experiments in this area are likely to focus more on the conditions required for
direct stimulation of the stem cells in specific tissues, than actual use of nuclear
transfer to activate novel developmental programs. These approaches to cellular
repair using adult stem cells will be greatly aided by an understanding of how
stem cells are established during embryogenesis.

Another strategy for cell-based therapies would be to identify methods by
which somatic cells could be "de-differentiated" and then "re-differentiated"
along a particular path. This would eliminate the need to use cells obtained from
embryos. Such an approach would permit the growth of specialized cells compatible with a specific individual person for transplantation. Although at the current time this strategy is highly speculative, ongoing research in animal systems
may identify new approaches or new molecular targets that might make this approach feasible.

It will be of great importance to understand through experiments in animals
how the environment of the egg reprograms a somatic cell nucleus. What cellular mechanisms can be elucidated? What components are involved in these
processes? Can we direct cells along particular developmental pathways in the
laboratory and use these cells for therapy? The capacity to grow human cells of
different lineages in culture would also dramatically improve prospects for effective somatic gene therapy.

Assisted reproduction

Another area of medicine where the knowledge gained from animal work has potential application is in the area of assisted reproduction. Assisted reproduction technologies are already widely used and encompass a variety of parental and biological situations, that is, donor and recipient relationships. In most cases, an infertile couple seeks remedy through either artificial insemination or in vitro fertilization using sperm from either the male or an anonymous donor, an egg from the woman or a donor, and in some cases surrogacy. In those instances where both individuals of a couple are infertile or the prospective father has nonfunctional sperm, one might envision using cloning of one member of the couple's nuclei to produce a child.

Although this constitutes an extension of current clinical practice, aside from the serious, moral, and ethical issues surrounding this approach, there are significant technical and medical causes for caution, some of which were described in the research questions enumerated above.

In most situations of assisted reproduction, other than the intentional union of the gametes by in vitro techniques, the fertilized egg and initial cells of the early embryo are not otherwise manipulated. In some rare cases, such as preimplantation genetic diagnosis, the embryo is manipulated by the removal of one of the identical cells of the blastomere to test its genetic status. In contrast, if nuclear transfer were to be used as a reproductive option, it would entail substantially more invasive manipulation. Thus far, the animal cloning of Dolly is a singular success, one seemingly normal animal produced from 277 nuclear transfers. Until the experiment is replicated the efficiency, and even the validity, of the procedure cannot be fully determined. It is likely that the mere act of manipulating a nucleus and transferring it into an egg could decrease the percentage of eggs that go on to develop and implant normally, as well as increase the rate of birth defects.

Cloning and genetic determinism

The announcement of Dolly sparked widespread speculation about a human child being created using somatic cell nuclear transfer. Much of the perceived fear that greeted this announcement centered around the misperception that a child or many children could be produced who would be identical to an already existing person.

This fear reflects an erroneous belief that a person's genes bear a simple relationship to the physical and psychological traits that compose that individual. This belief, that genes alone determine all aspects of an individual, is called "genetic determinism." Although genes play an essential role in the formation of physical and behavioral characteristics, each individual is, in fact, the result of a complex interaction between his or her genes and the environment within which they develop, beginning at the time of fertilization and continuing throughout life. As social and biological beings we are creatures of our biological, physical, social, political, historical, and psychological environments. Indeed, the great lesson of modern molecular genetics is the profound complexity of both gene–gene interactions and gene–environment interactions in the determination of whether a specific trait or characteristic is expressed. In other words, there will never be another you.

While the concept of complete genetic determinism is wrong and overly simplistic, genes do play a major role in determining biological characteristics including a predisposition to certain diseases. Moreover, the existence of families in which many members are affected by these diseases suggests that there is a single gene that is passed down with each generation that causes the disease. When such a disease gene is identified, scientists often say they have "cloned the gene for" breast cancer, for instance, implying a direct cause and effect of gene and disease. Indeed, the recent efforts of the Human Genome Project have led to the isolation of a large number of genes that are mutated in specific diseases, such as Duchenne Muscular Dystrophy, and certain types of breast and colon cancer.

However, recent scientific findings have revealed that a "one-gene, one-disease" approach is far too simplistic. Even in the relatively small list of genes currently associated with a specific disease, knowing the complete DNA sequence of the gene does not allow a scientist to predict if a given person will get the disease. For example, in breast cancer there can be many different changes in the DNA, and for some specific mutations there is a calculated risk of developing the disease, while for other changes the risk is unknown. Even when a specific genetic change is identified that "causes" the disease in some people, others may be found who have the same change but do not get the disease. This is because other factors, either genetic or environmental, are altered that mask or compensate for "the" disease gene. Thus even with the most sophisticated understanding of genes, one cannot determine with certainty what will happen to a given person with a single change in a single gene.

Once again, the reason rigid genetic determinism is false is that genes interact with each other and with the environment in extremely complex ways. For example, the likelihood of developing colon cancer, a disease with a strong hereditary component and for which researchers have identified a single "causative" gene, is also strongly influenced by diet. When one considers a human trait that is determined by multiple genes, the situation becomes even more complex. The number of interactions between genes and environment increases dramatically. In fact, the ability to predict what a person will be like knowing only their genes becomes virtually impossible because it is not possible to know how the environment and chance factors will influence the outcome.

Thus the idea that one could make through somatic cell nuclear transfer a team of Michael Jordans, a physics department of Albert Einsteins, or an opera chorus of Pavarottis, is simply false. Knowing the complete genetic makeup of an individual would not tell you what kind of person that individual would become. Even identical twins who grow up together and thus share the same genes and a similar home environment have different likes and dislikes, and can have very different talents. The increasingly sophisticated studies coming out of human genetics research are showing that the better we understand gene function, the less likely it is we will ever be able to produce at will a person with any given complex trait.

Conclusions

The term "clone" has many meanings but in its simplest and most scientific sense it means the making of identical copies of molecules, cells, tissues, and even entire animals. The latest news about cloning Dolly the sheep involved somatic cell nuclear transplant cloning. In this process the nucleus from an adult somatic cell is transplanted into an enucleated ovum to produce a developing animal that is a "delayed" genetic twin of the adult.

There are many applications that nuclear transfer cloning might have for biotechnology, livestock production, and new medical approaches. Work with embryonic stem cells and genetic manipulation of early embryos in animal species (including nuclear transfer) is already providing unparalleled insights into fundamental biological processes and promises to provide great practical benefit in terms of improved livestock, improved means of producing pharmaceutical proteins, and prospects for regeneration and repair of human tissues.

However, the possibility of using human cloning for the purposes of creating a new individual entails significant scientific uncertainty and medical risk at this time. Potential risks include those known to be associated with the manipulation of nuclei and eggs and those yet unknown, such as the effects of aging, somatic mutation, and improper imprinting. These effects could result in high rates of failed attempts at pregnancy as well as the increased likelihood of developmentally and genetically abnormal embryos.

Notes

1. Much of this appendix is derived from the material contained in two commissioned papers provided by Janet Rossant, Samuel Lunenfeld Research Institute, Mount Sinai Hospital, Toronto; and by Stuart Orkin, Children's Hospital, and Dana Farber Cancer Institute, Boston.

2. J. B. Gurdon, "The Developmental Capacity of Nuclei Taken From Intestinal Epithelium Cells of Feeding Tadpoles," *Journal of Embryology and Experimental Morphology* 10 (1962): 622–40; and R. Briggs and T. J. King, "Transplantation of Living Nuclei From Blastula Cells Into Enucleated Frog's Eggs," *Proceedings of the National Academy of Sciences* (USA) 38 (1952): 455–63.

3. Gurdon, "The Developmental Capacity of Nuclei," 1962.

4. J. B. Gurdon, R. A. Laskey, and O. R. Reeves, "The Developmental Capacity of Nuclei Transplanted From Keratinized Skin Cells of Adult Frogs," *Journal of Embryology and Experimental Morphology* 34 (1975): 93–112.

5. H. M. Blau, "Differentiation Requires Continuous Active Control," *Annual Review of Biochemistry* 61 (1992): 1213–30.

6. H. M. Blau, G. K. Pavlath, E. C. Hardeman, C. P. Chiu, L. Silberstein, S. G. Webster, S. C. Miller, and C. Webster, "Plasticity of the Differentiated State," *Science* 230 (1985): 758–66.

7. M. H. Baron and T. Maniatis, "Rapid Reprogramming of Globin Gene Expression in Transient Heterokaryons," *Cell* 46 (1986): 591–602.

8. H. Weintraub, "The MyoD Family and Myogenesis: Redundancy, Networks, and Thresholds," *Cell* 75 (1993): 1241–44.

9. C. F. Graham, "The Fusion of Cells With One- and Two-Cell Mouse Embryos," *Wistar Institute Symposium Monographs* 9 (1969): 19–35.

10. J. McGrath and D. Solter, "Inability of Mouse Blastomere Nuclei Transferred to Enucleated Zygotes to Support Development In Vitro," *Science* 226 (1984): 1317–19.

11. J. Rossant and R. A. Pederson, *Experimental Approaches to Mammalian Embryonic Development* (Cambridge: Cambridge University Press, 1986).

12. S. M. Willadsen, "Nuclear Transplantation in Sheep Embryos," *Nature* 320 (1986): 63–65.

13. R. S. Prather, M. M. Sims, and N. L. First, "Nuclear Transplantation in Early Pig Embryos," *Biology of Reproduction* 41 (1989): 414–18.

14. H. T. Cheong, Y. Takahashi, and H. Kanagawa, "Birth of Mice After Transplantation of Early Cell-Cycle-Stage Embryonic Nuclei into Enucleated Oocytes," *Biology of Reproduction* 48 (1993): 958–63.

15. X. Yang, S. Jiang, A. Kovacs, and R. H. Foote, "Nuclear Totipotency of Cultured Rabbit Morulae to Support Full-Term Development Following Nuclear Transfer," *Biology of Reproduction* 47 (1992): 636–43.

16. P. Collas and F. L. Barnes, "Nuclear Transplantation by Microinjection of Inner Cell Mass and Granulosa Cell Nuclei," *Molecular Reproduction and Development* 38 (1994): 264–67; and L. C. Smith and I. Wilmut, "Influence of Nuclear and Cytoplasmic Activity on the Development In Vivo of Sheep Embryos After Nuclear Transplantation" *Biology of Reproduction* 40 (1989): 1027–35.

17. M. Sims and N. L. First, "Production of Calves by Transfer of Nuclei From Cultured Inner Cell Mass Cells," *Proceedings of the National Academy of Sciences* (USA) 91 (1994): 6143–47.

18. J. Fulka, N. L. First, and R. M. Moor, "Nuclear Transplantation in Mammals: Remodeling of Transplanted Nuclei Under the Influence of Maturation Promoting Factor," *BioEssays* 18 (1996): 835–40.

19. R. S. Prather and N. L. First, "Cloning Embryos by Nuclear Transfer," *Journal of Reproduction and Fertility.* Suppl 41 (1990): 125–34.

20. K. H. Campbell, P. Loi, P. Cappai, and I. Wilmut, "Improved Development to Blastocyst of Ovine Nuclear Transfer Embryos Reconstructed During the Presumptive

S-Phase of Enucleated Activated Oocytes," *Biology of Reproduction* 50 (1994): 1385–93.

21. Cheong et al., "Birth of Mice After Transplantation," (1993); P. Collas, J. J. Balise, and J. M. Robl, "Influence of Cell Cycle Stage of the Donor Nucleus on Development of Nuclear Transplant Rabbit Embryos," *Biology of Reproduction* 46 (1992): 492–500.

22. K. H. Campbell, J. McWhir, W. A. Ritchie, and I. Wilmut, "Sheep Cloned by Nuclear Transfer From a Cultured Cell Line," *Nature* 380 (1996): 64–66.

23. I. Wilmut, A. E. Schnieke, J. McWhir, A. J. Kind, and K. H. Campbell, "Viable Offspring Derived From Fetal and Adult Mammalian Cells," *Nature* 385 (1997): 810–13.

24. R. M. Schultz, "Regulation of Zygotic Gene Activation in the Mouse," *BioEssays* 15 (1993): 531–38.

25. P. Braude, V. Bolton, and S. Moore, "Human Gene Expression First Occurs Between the Four- and Eight-Cell Stages of Preimplantation Development," *Nature* 332 (1988): 459–61.

26. D. Solter, "Differential Imprinting and Expression of Maternal and Paternal Genomes," *Annual Review of Genetics* 22 (1988): 127–46.

27. R. H. Fundele and M. A. Surani, "Experimental Embryological Analysis of Genetic Imprinting in Mouse Development," *Developmental Genetics* 15 (1994): 515–22.

28. L. L. Mantell and C. W. Greider, "Telomerase Activity in Germline and Embryonic Cells of *Xenopus*," *EMBO Journal* 13 (1994): 3211–17.

29. M. J. Weiss and S. H. Orkin, "In Vitro Differentiation of Murine Embryonic Stem Cells: New Approaches to Old Problems," *Journal of Clinical Investigation* 97 (1995): 591–95.

30. F. H. Gage, J. Ray, and L. J. Fisher, "Isolation, Characterization, and Use of Stem Cells From the CNS," *Annual Review of Neuroscience* 18 (1995): 159–192.

Index

Abortion, 5, 10–11, 13, 21–22, 24, 27–28, 52, 59, 61, 70, 72, 77, 95, 96, 130, 170, 176, 181–82, 186, 213, 224 n. 10, 224 n. 13, 224 n. 16, 240 n. 15, 256
Abram, Morris, 164
ADA. *See* Americans with Disabilities Act
Adoption, 31
Allen, Woody, 112
American Medical Association, 216
American Society for Reproductive Medicine, 161
Americans with Disabilities Act, 241 n. 47
Andrews, Lori, 5, 161
Annas, George 10, 136, 172, 185–87
Assisted hatching, 123, 159
Audi, Robert, 244 n. 30
Australia, 159, 161, 211
Australian Senate Select Community, 77
Ayalas family, 99

Baby M, 135
Baier, Annette, 195
Beddington, Rosa, 236 n. 5
Benda, Ernst, 212
Biographical v. biological life, 24, 224 n. 8

Birth control, 129. *See also* Contraception
Birth defects, 5, 61, 255, 281
Bladerunner, 94, 112
Blastomere separation, 8, 10, 87, 237 n. 61, 262–63, 270
Bone marrow transplantation, 30, 99, 279
Bonnicksen, Andrea, 128, 220
Boys from Brazil, 117
Bragdon v. Abbott, 241 n. 47
Briggs, Robert, 2, 272
Britain's Human Fertilization and Embryology Act of 1990, 68, 213
British Human Fertilization and Embryology Authority, 158
Brock, Dan, 13, 93
Brown, Louise, 2, 107, 154
Brave New World. See Huxley, Aldous

Cahill, Lisa Sowle, 62, 66, 229 n. 8
California, 207
Callahan, Daniel, 30, 50, 56, 74–76, 78
Campbell, Courtney, 2, 11–12, 32–34, 76, 78, 197–98
Campbell, K.H.S., 247 n. 43
Canada, 211

Cancer(s), 5, 30, 56, 59, 61, 278, 282
Caplan, Arthur, 10, 172, 185–87
Carter, Jimmy, 84
Casuistry, 12, 35, 67–70, 72, 77, 80–81, 229 n.
    17, 230 n. 41
  geometric casuistry, 70–71
  high, 69
Catholic Church, 31, 75, 82, 151, 153, 184,
    188, 230 n. 25
Charo, R. Alta, 13, 75, 78–79, 82, 128,
    184–86, 193, 225 n. 35
Children
  as objects, 11, 265. See also Objectification
  and the right to an open future, 103–6,
    126–27
China, 212
Chirac, Jacques, 212
Christianity, 188, 190
Clinton, William 1, 3, 6–7, 50, 94, 128, 147,
    153, 202–203, 206, 211, 256
Cloning
  diagrams of, 8, 9
  federal funding of, 14–15, 94, 130–31, 160,
    203–205, 265, 267
  history of, 2, 222 n. 2, 264, 271–77
  laissez faire approaches to, 148, 161
  and nightmare scenarios, 13–14, 94, 112,
    117, 219
  private funding of, 94, 130, 147
  ratio of transferred embryos to births in, 93,
    108, 123–24, 276, 281
  symbolic arguments about, 33, 146, 178
  types of, 7–9, 269–270
Cloning Prohibition Act of 1997, 202–203
Cloning Prohibition and Research Protection
    Act, 210
Cohen, Cynthia, 148, 155–56
Coleman, June, 249 n. 89
Committee for Life Sciences, 212
Commodification. See Objectification
Common good, 180, 190, 192–93, 197–98,
    200
Communitarianism, 184
Congress. See United States Congress
Connecticut, 208
Consequentialism, 71, 149
Consequentialist, 181
Contraception, 21, 24, 56–59, 61, 95, 255
Corea, Gena, 62
Council of Europe Protocol, 94, 211–12,
    247 n. 45
Council for Responsible Genetics, 211
Crawford, Cindy, 117

Davis, Dena, 71–73, 76–77, 126, 149
Dawson, Karen, 233 n. 7
DeCorduba, Antonius, 70
Deech, Ruth, 31
Djerassi, Carl, 138
Delaware, 208
Denmark, 212
Department of Health and Human Services, 6
Dolly, 1–2, 4, 6, 9, 93, 102, 108, 110, 122–23,
    128, 135, 146, 213, 215, 264–65, 271,
    276, 277, 281, 283
Donor gametes. See Egg donation; Sperm do-
    nation
Dorff, Elliott, 133, 136
Double effect, 70–72, 230 n. 25
Drane, James, 232 n. 63
DuBose, Edwin, 232 n. 63
Dworkin, Ronald, 29, 95

EAB. See Ethics Advisory Board
Edwards, Robert, 153
Egg donation, 63, 98, 114, 148, 227 n. 20,
    255–57, 281
Einstein, Albert, 45–46, 100–101, 111, 283
Elias, Sherman, 10, 172, 185–87
Elster, Nanette, 5
Embryo(s)
  freezing, 3, 30, 31, 77, 152, 176
  reduction. See Selective reduction
  research,
    federal funding of, 14–15, 50, 57, 86, 94,
      130–31, 145, 148, 160, 180–81, 185,
      203–205, 242 n. 9, 251, 253, 255,
      257–58, 260–62, 265, 267
    private funding of, 94, 130, 145, 147
    symbolic arguments about, 24, 29, 33, 51,
      53–56, 58, 76, 78, 146, 178
    with research embryos, 39, 50–51, 55, 63,
      66–68, 72–74, 102, 255–56, 265
    with spare embryos, 11, 32, 39–40, 50–51,
      54, 72, 74, 77, 152, 169, 255–56
  splitting, 7, 94, 98, 107 See also Blastomere
    separation
  twinning, See Blastomere separation
Engelhardt, H. Tristram, Jr., 165
Ethics Advisory Board, 3–4, 28, 146, 154–56,
    259
European Commission, 212
Evans, Donald, 68

FDA. See Food and Drug Administration
Faden, Ruth, 237 n. 8

Farley, Margaret, 61
Federal funding. *See* Embryo research; Cloning
    research
Feinberg, Joel, 29, 52, 84, 104–106, 126
Fertilization and Embryology Act, 31
Fetal tissue transplantation, 180, 251
FLO. *See* Future like ours
First, Neal, 2, 275
Food and Drug Administration, 148
Forster, Heidi, 16, 201
France, 68, 212
Frankenstein, 219
Frankensteinian, 33
Frist, Bill, 199, 201
Future like ours, 26, 27, 224 n. 11

GAEIB. *See* Group of Advisors on the Ethical
    Implications of Biotechnology
Gamete donors. *See* Egg donation; Sperm do-
    nation
Gandhi, Mohandas, 100, 101
Gene therapy, 116, 132, 204, 280
Genetic
    defects, 3, 99, 159, 181
    determinism, 6, 101, 104–105, 113, 125–26,
        281–82
    engineering, 21, 28, 52, 164, 210
    lottery, 41, 48, 116
    uniqueness, 13, 83, 96, 103–104, 170,
        217–18
George Washington University Medical Center,
    8, 107, 223 n. 15
Germany, 68, 212
Geron Corporation, 4, 146–47
G.I.F.T., 61
Glover, Jonathan, 85
Gold, E. Richard, 43
Green, Ronald, 13–14, 78, 114
Group of Advisors on the Ethical Implications
    of Biotechnology, 212
Gurdon, J. B., 272–73

HFEA. *See* Human Fertilization and
    Embryology Authority
Haldane, J.B.S., 2
Hall, Jerry, 2
Hare, R. M., 224 n. 12
Harkin, Tom, 201
Healy, Bernadine, 230 n. 39
Heller, J. C., 237 n. 8
Heyd, David, 71, 79, 119, 230 n. 41, 231 n. 41
Hitler, Adolph, 94, 112

Holocaust, 135
Holy See, 211
Hubbard, Ruth, 57, 59
HUGO. *See* Human Genome Organization
Human embryo. *See* Embryo
Human Fertilization and Embryology Act, 31
Human Genome Organization (HUGO), 221
Human Genome Project, 41, 116, 282
Human Cloning Prohibition Act, 204–205
Hungary, 68
Hussein, Saddam, 117
Husted, G. L. and J. H., 218
Huxley, Aldous, 94, 112, 237 n. 6
Hyperovulation, 61, 77, 257
Hyperstimulation. *See* Hyperovulation

ICSI. *See* Intracytoplasmic sperm injection
Illinois, 209
Informed consent, 31–32, 39, 60, 102, 109,
        122, 164, 181, 242 n. 9, 253, 255,
        256–57, 260, 268
Institutional Review Board, 32, 37–39, 166,
        242 n. 9, 254, 259–60,
Intracytoplasmic sperm injection, 27, 114, 123,
        135, 158–59
I.R.B. *See* Institutional Review Board
Islam, 188, 190

Japan, 211
Jewish. *See also* Judaism
    teachings, 184
    tradition, 14, 133, 136
Johnson, T. R., 43
Jonas, Hans, 103–106
Jonsen, Albert, 68, 70
Jordan, Michael, 283
Joyce, E., 232 n. 4
Judaism, 188, 190
Justice 62, 81, 139, 141, 181, 187, 194, 195,
        243 n. 1

Kahn, Jeffrey P., 238 n. 27
Kant, Immanuel, 43
Kantian, 21, 71, 99
Kass, Leon, 2–3
Katz, Jay, 164
Kavka, Gregory, 237 n. 8
Keenan, James, 12, 67, 149, 150, 153, 229 n. 8
King, Patricia, 65–66, 78, 153, 228 n. 33
King, Thomas, 2, 272
Kinship, 12, 55, 219

Klotzko, Arlene, 68
Kolata, Gina, 77, 222 n. 2
Kopfensteiner, Thomas, 229 n. 12
Krimsky, Sheldon, 57, 59
Kuhn, Thomas, 73

Ladd, John, 150
Lauritzen, Paul, 1, 42, 228 n. 33, 229 n. 8
Lederberg, Joshua, 2
Leguin, Ursula, 237 n. 6
Levinas, Emmanuel, 137
Levin, Ira, 112
Lewontin, Richard, 125
London, Alex John, 15–16, 162

Macklin, Ruth, 215
Mahowald, Mary, 58
Marquis, Don, 24, 26–27, 224 n. 10
Marxism, 184
Massachusetts, 234 n. 19, 238 n. 31
Mayor, Federico, 212
McClamrock, Ron, 237 n. 8
McCormick, Richard A, 233 n. 7
Meilaender, Gilbert, 55, 225 n. 1
Mill, J. S., 95
Miller, Richard, 229 n. 19
Michigan, 208
Minnesota, 209
Missouri, 207
Moral relativism, 74
Moreno, Jonathan, 15–16, 162
Mori, Maurizio, 69, 72, 79, 151
Mozart, Wolfgang, 100–101
Multiple births. See Multiple gestation
Multiple gestation, 61, 157–58, 270
Murray, Thomas, 140, 194

N.A.B.E.R. See National Advisory Board on
    Ethics in Reproduction
National Advisory Board on Ethics in
    Reproduction, 161
National Commission for the Protection of
    Human Research Subjects of
    Biomedical and Behavior Research, 3,
    68, 79
Navarre, Peter of, 70
Nazism, 117, 153
New Jersey, 209
New York, 210
New York State Task Force on Life and Law,
    242 n. 48

New York Times, 77, 132, 138–39, 238 n. 19
N. I. H. Revitalization Act, 4
Nobel Prize Sperm Bank, 112, 118
Non-identity argument, 107–8, 119–20
    responses to, 120–22, 236 n. 29, 237 n. 8,
    249 n. 82
Noonan, John, 81, 232 n. 4
Nuffield Council of Bioethics, 213

Objectification, 13, 48, 98, 137, 146
Office of Technology Assessment, 232 n. 4
Oocyte donation. See Egg donation
Ozick, Cynthia, 137

P.V.S. See Persistent vegetative state
Parfit, Derek, 107–108, 119
Parthenogenesis, 4, 64–65, 228 n. 33, 251, 256,
    258–60, 263, 278
Pauling, Linus, 118
Pavarotti, Luciano, 283
Pence, Gregory E., 237 n. 6
Persistent vegetative state, 22, 83
Picasso, Pablo, 53
Pitt, Brad, 117
Poland, 68
Preimplantation genetic diagnosis, 4, 57–58,
    115, 168, 261, 263, 281
President, 131, 162, 186, 199, 223 n. 13. See
    also Carter, Jimmy; Clinton, William;
    Reagan, Ronald; Roosevelt, Franklin
President's Commission on Ethical Problems
    and Biomedical and Behavioral
    Research, 164, 173
Primitive streak, 35, 51, 57, 182–83, 186, 254,
    260, 262
Presley, Elvis, 117
Procreative liberty, 31, 52, 56, 97–98, 103, 113,
    213–16, 220
Prohibition on Cloning of Human Beings Act
    of 1998, 204

Ramsey colloquium, 50
Ramsey, Emily, 16, 201
Ramsey, Paul, 38, 50
Rawlsian, 166
Reagan, Ronald, 4, 84
Reichlin, Massimo, 85, 232 n. 4
Reproductive
    freedom. See Procreative liberty
    liberty. See Procreative liberty
Resolve, 155

Retortion, 73–74, 80, 150
Roberts, Melinda, 237 n. 8, 249 n. 82
Robertson, John, 28, 56, 73, 76, 119–120,
    136–37, 215, 217, 220, 224 n. 11
Roosevelt, Franklin, 84
Roslin Institute, 1, 4, 83, 264–65
Rosner, Mary, 43
Royal, Teri, 118
Russo, Eugene, 234 n. 19
Ryan, Maura, 12, 50

Sacred Congregation for the Doctrine of the
    Faith, 240 n. 15
Safire, William, 132
Sanctity of human life, 55–56, 190
Santer, Jacques, 212
Schweitzer, Albert, 100–101
Seed, Richard, 130, 146–47
Selective reduction, 78, 158
Seller, Mary, 157
Sentience, 23–24, 34–35, 53, 171, 182, 233 n.
    12
Shapiro, David, 213
Shapiro, Harold, 7, 10, 245 n. 41
Silver, Lee, 60, 223 n. 10
Sims, M., 275
Singer, Peter, 85, 124
Slippery slope, 54, 67, 71–72, 78–79, 137
Spain, 68, 212
Spallone, Patricia, 62
Sperm donation, 98, 114–15, 281
Star Trek, 87
Steinbock, Bonnie, 11–12, 21, 51–53, 55–58,
    71–72, 75, 149, 215–16, 223 n. 12, 224
    n. 17
Stem cells, 4, 15, 132, 146, 149, 156, 168, 234
    n. 19, 238 n. 19, 261–62, 279–80, 283
Stillman, Robert, 2
Stiltner, Brian, 16, 178
Stock, Gregory, 132–33
Stolberg, Sheryl Gay, 132
Supreme Court. See United States Supreme
    Court
Surrogate motherhood, 95, 114, 135, 148, 160,
    176, 281

Tauer, Carol, 14–15, 71–74, 145, 231 n. 59
Taunton-Rigby, Allison, 238 n. 31
Telomeres, 278
Tendler, Moshe, 133, 135

Tooley, Michael, 84, 233 n. 10
Totipotency, 234 n. 19, 271, 279
Toulmin, Stephen, 68, 70
Tribe, Laurence, 176
Trounson, Alan, 158
Tucker, Michael, 158
Twinning, 8, 220. See also Blastomere separa-
    tion

UNESCO, 211–12
United Nations, 59
United States Congress, 1–7, 16, 130, 147,
    167, 199, 202–07
United States House of Representatives. See
    United States Congress
United States Senate. See United States
    Congress
United States Supreme Court, 215–16

Van Blerkom, Jonathan, 156
Varmus, Harold, 5, 109, 180, 202
Vasquez, Gabriel, 70
Veatch, Robert, 223 n. 2
Vereecke, Louis, 229 n. 11

Wade, Nicholas, 238 n. 19
Walzer, Michael, 195
Warnock Committee, 28
Warnock, Mary, 248 n. 56
Warren, Mary Anne, 22
Washington Post, 50, 154
Watson, James, 2
Weber, Max, 40, 42, 46
Wells, Deane, 85
Willadsen, Steed, 2 193, 274
Wilmut, Ian, 1–2, 93–94, 103, 108, 211, 264,
    271, 276
Wolf, Susan, 220
Wolterstorff, Nicholas, 244 n. 30
World Health Organization, 94
World population, 116

Z.I.F.T., 61
Ziman, John, 37
Zoloth, Laurie, 14, 132
Zona
    drilling, 232 n. 4
    removal. See Assisted hatching